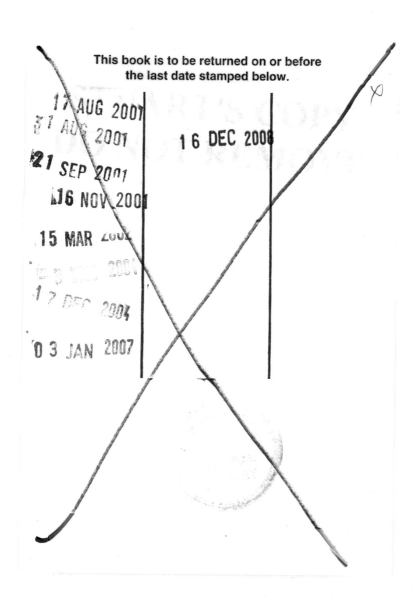

**This book is to be returned on or before
the last date stamped below.**

17 AUG 2001
31 AUG 2001
21 SEP 2001
16 NOV 2001

15 MAR 2002

17 DEC 2004

03 JAN 2007

16 DEC 2008

INCONTINENCE

This book is dedicated to the memory of Huw Williams
whose humanity, good humour and sagacity were a model for us all.

INCONTINENCE

EDITED BY

Malcolm Lucas ChM, FRCS
Consultant Urologist, Morriston Hospital, Swansea

Simon Emery MB, ChB, MRCOG
Consultant Obstetrician and Gynaecologist, Singleton Hospital, Swansea

John Beynon MS, FRCS
Consultant General and Colorectal Surgeon, Singleton Hospital, Swansea

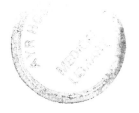

**Blackwell
Science**

© 1999 by
Blackwell Science Ltd
Editorial Offices:
Osney Mead, Oxford OX2 0EL
25 John Street, London WC1N 2BL
23 Ainslie Place, Edinburgh EH3 6AJ
350 Main Street, Malden
MA 02148 5018, USA
54 University Street, Carlton
Victoria 3053, Australia
10, rue Casimir Delavigne
75006 Paris, France

Other Editorial Offices:
Blackwell Wissenschafts-Verlag
GmbH
Kurfürstendamm 57
10707 Berlin, Germany

Blackwell Science KK
MG Kodenmacho Building
7–10 Kodenmacho Nihombashi
Chuo-ku, Tokyo 104, Japan

Iowa State University Press
A Blackwell Science Company
2121 S. State Avenue
Ames, Iowa 50014-8300, USA

First published 1999
Reprinted 2001

Set by Graphicraft Ltd, Hong Kong
Printed and bound in Great Britain
by MPG Books Ltd, Bodmin, Cornwall

A catalogue record for this title
is available from the British Library

ISBN 0–632–05003–9

Library of Congress
Cataloging-in-publication Data

Incontinence / editors, Malcolm
Lucas, Simon Emery, John
Beynon.
    p.   cm.
    ISBN 0–632–05003–9
    1. Urinary incontinence—
Treatment.   2. Fecal
incontinence—Treatment.
I. Lucas, Malcolm.
II. Emery, Simon, MB ChB.
III. Beynon, J. (John).
    [DNLM: 1. Urinary
Incontinence—therapy.
2. Fecal Incontinence—
therapy.   3. Urologic Surgical
Procedures—methods.
4. Gynecologic Surgical
Procedures—methods.
5. Colorectal Surgery—
methods.   WJ 146 I358 1999]
RC921.I5I46 1999
616.6—dc21
DNLM/DLC
for Library of Congress
                        98–49186
                        CIP

DISTRIBUTORS

Marston Book Services Ltd
PO Box 269
Abingdon, Oxon OX14 4YN
(Orders: Tel: 01235 465500
          Fax: 01235 465555)

USA
Blackwell Science, Inc.
Commerce Place
350 Main Street
Malden, MA 02148 5018
(Orders: Tel: 800 759 6102
               781 388 8250
          Fax: 781 388 8255)

Canada
Login Brothers Book Company
324 Saulteaux Crescent
Winnipeg, Manitoba R3J 3T2
(Orders: Tel: 204 837–2987)

Australia
Blackwell Science Pty Ltd
54 University Street
Carlton, Victoria 3053
(Orders: Tel: 3 9347 0300
          Fax: 3 9347 5001)

For further information on
Blackwell Science, visit our website:
www.blackwell-science.com

The Blackwell Science logo is a
trade mark of Blackwell Science Ltd,
registered at the United Kingdom
Trade Marks Registry

Contents

Contributors

John Beynon MS, FRCS
Consultant General and Colorectal Surgeon, Swansea NHS Trust, Singleton Hospital,
Swansea, SA2 8QA, UK

Alison F. Brading MA (Oxon), BSc, PhD
Professor of Pharmacology, University Department of Pharmacology, Mansfield Road,
Oxford, OX1 3QT, UK

Nicholas Carr MD, FRCS
Consultant General and Colorectal Surgeon, Swansea NHS Trust, Singleton Hospital,
Swansea, SA2 8QA, UK

Simon Emery MB, ChB, MRCOG
Consultant Obstetrician and Gynaecologist, Swansea NHS Trust, Singleton Hospital,
Swansea, SA2 8QA, UK

Robert Flynn MB, FRCS (Urol)
Specialist Registrar, Department of Urology, University Hospital of Wales, Heath Park,
Cardiff, CF4 4XW, UK

Lesley Irvine SRN, H.Ed.Cert
Clinical Nurse Specialist/Continence Advisor, Swansea NHS Trust, Singleton Hospital,
Swansea, SA2 8QA, UK

Jo Laycock PhD, FCSP
Chartered Physiotherapist, Culgaith Clinic, Pea Top Grange, Culgaith, Penrith, CA10 1QW,
UK

Malcolm Lucas ChM FRCS
Consultant Urologist, Morriston Hospital NHS Trust, Swansea, SA6 6NL, UK

Kirsten A. Major BA
Health Economist, Ayrshire and Arran Health Board, Boswell House, 10 Arthur Street,
Ayr, KA7 1QJ, UK

Ru McDonagh MD, FRCS
Consultant Urologist, Taunton and Somerset Hospital, Musgrove Park, Taunton, TA1 5DA,
UK

Ian W. Mills MA (Cantab), FRCS
Urological Research Fellow, University Department of Pharmacology, Mansfield Road, Oxford, OX1 3QT, UK

Henry Sells MB BS FRCS
Specialist Registrar in Urology, Bristol Royal Infirmary, Bristol, BS2 8HW, UK

Noreen R. Shields BA MSc
Social Scientist, Department of Public Health (Women's Health), Greater Glasgow Health Board, Dalian House, 350 St Vincent Street, Glasgow, G3 8YU, UK

Mark J. Speakman MB MS FRCS
Consultant Urologist, Taunton and Somerset Hospital, Musgrove Park, Taunton, TA1 5DA, UK

Tim Stephenson MS FRCS
Consultant Urologist, Department of Urology, University Hospital of Wales, Heath Park, Cardiff, CF4 4XW, UK

Preface

To suffer from either urinary or faecal incontinence is a demeaning and distressing experience that merits a standard of care and understanding from health professionals at least as high as other areas of medicine dealing with chronic debility. Sadly this is often not the case and there is a tendency for patients' needs to be met merely with unhelpful platitudes. Many specialists provide care for patients with incontinence yet have no particular interest in the subject and simply offer what they know. Fortunately this works for the majority but the rest are frequently left to fend for themselves, believing that nothing more can be done or that it is all just an inevitable part of growing old. Perhaps because nobody ever dies of incontinence and possibly because of its rather distasteful or embarrassing nature, incontinence has remained an area of low clinical priority and rarely features high on lists of health targets or planned service developments.

This book has been written for two reasons. Firstly, it is a training manual and practical guide aimed at the surgical trainee, continence nurse specialist or the working specialist who wishes to develop an incontinence practice. Although several excellent definitive textbooks already exist on most of the subjects covered in this book, there has been very little directed specifically at these readers. They have particular pressures on their time and need a straightforward and clear discussion of theory and common practice to help them prepare for postgraduate examinations or form the basis for sound clinical practice in day-to-day management.

Secondly, we wish to promote a cooperative team approach to incontinence management. Traditional clinical practice has evolved three separate clinical specialities who work within millimetres of each other within the pelvis. At best there has been occasional cooperation between them, but at worst a jealous guarding of territory in which each specialist denies or belittles the contribution of the other. The bladder/urethral outlet and the rectum/anal canal are analogous in many ways. The abnormalities that develop are similar, often coexist and the solutions we develop to correct them are based on the same underlying principles.

The urologist should realize that it is futile to perform a bladder neck suspension on a patient who strains so hard at stool that she will soon disrupt any attempt at fascial support or repair. Equally, the colorectal surgeon should know that a rectocoele repair may be followed by exacerbation, or emergence, of stress urinary incontinence and an increase in cystocoele. Gynaecologists must be aware of the impact that repair procedures may have on bladder, bowel and sexual function. To perform a urinary diversion on a patient with multiple sclerosis and ignore the coexisting problem of faecal incontinence would be to sadly neglect the best interests of the patient.

This book is based on a philosophy that we have worked with in Swansea for many years, where a common approach has been developed in which all three pelvic specialties recognize the importance and proximity of the others. We encourage our trainees to 'think horizontally' and have joint clinical meetings, protocols, clinics and shared operating where appropriate. This cooperative approach applies to other aspects of pelvic surgery as well as incontinence. We anticipate the emergence of surgeons who wish to become pelvic floor specialists and we should try to offer these individuals the opportunity to obtain a broad cross-boundary training. However, skill mixes are rarely complete and, although this book is largely Swansea based, we have called on the particular expertise of a number of respected colleagues to help us set the practical day-to-day work in an appropriate scientific, social and economic background.

The reader is urged particularly to read those parts of the book that might traditionally be perceived as being outside his or her field of work. Only by doing this will an appreciation of the importance of a cooperative and broad approach to pelvic floor dysfunction develop. We hope that the sections on research and audit and economic and business aspects will encourage a more innovative approach to clinical practice that will maximize the potential benefit from the available mix of local expertise. The book is deliberately didactic, generously illustrated and, for the most part, thinly referenced. Key references and recommended sources of further reading are collected together at the end of the book so that the flow is interrupted as little as possible.

If the reading of the book achieves half as much in building understanding and cooperation between our clinical disciplines, and between clinicians and scientists, as has its writing, then it should make a valuable and lasting contribution to the standards of patient care.

Whilst this book was in production an important international agreement on the nomenclature of drugs was announced by the Medicines Control Agency. This announcement was made too late to be implemented in this book.

MGL, SJE & JB
Swansea

Acknowledgements

The motivation for this book stems from a few of our teachers who instilled in us a conviction of the importance of cooperative working and learning that has grown with us into our clinical practice. We wish to mention in particular David Thomas and Nick Read, Geoffrey Chisholm, Adam Smith, Alan Brown, David Millar and Neil Mortensen.

Thanks are due to many individuals for supporting the preparation of this book. Mr Douglas Neil, Medical Photographer at Singleton Hospital for his photography and skills with image manipulation, Dr Bharat Patel, Consultant Radiologist for his help in providing defaecating proctography and endo anal ultrasound and colonic transit images. Mr Mike Nelson, Research Fellow in Colorectal Surgery, for his help with anorectal physiology images and video image capture of the videourodynamic images.

We thank our clinical colleagues and junior medical and secretarial staff for their forbearance in our occasional absence from the workface and frequent preoccupation with matters of writing style and publishing in the face of more pressing clinical matters. Finally, those who have suffered most from our neglect are those closest to us, and it is to our families that we offer our most heartfelt thanks.

1: Psychological Aspects of Incontinence

Henry Sells & Ru McDonagh

Incontinence in our society tends to be shrouded in secrecy and embarrassment because of the stigma associated with it. Consequently, as doctors and nurses, we may only see a fraction of those who are affected. Psychological, social and behavioural problems are unpredictable in each individual and some will find their life intolerable because of incontinence. The expected cause and effect relationship between incontinence and psychological problems is complicated and either can lead to the other. Incontinence can also affect those around the sufferer, including spouse, family and carers, and can lead to frustrations, fatigue and institutionalization for the subject. The complicated relationship between incontinence and psychosocial issues is reinforced by the variable success of psychological and behavioural techniques in the treatment of incontinence.

Psychosocial causes of incontinence

Some researchers have argued that psychosocial factors contribute to the development and maintenance of urinary incontinence. It has been suggested that urine loss due to detrusor instability without an anatomical or neurological cause should be viewed as a physical manifestation of emotional stress, personality disorder or an unsupportive environment.

Fliegner and Glenning (1979) concluded that urge incontinence is one of the commonest psychosomatic conditions in gynaecology and its treatment must be orientated with this in mind. This chapter shows that those patients with idiopathic detrusor instability suffer more anxiety and depression than their counterparts with stress incontinence. Freeman *et al.* (1985) found similar results but diverged from the usual reasoning that urge incontinence causes psychological problems, instead suggesting that underlying this relationship there is a personality type unable to express emotions and prone to somatic conversion, which might take the form of urinary incontinence.

Others have characterized urge incontinence as a stress reaction, the severity of which depends on the degree of emotional disturbance and its duration. Stresses such as marital problems, widowhood, family illness, accidents, unemployment and financial worries can all act as triggers that lead to incontinence (Frewen, 1978). Schwartz and Stanton (1950) identified five types of social situations among mental patients that acted as triggers for the majority of incontinent episodes: conflict, abandonment, isolation, being devalued and unconstructive episodes. Caregivers interviewed by Noelker (1987) reported more disruptive behaviour among incontinent older subjects. Again this can be interpreted as either the incontinence causing the behavioural problem or the behavioural problem leading to disrupted voiding behaviour.

Continence is a conditioned reflex acquired through social learning. Detrusor instability has been aetiologically linked to the loss of conditioned reflexes through self-induced or iatrogenic circumstances and also to the loss of cortical inhibition through ageing or central nervous system pathology (Williams & Pannill, 1982). Negative stimuli applied to a conditioned reflex inhibit its control. Thus negative stimuli such as lack of privacy, uncomfortable positions in voiding or using bedpans or bottles have a disruptive effect on voiding behaviour. Motivation is also important for patients to remain continent of faeces and urine and this diminishes with confusion, depression, dementia and sedation (Tarrier & Larner, 1983).

There appears to be enough evidence to count psychological causes among the many factors that lead to incontinence. Use of behavioural and psychological treatments in treating incontinence helps to confirm this. These are discussed later in the chapter.

Reluctance to seek help

The stigma attached to urinary incontinence makes it difficult to assess its prevalence; accordingly, studies have variable results. Further difficulties arise because of the different definitions of incontinence, brought about by differences in the population's perceptions. People who suffer involuntary loss do not necessarily regard themselves as incontinent and may only perceive a problem if they have public accidents rather than losing urine at home or into a pad (Herzog et al., 1989).

Quoted prevalence figures for overall incontinence vary from 10 to 51%, with females reporting a 1.5–2 times higher prevalence than males (Fliegner & Glenning, 1979; Breakwell & Walker, 1988). These figures clearly demonstrate that the vast majority of patients with incontinence are not being assessed for treatment. A study of perimenopausal women found that only one-quarter of those with incontinence had consulted a doctor (Reymert & Hunskaar, 1994).

Incontinence clearly embarrasses those who are affected and this has been shown to be a major factor in delay in seeking help. Many regard their symptoms as not serious enough or too infrequent to warrant treatment. Similarly, many regard it as a normal part of ageing. Older people have been shown to rank their symptoms in order of priority and may regard incontinence as insignificant compared with other more serious conditions. Those who do seek professional help often have their problems minimized, only serving to reinforce the idea that incontinence is typical of ageing and that treatment is not available (Ory *et al.*, 1986). This response may be due to the fact that physicians themselves have been shown to be reluctant to talk about faecal or urinary incontinence (Huppe *et al.*, 1992).

Gender is thought to play a major role in the help-seeking behaviour of those with incontinence. While prevalence is highest in women, their physicians have been primarily male. Women fear both the embarrassment of discussing personal problems with a man and the possibility of an internal examination. Many older women passively acknowledge the presence of 'women's problems' and regard the leaking of urine as another inevitable 'curse' (Wells, 1984). Rather than see a health professional, older incontinent individuals will change their daily routines and the amount that they drink in order to conceal their accidents. However, males are by no means free from the burdens of gender when presenting with incontinence, with evidence that men are more reluctant to seek help because they regard it as a 'woman's problem' (Norton, 1986).

A study of female patients of all ages attending a urodynamic clinic showed that 40% delayed seeing their GP for up to 1 year, one-third for 1–5 years and one-quarter for over 5 years (Norton *et al.*, 1988). The length of delay was significantly associated with age, those over 65 being twice as likely as those under 35 to wait more than 5 years. Married women were also more likely to delay seeking help than unmarried women. The reasons given for delay incorporate those mentioned above, with the most common reasons being embarrassment at discussing the problem with their doctor and hope that the problem would get better on its own. Unsurprisingly, fear of operation was given as a reason for delay much more commonly in older patients. The length of delay was not correlated to the distress that the women were suffering because of their symptoms, which suggests that large numbers of the worst-affected patients may take years to present or do not present at all.

Although it is difficult to overcome the stigma that patients attach to incontinence, we can encourage women to reduce the delay before seeking medical help. Patients need to be informed that help for incontinence is available and that many symptoms can be helped or completely alleviated without surgery. As the prevalence is so high in the community, we should be encouraged to actively elicit urinary complaints at consultation, as many incontinent patients are unable to initiate discussion themselves.

Psychosocial consequences of incontinence

Involuntary loss of urine has far-reaching effects on a person's life, involving mental well-being, social life, ability to continue working and relationships with family and friends. All come under the psychosocial umbrella. These wide-ranging categories cover most aspects of a person's life but are all closely interrelated. The studies that address the psychosocial implications can be divided into two groups: those looking at behavioural and social consequences, and those looking at psychological consequences. In this section we also look at how different types of incontinence and demographics govern any morbidity.

Behavioural and social consequences

Many studies have been published that attempt to quantify the effect that incontinence has on the population, both men and women, living both in the community and in institutions. Predictably in a condition where definitions vary, the results change with each study. Overall, however, 12–52% of people with incontinence report interference with social activities (Wyman *et al.*, 1990). Grimby *et al.* (1993) compared the overall quality of life of a group of incontinent women with an age-matched continent group using a validated generic measure, the Nottingham Health Profile (NHP). The incontinent group were found to be significantly more socially isolated than the continent group. Two reasons for restriction of social activities and interactions are embarrassment about smells and concerns about possible accidents. Interviews with incontinent older adults living in residential facilities indicated that they rarely left their apartments for fear of accidents and also that those who could not control wetness and smells in public were shunned by their social groups (Breakwell & Walker, 1988).

McGrother *et al.* (1987) confirmed that an older incontinent group was three times as likely to have less than one social interaction per day compared with a continent group, while a similar study of older community dwellers could find no significant difference between the social interactions of incontinent and continent groups (Herzog *et al.*, 1988). This may be explained by the different methods of measurement: while those who are incontinent may withdraw from certain types of social interaction, they may also require more assistance because of their incontinence, thereby increasing interactions with carers or caring relatives. This was confirmed by Vetter *et al.* (1981) who showed that incontinence increased the frequency of contact with relatives while decreasing contact with friends.

Seemingly bizarre behaviours are adopted to try to conceal incontinence: frequent checking of clothing for wet patches, frequent visits to the bathroom to try to avoid leaks and attempts to mask any smell of urine with excessive perfumes. Life is further complicated by the need to know where toilets are located when away from home and the need to carry dry clothes and pads. This leads to restrictions in shopping, travelling, holidays, church-going and any other activities outside the home (Wyman *et al.*, 1990). In addition it has been shown that incontinent women were less able to lift or carry and over half said their incontinence was affecting their work (Norton *et al.*, 1988).

Due to the nature of the disease, in which urine tends to leak with certain physical activities, those with stress incontinence have been shown to shy away from such activities. However, those with urge incontinence also avoid these activities, presumably because participation takes them away from accessible toilets and also because they are usually among other people (Wyman *et al.*, 1990). It has been shown that both urinary and faecal incontinence lead to decreased sexual activity, particularly in those subjects who are unmarried or under 65 years (Huppe *et al.*, 1992). Hunskaar and Sandvik's (1993) study of 150 community-dwelling men showed that they were restricted in a significant number of the social activities listed on a questionnaire. Most commonly affected was travelling, followed by going to the cinema, wearing desired clothes, heavy lifting, sports, visiting friends and work.

It is still debated whether children with nocturnal enuresis exhibit more behavioural problems than do children without enuresis. What is now clear, however, is that any psychological stress is a result of enuresis rather than a cause (Norgaard *et al.*, 1997). However, difficulties do arise between the child and its parents and friends. If parents choose to punish the child to stop it happening again, this reduces parent–child interaction and can contribute to a stressful home environment. Siblings may be embarrassed or angered or their activities limited by the child's enuresis. Further isolation of the child results from reluctance to go on camping trips, stay at friends' houses or even to have friends in their room because of the fear of detection via odours or plastic sheeting (Warzak, 1993). Faecal incontinence has also been shown to produce psychosocial and behavioural problems in children, and three distinct coping strategy phases have been described: withdrawal, denial or secretiveness and eventual acceptance (Ludman & Spitz, 1996). The success of these stratagies has been shown to vary with family and social environments.

Psychological consequences

These social, sexual and behavioural restrictions all contribute to the psychological problems resulting from incontinence. Incontinent persons may never feel at ease due to the threat of an incontinent episode occurring. The embarrassment associated with their condition may lead to lowered self-esteem and self-confidence and the feeling of vulnerability. Feelings of control or mastery are typically affected by losing control at critical life situations, and experiencing a leak of urine during such a situation can have long-lasting effects (Herzog *et al.*, 1989). Many view incontinence as a natural part of ageing and for them its onset heralds further deterioration in health.

Proving a relationship between incontinence and psychological distress has been difficult. Herzog *et al.* (1989) observed a weak but statistically significant relationship, although some of this has been put down to the poorer general health of the incontinent population. Wyman *et al.*'s (1990) analysis of published studies shows that varying proportions of the incontinent population suffer increasing social isolation, a moderate to severe impact on daily life, and negative self-image and perceptions. Part of the problem in drawing conclusions from the many studies is the lack of validated instruments and studies containing large numbers of patients.

Using the NHP, Grimby *et al.* (1993) found that incontinent women scored higher in the emotional disturbance dimension than a continent control group. Kelleher *et al.* (1993) found that the overall NHP scores were higher in incontinent vs. continent subjects, indicating a worse overall quality of life. A study of 411 incontinent people from Sweden using the Short Form 36, another validated generic questionnaire, showed that they were significantly worse off than the general population in each of the eight domains and, furthermore, that their morbidity correlated well with their symptom severity (Johannesson *et al.*, 1997). Interestingly, a study examining faecal incontinence using the Hospital Anxiety and Depression questionnaire showed subjects to be no worse off than controls, though scores were improved in those who underwent successful treatments (Fisher *et al.*, 1989).

Two studies that evaluated the effects of urinary incontinence produced no difference between continent and incontinent groups (Simons, 1985; Breakwell & Walker, 1988). This appears especially true when addressing incontinence in housebound people, suggesting that social restrictions are a major cause of any psychological problems caused by incontinence. However, there does appear to be a subset of individuals who have severe anxiety and depression associated with their incontinence. Macaulay *et al.* (1987) found that a group of 211 incontinent patients had anxiety scores higher than the general population, but also identified a subgroup of 25% whose incontinence rendered their lives intolerable. This subgroup demonstrated obsessionality scores equivalent to psychiatric in-patients and phobic and anxiety scores higher than psychiatric in-patients.

A specific Incontinence Stress Index developed at Pennsylvania State University indicated that patients exhibited both retarded and agitated symptoms of depression, reported feelings of abandonment and had anxieties related to their incontinence (Yu & Kaltreider, 1985). A circular sequence of events may occur, involving fear, shame or embarrassment in discussing the problem with anyone and leading to further isolation, loss of self-esteem, and psychological symptoms such as depression, apathy or anger.

Studies examining the treatment of incontinence tend to avoid psychosocial outcome measures and concentrate on cure rates or complications.

Unfortunately, this slows the development of a well-constructed, disease-specific questionnaire for incontinence. Although we have discusssed the use of validated generic questionnaires above, disease-specific questionnaires are more responsive as they only target relevant issues. The disadvantage of disease-specific questionnaires is the longer and more difficult validation process. The development of such a measure will standardize studies measuring the psychosocial consequences of incontinence as well those looking at treatment outcomes. It may be found in the future that use of the new generation of individual quality-of-life measures, such as the SEIQol-DW (schedule for the evaluation of individual quality of life – direct weighting), may be more appropriate (Hickey *et al.*, 1996).

Other factors influencing psychosocial consequences

We have seen how the psychosocial impact of incontinence varies between wide groups of the population. Many studies have tried to detect which factors determine how the incontinent person is affected.

Despite the predominant use of specific non-validated questionnaires, studies suggest that urge incontinence causes greater psychosocial impact than stress incontinence (Sutherst, 1979; Iosif *et al.*, 1981). Wyman *et al.* (1987) issued a specific incontinence impact questionnaire to 69 women with incontinence of mixed aetiology who had undergone urodynamic studies. The questionnaire addressed three broad categories: activities of daily living, social interactions and self-perception. Subjects with sphincteric incompetence had significantly lower impact scores than those with detrusor instability. Similar differences between the two groups were found using the NHP, the group with detrusor instability scoring significantly higher than the group with stress incontinence in the emotional disturbance dimension (Grimby *et al.*, 1993). This may be because those with detrusor instability are less able to predict incontinent episodes or have more precipitating factors for leakages. This leads to less feelings of control over bladder function and more restrictions in everyday life. Those with stress incontinence tend to have a better idea of when and where leakages will occur and can make arrangements to avoid these situations accordingly.

The correlation between the impact of incontinence and number of incontinent episodes and quantity of fluid loss (measured by weighing pads) was positive and statistically significant but modest. This suggests that it is the state of being incontinent rather than its severity that determines the impact of many of the restrictions. This becomes relevant in treatment aims: a significant reduction in severity of incontinence may not produce a corresponding reduction in restrictions and complete cure may be the only way to improve perceived impact significantly. In contrast, a study looking at children with faecal incontinence showed that the degree of mental health symptoms correlated well with the degree of soiling. Again this is important when considering treatment aims (Diseth & Emblem, 1996).

The higher impact of urge incontinence was confirmed by Hunskaar and Vinsnes (1991) who assessed 76 incontinent community-dwelling women using another generic, validated, quality-of-life measure, the Sickness Impact Profile. These authors also looked at the impact on different age groups. In the group with stress incontinence, the elderly subjects had significantly less dysfunction than the middle-aged subjects. This was most apparent in the Emotional Behaviour and Recreation and Pastimes domains, which addressed such items as discomfort, hopelessness, physical recreation and going out for entertainment. In these domains, the middle-aged group with stress incontinence was affected more than the groups with urge incontinence. In contrast, there was no significant difference between the two age groups with urge incontinence. It is apparent that stress incontinence can be extremely debilitating to the social life and recreation of younger sufferers, while their older counterparts have either adapted their lifestyles to avoid any disruption or are not taking part in as many activities due to the constraints of age. The same study confirmed a weak correlation between both frequency of incontinent episodes and amount of urine leaked. The impact scores were not correlated to duration of incontinence, i.e. the problem does not get smaller with time. This indicates that adaptation of lifestyle, as occurs in the elderly group with stress incontinence, does not take place in the other groups or that adaptation takes place very early on.

In summary, the only variable that has been shown to have a predictable effect on psychological impact is the mechanism of incontinence. The lack of any other predictive factors illustrates the heterogeneity of response to urinary incontinence and indicates that perception of the severity of incontinence is unique to each individual.

Effects on carers

The consequences of incontinence reach further than the affected individuals themselves. The condition creates effects that spill over to family, friends or caregivers. In a study comparing the family caregivers of continent and incontinent people, Noelker (1987) found that the presence of incontinence was associated with more stress: the caregiver shouldered the burden of care and exhibited deterioration in health and of family relationships. It should not be forgotten that the spouse is often the caregiver and that this is the relationship most often affected. This relationship is also affected by any sexual difficulties caused by incontinence. Another indication of the effects of incontinence on the whole family is the fact that it frequently precipitates or contributes to the decision to seek care for the affected person. Along with confusion and ambulatory problems, incontinence is one of the three factors most often responsible for the decision to place the sufferer in long-term residential care. Incontinence may be one of the factors that finally contributes to the family caregiver's breaking point.

Learning point: Reasons to enter long-term care
   Confusion
   Ambulatory difficulty
   Incontinence

    Attitudes to incontinence may also affect non-family caregivers. The care of the incontinent patient involves time-consuming changes of clothing and linen, the prolonged and difficult treatment of decubitus ulcers and other unpleasant tasks; it has been shown that nurses may have negative feelings towards incontinence that are displaced on to the patient (Wells, 1984). It has also been observed that incontinence is destructive of staff morale and that the regular care of incontinent patients quickly brings on 'burn-out' of personnel (Anderson, 1971). The process of cleaning up after episodes of urinary and faecal incontinence is demanding on staff time and demoralizing for staff and patient. This leads to attempts to forestall any incontinence by excessive watchfulness of the patient and by a willingness to accept false alarms and toilet the patient at the slightest sign (Tarrier & Larner, 1983).

    A survey of 156 nurses was carried out to measure staff stress in relation to incontinence (Yu & Kaltreider, 1985). Analysis of staff reactions showed that 50% felt frustrated, tired, discouraged and irritable some of the time, and one-third felt depressed about their work due to incontinence. Some felt that they wanted to resign due to the extra work involved in looking after incontinent patients. These negative feelings can lead to guilt or even 'reaction formation', in which nurses compensate for conscious or unconscious frustrations by over-indulgence, ultrapermissiveness or over-caring.

Psychological factors in the treatment of incontinence

Although sensory urgency can often be treated by pelvic exercise or surgery, urge incontinence or incontinence of mixed aetiology is more difficult to treat with drugs or surgery. As most patients with incontinence have urge-type leakage, other treatments have been explored including the use of behavioural or psychological techniques. Frewen (1978) claimed an 82% cure rate for incontinence using a programme of in-patient treatments comprising a bladder diary, bladder retraining, anxiolytic and anticholinergic drugs and supportive care. Bladder retraining involves gradual postponing of voiding at first desire and enforced voiding at set times. However, none of the factors was isolated as a therapeutic measure on its own. The techniques of biofeedback and social reinforcement have both been successful in treating faecal incontinence, although the results are expressed in reduction of incontinent episodes rather than cure rates (Tarrier & Larner, 1983; Ho *et al.*, 1996).

A trial to assess the efficacy of psychological treatments randomized patients to psychotherapy, bladder training or medication (Macaulay *et al.*, 1987). Those in the psychotherapy group underwent counselling and anxiety-relieving techniques with a psychiatrist. Those in the bladder training group were trained by a nurse to ignore cues from the bladder at first sensation and to void at set times. The control group was given propantheline (anticholinergic) for 3 months. In the psychotherapy group there were statistically significant improvements in nocturia, the number of incontinent episodes and urgency, although surprisingly there were no significant changes in psychological measures before and after treatment. Those in the bladder training group had a significant decrease in mean detrusor pressure rise and an increase in volume at first desire to void (FDV), but no significant change in urgency, nocturia and incontinence. Urinary frequency improved as did psychometric profile, with a significant reduction in anxiety and depression. The results of the group given propantheline were similar to those in the group receiving psychotherapy, with some increase in FDV and bladder capacity and slight improvement in frequency. The results confirm that psychotherapy can be an effective treatment for incontinence due to detrusor instability. Interestingly, improvements in the psychoneurotic profile were seen in the group with bladder training but not the group given psychotherapy. This again demonstrates the complex relationship between urinary incontinence and psychological measures, although this study did produce positive results in a difficult treatment group.

In summary, there seems to be a distinct subgroup in whom incontinence brings on severe anxiety, fear and depression. A 'middle-ground' group seems to show variable anxieties and impact on everyday life above that of the normal population. Finally, in the old, frail and housebound and especially those receiving care for mental or physical impairments, incontinence does not cause negative psychological effects.

Summary

We have shown that a complex relationship exists between urinary incontinence and psychosocial morbidity. The psychosocial consequences of incontinence fall into groups of severity; these groups can be predicted to a certain extent by the type and severity of incontinence and the age and sex of the affected person. The embarrassment caused by incontinence may lead to behaviour changes or social isolation and a reluctance to come forward for help. This in turn leads to anxiety, loss of confidence and depression and effects can spill over to carers or family. Further reluctance to seek help stems from fear of operations and the perception that surgery is the only treatment available. Clinicians need to actively seek out symptoms of incontinence and ensure that sufferers are aware that drugs, pelvic floor treatments, behaviour therapies and psychotherapy can provide successful non-operative treatment. Studies on new treatments for incontinence need to look at psychometric outcomes as well as cure rates and complications, and the development of a validated specific scoring system will standardize and facilitate this assessment.

2: Structure and Function in Continence and Incontinence

Robert Flynn

The process of urine and faecal storage within a compliant muscular reservoir and intermittent voiding in times and places that fit with social conventions is, arguably, better developed in humans than any other mammal. It is helpful to think of the bladder–urethral sphincter and rectum–anal canal as a functional whole, in which storage is dependent on outlet pressure exceeding reservoir pressure and emptying is dependent on the reverse. Although simplistic in concept, it is a principle that underpins all our understanding of continence and the solutions we develop when 'things go wrong'. The situation is, of course, more complex than these concepts would suggest and a clear grasp of the anatomy and physiology of the pelvic floor, bladder, urethra, rectum and anus is essential before the pathological mechanisms that result in incontinence can be understood.

This chapter describes the anatomical and pathological principles of normal function and presents a classification of incontinence, with an explanation of the common abnormalities; however, congenital malformations such as extrophia vesicae, epispadias, cloacal abnormalities and acquired leakage due to urinary and faecal fistulae are excluded.

Structure and function of the pelvic floor

The pelvic floor supports the pelvic and abdominal contents. It consists of three layers, the endopelvic fascia, the levator ani muscles and the perineal membrane. The most cranial layer of the pelvic floor is the endopelvic fascia (Fig. 2.1), which connects the pelvic viscera to the pelvic sidewalls. It consists of fibromuscular tissue, which is thickened in various areas to produce what are referred to as ligaments. The uterus, cervix and upper third of the vagina are attached to the pelvic sidewall by broad sheets of endopelvic fascia known as the cardinal and uterosacral ligaments (Fig. 2.2). These ligaments originate from the region of the greater sciatic foramen and the lateral aspect of the sacrum. In the erect position these ligaments run almost vertically and suspend their attached structures. The middle third of the vagina is attached to the pelvic sidewall by the pubocervical and rectovaginal fasciae, which insert into the arcus tendineus fascia pelvis and are in continuity with the uterosacral and cardinal ligaments. They provide a horizontal sheet of

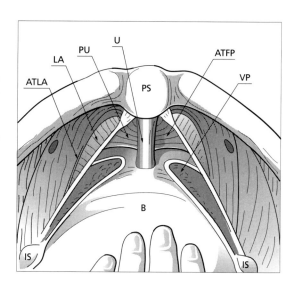

Fig. 2.1 A view into the female pelvis showing the relationship of the pelvic ligaments to the arcus tendineus fascia pelvis (ATFP). The bladder (B), pubic symphysis (PS), ischial spine (IS), and levator ani (LA) covered by obturator fascia are shown, as well as, arising from the arcus tendineus levator ani (ATLA), the pubourethral-supporting fascia (PU), urethra (U), and vesicopelvic fascia (VP). After Delancey.

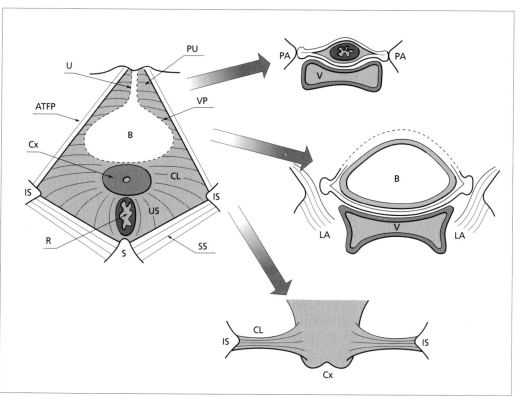

Fig. 2.2 Schematic diagram showing the relationship of the pubourethral-supporting ligaments, the paravesical fascia, the cardinal ligaments and the uterosacral ligaments, which are all condensations of the endopelvic fascia. Alongside are transverse sections through the vagina and fascial layers at three levels of the vagina to show how the two layers of the endopelvic fascia encircle the midline structures. Abbreviations as for Fig. 2.1 plus vagina (V), rectum (R), cervix (Cx), pubic arch (PA), cardinal ligament (CL), uterosacral ligament (US), sacrum (S) and sacrospinous ligament (SS).

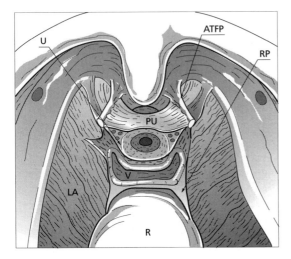

Fig. 2.3 A cross-section through the vagina and urethra just below the bladder neck showing the arcus tendineus fascia pelvis (ATFP), urethra (U), pubourethral-supporting fascia (PU), levator ani (LA), vagina (V), rectum (R) and rectal pillars (RP). After Delancey.

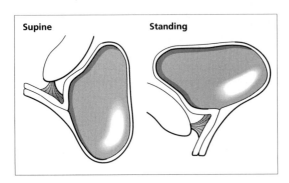

Fig. 2.4 A sagittal section through the pelvis showing that the bladder neck lies higher than the pubourethral fascia in the standing position.

support for the bladder. The urethra is intimately attached to the anterior wall of the lower third of the vagina in the female and hence the support of the lower third of the vagina is identical to that of the urethra. The paravaginal fascial attachments (Fig. 2.3) connect the periurethral tissues and the anterior vaginal wall to the arcus tendineus fascia pelvis. The urethra is not firmly attached to the symphysis pubis by the pubourethral ligaments as previously thought. Indeed the bladder neck lies above the attachment of the pubourethral ligaments in the healthy female and is mobile and under voluntary control by contraction of the levator ani (Fig. 2.4).

There is an argument that the levator ani muscle contributes most of the support to the pelvic organs by closing off the pelvic opening and creating a structure upon which the organs can lie, whereas the pelvic ligaments probably give an added support. In health, the pelvic ligaments are unlikely

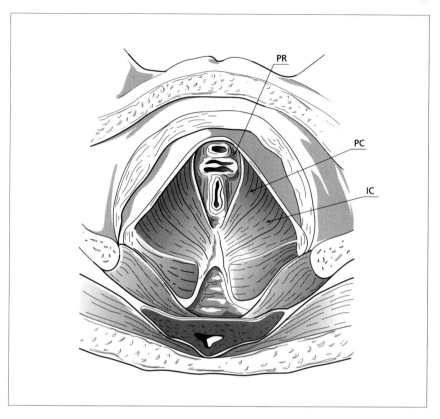

Fig. 2.5 A view into the female pelvis with the bladder and rectum removed to show the three components of the levator ani: puborectalis (PR), pubococcygeus (PC) and ileococcygeus (IC).

to be continually under strain. This concept is supported by the observation that fibrous tissue responds poorly to continual stress and eventually exceeds a given limit and stretches. In contrast, however, muscle is capable of providing renewable and flexible support. Clearly an intimate relationship exists between the pelvic floor musculature and the endopelvic fascia that is not fully understood.

The levator ani consists of three components, the puborectalis, pubococcygeus and iliococcygeus muscles (Figs 2.5 & 2.6). The puborectalis and pubococcygeus form a U-shaped band of muscle that arises from the pubic bones and forms a sling about the rectum and inserts into the coccyx. The puborectalis muscle forms a muscular sling around the anorectal junction and due to its attachment anteriorly to the pubic bone creates an angulation between the anal canal and the rectum. At rest the anorectal angle is 90°; however, during straining and defaecation the angle increases to about 135°, which

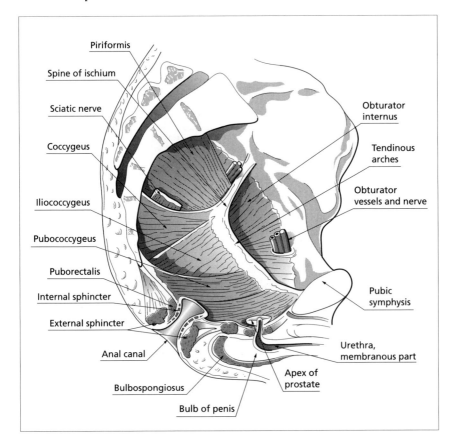

Fig. 2.6 A sagittal section of the pelvis to show the levators in a male.

assists the passage of stool, (Fig. 2.7). The puborectalis is closely related to the deep part of the external anal sphincter and some of its fibres enter the wall of the anal canal to contribute to its longitudinal muscle layer. The iliococcygeus arises from the arcus tendineus levator ani as it runs over the obturator internus from the pubic bone to the ischial spine. These muscles create a type of 'hammock' and in health are maintained in a state of tonic contraction and support the abdominal and pelvic viscera. It is through this hammock of muscle that the urethra, vagina and anal canal pass. In contrast to the urethral rhabdosphincter, which is composed predominantly of small-diameter slow-twitch (type I) fibres, the levator ani muscle is a mixture of approximately 70% slow-twitch and 30% fast-twitch (type II) fibres. Fibre type reflects function in that the slow-twitch fibres rely on aerobic metabolism and maintain tone, whereas the fast-twitch fibres rely on anaerobic metabolism and are mainly active in responding to sudden increases in intra-abdominal pressure.

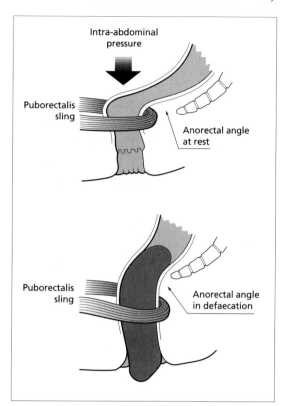

Fig. 2.7 Anorectal angle at rest
and during defaecation.

The final and most caudal layer of the pelvic floor is a fibromuscular sheet
known as the perineal membrane or urogenital membrane (Fig. 2.8). This lies
immediately below the levator ani. In the male it forms a complete sheet of
tissue that spans the anterior triangle of the pelvic outlet. In the female it is an
incomplete layer at the level of the hymenal ring, through which the vagina
passes. It attaches the edge of the vagina to the ischiopubic ramus and gives
support to the 'perineal body', a diffuse fascial thickening that lies between
the genital hiatus and the anus. The smooth and striated muscle components
of the perineal membrane contribute to its resting tone and the striated
muscle contributes to urethral function.

Structure and function of the anus

The anal canal forms a slit in the sagittal plane as it normally remains closed
at rest. The canal extends from the anorectal ring to the anal verge and measures 3–5 cm. The walls are closely opposed with mucosal folds (columns of
Morgagni) that extend from the anal valves at the dentate line (Fig. 2.9). The
circular muscle of the rectum thickens to form the internal anal sphincter that

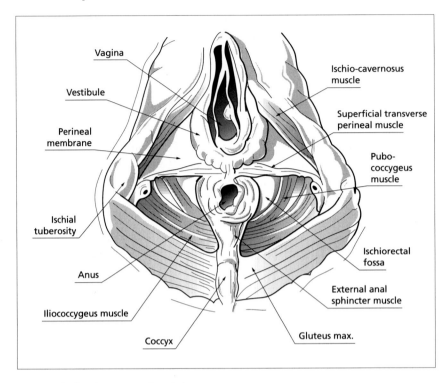

Fig. 2.8 The female perineum from below.

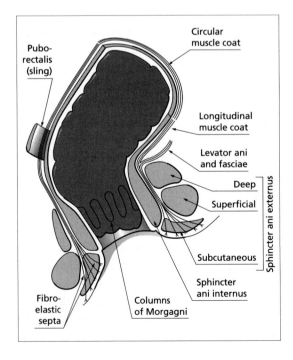

Fig. 2.9 A section through the anal canal and lower rectum.

contributes about 80% of the resting sphincter pressure. The pressure in the canal increases distally and is maximal at about 2 cm from the anal verge due to the external anal sphincter. Squeeze pressure is produced by voluntary contraction of the external anal sphincter and puborectalis and can double the normal resting pressure. It is increasingly recognized that there is an important association between faecal soiling, anal sphincter damage and obstetric injury. Coughing and the Valsalva manoeuvre both lead to increased electrical activity within the external anal sphincter. The vascular cushions of the anal canal contribute significantly to continence. During straining venous blood flow from these spaces stops, resulting in swelling of these cushions which then act as a kind of gasket.

Continence is preserved as long as anal pressure exceeds rectal pressure; the mechanisms controlling anal pressure have already been mentioned. Rectal factors play a role in continence also. The rectum is usually empty, the main reservoir for faeces being the transverse colon. Colonic contents will be delivered to the rectum at variable rates specific to an individual and the rectum then functions as a reservoir. The first sensation of rectal filling occurs at about a volume of 50 ml, the maximum tolerated volume being about 200 ml. Rectal compliance varies and is reduced in certain diseases such as Crohn's disease and radiation proctitis.

Structure and function of the bladder and urethra

Functionally, the detrusor can be divided into a body and base, although no such anatomical or histological division exists. The body is the muscular component largely responsible for the reservoir and pump functions of the bladder. The organization of the individual fibres is relatively random, the bundles continually branching with no discrete layers as such. As the healthy bladder fills it does so with practically no rise in intravesical pressure. The interwoven arrangement of the muscle bundles allows the detrusor body to contract in unison and thus produce efficient voiding. The predominant innervation of the detrusor body is cholinergic, although adrenergic (mainly β) receptors are also found here.

The detrusor base includes the continuation of body fibres on to the trigone and distally into the urethra. The detrusor base is relatively fixed and non-distensible during storage but is transformed into a funnel by the contracting detrusor during voiding (Fig. 2.10). The extension of the distal ureteral musculature into the trigone provides an anchor to the terminal ureter. Craniolateral extensions of the detrusor base both longitudinally and helically into the distal ureter prevent vesicoureteric reflux by closure of the orifice when the sheath contracts with the base during voiding. The predominant innervation is α-adrenergic, but there is some sparse cholinergic innervation.

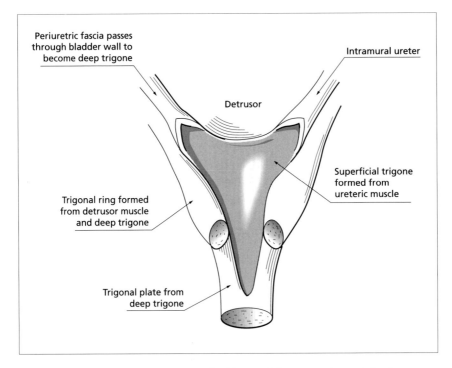

Periuretric fascia passes
through bladder wall to
become deep trigone

Intramural ureter

Detrusor

Superficial trigone
formed from
ureteric muscle

Trigonal ring formed
from detrusor muscle
and deep trigone

Trigonal plate from
deep trigone

Fig. 2.10 The female trigone with the superficial layer and deeper ring that encircles the bladder neck.

The urethra is a multilayered muscular tube that provides a conduit for urine to pass to the exterior and also plays a role in continence. In the male it is of far greater length than in the female, where it measures approximately 3–4 cm. The urethra consists of three layers, the mucosal, submucosal and muscular layers. In both males and females the mucosa is folded in longitudinal layers that allow for considerable distensibility, just as in the rectum. The submucosa consists of a rich vascular plexus that may act as a cushion to promote mucosal coaptation (Fig. 2.11) and hence aid in the maintenance of continence. The muscular elements differ considerably in both sexes and are described separately below.

There are smooth and striated muscle elements in the female urethra. The smooth muscle is predominantly arranged longitudinally and is in continuity with the detrusor and probably acts to shorten the urethra. The striated fibres, otherwise known as the rhabdosphincter, surround the smooth muscle elements (Fig. 2.12). The striated fibres consist of two different portions. The upper portion surrounds the upper two-thirds of the urethra and consists of circularly orientated fibres, although they do not form a complete circle being

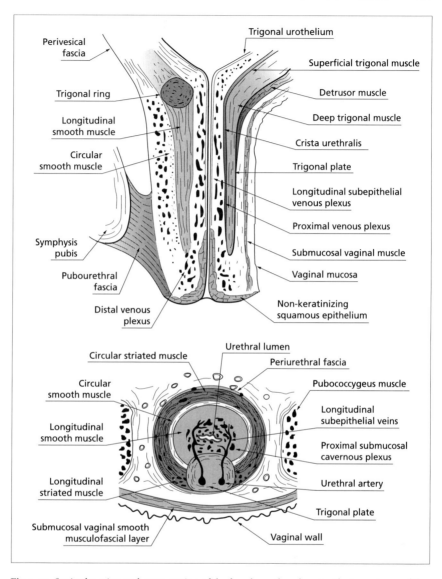

Fig. 2.11 Sagittal section and cross-section of the female urethra showing the importance of the vascular plexus.

deficient posteriorly. The second portion consists of two strap-like bands that lie adjacent to the lumen of the lower third of the urethra (Fig. 2.13) and arch over the anterior surface. One of these bands originates in the vaginal wall and is called the urethrovaginal sphincter muscle; the other originates near the ischiopubic ramus and is known as the compressor urethrae. The precise function of these two strap muscles is not fully understood.

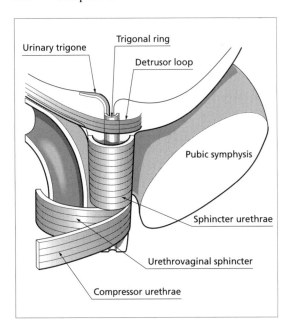

Fig. 2.12 The female urethral sphincter mechanism showing detrusor and trigonal fibres at the bladder neck, the circular muscle of the sphincter urethrae and the strap-like muscles of the distal urethra.

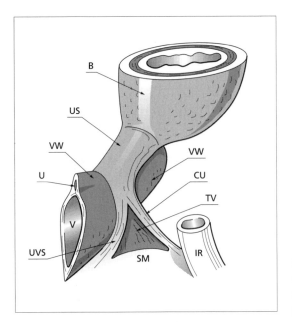

Fig. 2.13 The relationship of the strap muscles of the urethra to the vaginal introitus and the perineal body.

In the male the urethra is divided into four anatomical regions, the pre-prostatic, prostatic, membranous and penile urethra (Fig. 2.14). The prepro-static urethra measures about 1 cm and runs from the bladder neck to the prostatic urethra. It is surrounded by a complete ring of smooth muscle and

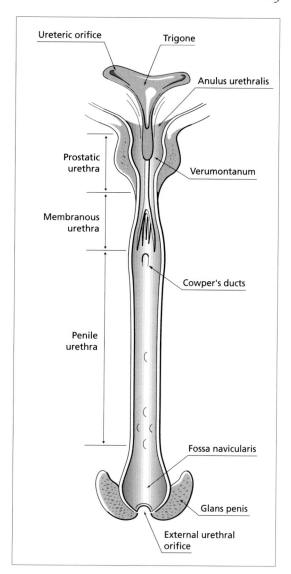

Fig. 2.14 The posterior wall of the male urethra.

can maintain continence in some men in whom the rhabdosphincter has been destroyed and allows antegrade ejaculation. The prostatic urethra extends the length of the prostate, terminating at the apex. It is surrounded by a thin layer of smooth muscle that extends throughout the prostate and its capsule. Endoscopically, it terminates just distal to the verumontanum where the membranous urethra commences. At this level on its anterior surface the urethra is surrounded by a layer of circularly orientated striated fibres in a horseshoe conformation known as the rhabdosphincter. The periurethral striated fibres of the pelvic floor lie external to this.

The predominance of slow-twitch fibres in the rhabdosphincter is consistent with its role in maintaining tone, whereas the fast-twitch fibres of the pelvic floor musculature allow rapid recruitment of motor units to counteract sudden changes in abdominal pressure.

Neural control of the lower urinary tract, pelvic floor and anal canal

Conceptually, bladder function can be usefully divided into two phases, storage and voiding. While peripheral autonomic nerves and those somatic fibres that supply the urethral rhabdosphincter are the final pathways of control, it is obvious the higher centres play a major role, both inhibitory and facilitatory, in modifying the various aspects of bladder control. The brainstem, namely the pontine–mesencephalic grey matter, consists of nuclei containing motor neurones that are the origin of the final common pathway to the bladder. This area is known as Barrington's centre after the experimental work by this neurophysiologist in the early part of this century. He described experimentally produced lesions and reflexes in a cat model, many of which have been adapted to explain human bladder function. Transection above Barrington's centre leads to detrusor hyperreflexia, transection below it leads to disturbances of bladder emptying, while stimulation of this area causes bladder contraction and relaxation of the urethral rhabdosphincter. Higher centres, including the cerebellum, basal ganglia, thalamus, hypothalamus and cerebral cortex, have input into this brainstem nucleus. The influence of the cerebral cortex and basal ganglia appear to be mainly inhibitory. The combination of animal work (mainly cat models) and clinical experience provides us with the current working models for neurological dysfunction.

The main cerebral areas involved with control of micturition appear to be the superiomedial portion of the frontal lobes and the genu of the corpus callosum. Once again these are predominantly inhibitory, which is in keeping with the common clinical finding of uninhibited detrusor contractions in patients with cortical lesions, e.g. epilepsy and following cerebrovascular accidents. The cortical area concerned with innervation of the urethral rhabdosphincter is located separately on the medial aspect of the sensorimotor cortex.

The bladder and urethra are supplied by branches of the pelvic plexus (Fig. 2.15). This plexus lies deep in the pelvis on either side of the pelvic organs in a fascial sheath running from the lateral pelvic wall to the base of the bladder. It is formed by contributions from the pelvic (parasympathetic), hypogastric (sympathetic) and somatic nerves. The cell bodies of the pelvic nerves arise in the intermediolateral column of grey matter in the S2–S4

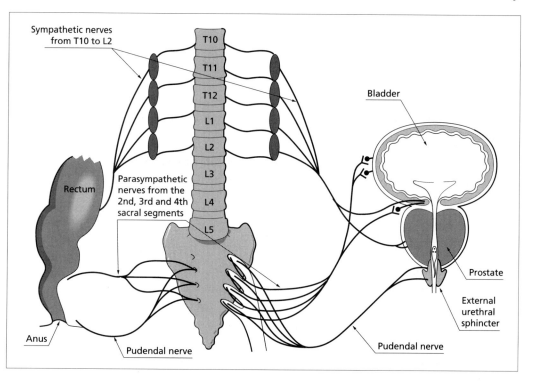

Fig. 2.15 The major innervation pathways at the pelvic level that are basic to control of micturition and continence. The exact combinations of afferent and efferent activity during each phase of a filling and voiding cycle remains unclear, although the importance of the integrity of these pathways is well known.

segments of the spinal cord; the cell bodies of the hypogastric nerves lie in the intermediolateral column of grey matter in the T10–L2 segments of the spinal cord. The autonomic supply to the urethra travels via an intrapelvic route from the pelvic plexus to the bladder and urethra. The autonomic neurones are divided into preganglionic and postganglionic fibres. Typically, in the parasympathetic system ganglia are located in or near the innervated organ and in the lower urinary tract there are numerous intramural ganglia in the wall of the bladder from which arise the postganglionic parasympathetic nerves (short neurones). This is in contrast to the sympathetic system where the ganglia tend to be remote from the organ they supply, i.e. the cell bodies of the postganglionic neurones to the bladder lie in the hypogastric plexus.

The cell bodies of the somatic nerves supplying the urethral rhabdosphincter lie in the anterior horn of S2–S4 (anatomically located at vertebral levels T12–L1) in a site known as Onuf's nucleus. Elbadawi and Schneck (1974) have demonstrated in many mammals the existence of a triple (parasympathetic–

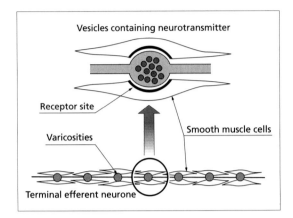

Fig. 2.16 The neuromuscular junction within the detrusor.

sympathetic–somatic) innervation to the urethral rhabdosphincter. However, debate continues as to whether the fibres supplying the rhabdosphincter run with the pudendal nerve via an extrapelvic route or via a parallel intrapelvic pathway. Recent evidence strongly suggests that there is an intrapelvic somatic pathway derived from the S2–S4 sacral roots that is distinct from the pudendal nerve, which supplies the levator ani and the urethra (Borirakchanyavat *et al.*, 1997). Preservation of the intrapelvic nerve supply is critical for maintaining the somatic innervation of the urethra during radical pelvic surgery.

The neuromuscular junction of smooth muscle differs from that of striated muscle. The terminal branches of the efferent autonomic nerves run within the smooth muscle bundles and possess a series of swellings called varicosities that contain neurotransmitters (Fig. 2.16). The net effect is that a single nerve fibre subserves a group of muscle cells. There are three main types of vesicles: (i) agranular, which are cholinergic; (ii) small dense-cored, which are adrenergic; and (iii) large dense-cored, the contents of which are uncertain.

The traditional description of autonomic nerve transmission suggested that parasympathetic nerves release acetylcholine, which acts on nicotinic receptors in the ganglia and muscarinic receptors at the neuromuscular junction, and that sympathetic nerves release noradrenaline. However, control is unlikely to be this simple and it is now known that many substances are co-released and various neuropeptides have been identified in the bladder (Table 2.1). The search for these neurotransmitters was driven by the recognition of the phenomenon of atropine resistance, a finding that the contraction induced by cholinergic fibres could not be totally eliminated by

Table 2.1 Neurotransmitter substances identified in the bladder.

Acetylcholine

Noradrenaline

Adenosine triphosphate

Prostaglandins F_2, E_1, E_2

Peptides
  Substance P
  Neuropeptide Y
  Vasoactive intestinal polypeptide
  Somatostatin
  Enkephalins
  Calcitonin gene-related peptide

atropine. Substance P and neuropeptide Y, which contract the bladder, and vasoactive intestinal polypeptide, which relaxes the bladder, are examples of such neuropeptides. Substance P appears to be a predominantly sensory neurotransmitter. The co-release of these neuropeptides may well alter the nature or the intensity of the classic transmitters.

The afferent innervation of the bladder is less well understood. Information arises from mechanoreceptors and from pain and temperature receptors in the bladder; some Pacinian corpuscles have also been identified. The sensory fibres appear to run with the parasympathetic, sympathetic and somatic nerves, and arrive at the cord at the same level as the efferent fibres.

Normal filling and voiding

In an attempt to unify the available data, the normal control of storage and voiding of urine can be summarized as follows. Normal storage depends on adequate bladder compliance and stability, competence of the vesicoureteral junctions and the vesical outlet, and appropriate bladder sensation. Normal compliance (dV/dP) means that at natural filling rates intravesical pressure remains low, primarily due to the passive elastic and viscoelastic properties of the smooth muscle and bladder wall connective tissue (Fig. 2.17). Detrusor stability depends upon intrinsic properties of the muscle cell itself and the suppression of neuroexcitatory influences. At a critical bladder volume close to capacity the desire to void is appreciated and in health voiding can be wilfully postponed if conditions are not appropriate. Efferent activity to the internal sphincter increases as bladder filling proceeds, leading to an increase in outlet resistance mediated by excitatory α-adrenergic sympathetic activity.

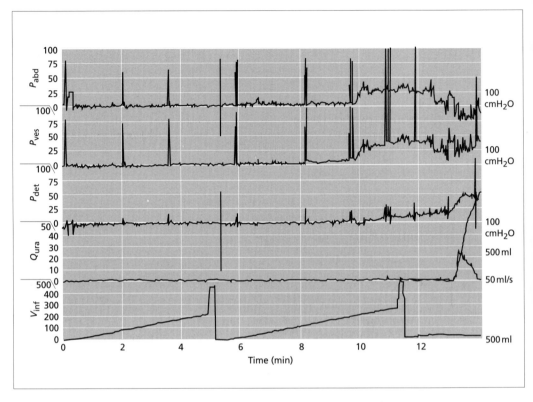

Fig. 2.17 A normal filling cystometrogram, in which the detrusor pressure remains the same due to its viscoelasticity up until the point where it contracts during a voluntary void.

Contraction of the internal sphincter not only keeps the detrusor base flat or 'unfunnelled' but also ensures closure of the ureters by contraction of the periurethral sheaths. There may be a sympathetic reflex which in response to bladder stretching gives rise to suppression of bladder contractility by inhibition of parasympathetic efferents and stimulation of β-adrenergic receptors in the detrusor body. The maintenance of a higher intraurethral than intravesical pressure is assisted by the intra-abdominal location of the sphincter zone, thus allowing pressure transmission to this zone also.

Eventually, a sensation of bladder fullness is responsible for the initiation of voluntary voiding. Voiding is then mediated via a strong parasympathetic discharge in the pelvic nerves, whose cell bodies lie in the sacral spinal cord but are under higher control, and by simultaneous suppression of α-adrenergic sympathetic influence to produce relaxation of the internal sphincter and a funnelling of the detrusor base. The urethral rhabdosphincter remains inactive throughout the voiding phase.

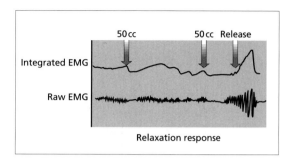

Fig. 2.18 The rectoanal inhibitory reflex caused by sudden inflation of a balloon in the rectal lumen. EMG, electromyograph.

Neural control of anorectal function

The striated muscles of the pelvic floor are innervated by the pudendal nerves (see Fig. 2.15). The external anal sphincter is supplied by inferior haemorrhoidal branches of the pudendal nerve, although branches also come directly from the fourth sacral nerve. The puborectalis is supplied by branches from the pelvic plexus superiorly and by perineal branches of the pudendal nerve inferiorly. The internal anal sphincter is tonically active and under both excitatory (sympathetic L_1–L_2) and inhibitory (parasympathetic S_2–S_4) control. The rectum has a poor supply of intraepithelial receptors but is sensitive to distension. That patients who have had their rectum excised and an ileal pouch formed can experience a sensation of fullness (and indeed can discriminate flatus from faeces) suggests that it may be receptors lying outside the rectal wall and in the pelvic floor that are responsible for this sensation.

However, the anal canal has a rich sensory nerve supply. The anal transitional zone extends for 2 cm, from the squamous mucosa of the perianal skin to the columnar mucosa of the rectum, and plays a critical role in the sensory function of the anal canal. The anal canal is normally closed and thus prevents rectal contents coming in contact with the sensitive anal transitional zone epithelium. When the rectum distends to 20–40 ml the internal sphincter relaxes while the external sphincter contracts, thus maintaining continence. This process has been referred to as 'sampling' or the rectoanal inhibitory reflex (Fig. 2.18) and allows the discrimination of flatus from faeces. With progressive rectal distension defecation becomes inevitable. In faecal impaction there is chronic inhibition of this reflex and this leads to stool in the anal canal and a patulous anus. Upper motor neurone lesions lead to loss of voluntary control of defecation; however, the anal reflexes are preserved, enabling control by reflex evacuation with regular enemas.

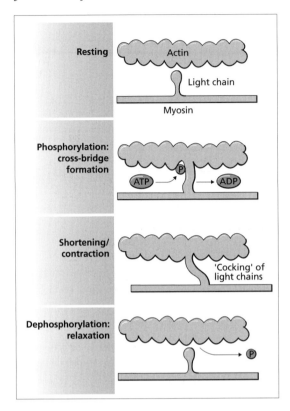

Fig. 2.19 The process of phosphorylation of myosin by ATP, resulting in a change in conformation of the cross-bridges between actin and myosin filaments and thus shortening of the muscle.

Detrusor physiology

Smooth muscle is composed of cytoskeleton and contractile proteins. The mechanical properties of smooth muscle depend on interaction between the contractile proteins. Ultrastructural examination of smooth muscle reveals thin, intermediate and thick filaments. The thin filaments represent actin and the thick filaments myosin, the main contractile proteins. The intermediate filaments represent either desmin or vimentin, which provide the cytoskeleton for the smooth muscle cell. Interaction between actin and myosin is responsible for smooth muscle contraction and hence voiding (Fig. 2.19). Following phosphorylation of myosin by ATP, attachments form between the globular head of the myosin light chain and actin. The conformational changes that occur with the phosphorylation of myosin give rise to a sliding of the filaments or cycling of the cross-bridge mechanism that leads to mechanical shortening of the filaments. With dephosphorylation these cross-bridges are broken down and smooth muscle relaxation occurs. However, one way in which smooth muscle differs from striated and cardiac muscle is that it can maintain tone with a low expenditure of ATP and hence energy.

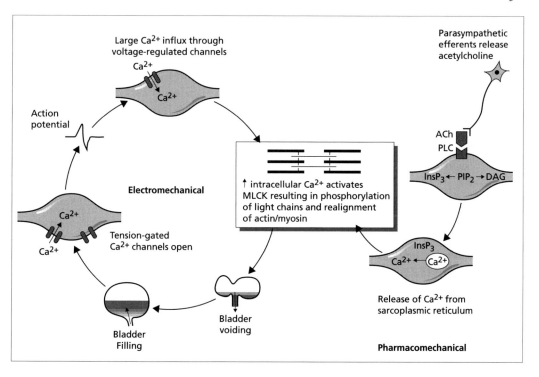

Fig. 2.20 The intracellular processes that permit electromechanical and pharmacomechanical coupling in a detrusor cell. See the text for abbreviations.

This has been attributed to the development of a latch state, a process whereby cross-bridges are dephosphorylated while still attached but have a lower detachment rate than phosphorylated cross-bridges.

Smooth muscle contraction can be initiated either by electromechanical or pharmacomechanical coupling. A change in intracellular Ca^{2+} is the primary mechanism by which excitation–contraction coupling occurs and unlike other smooth muscle the transmission of impulses does not rely on the presence of gap junctions. In smooth muscle three mechanisms for increasing intracellular Ca^{2+} have been described: the influx of extracellular Ca^{2+} through voltage-regulated channels and receptor-operated/ligand-gated channels and the release of intracellular Ca^{2+} from the sarcoplasmic reticulum (Fig. 2.20).

Electromechanical coupling is a process whereby a change in the resting membrane potential of the cell opens voltage-gated channels and hence allows the movement of ions into and out of the cell. The resting membrane potential (normally around −50 to −60 mV) is maintained largely by the high intracellular concentration of K^+ ions. Maintenance of the gradient is an energy (ATP)-dependent process. While these channels are frequently represented as openings in the membrane, it is more appropriate to regard them as energy barriers to the flow of ions. Depolarization of the cell (which makes the interior of the cell less negative) causes the muscle to contract and is mediated by an influx of Ca^{2+}. This can be initiated by distension of the bladder, neurotransmitters or a variety of drugs. The initial influx of Ca^{2+} causes the additional release of intracellular Ca^{2+}. Once a threshold concentration of Ca^{2+} is reached muscle contraction occurs. Similarly, repolarization causes muscle relaxation and is mediated by a rapid efflux of K^+. Theoretically, intervention with Ca^{2+} channel blockers (e.g. verapamil) or K^+ channel openers (e.g. pinacidil) could relax bladder muscle; however, they have not proved useful in clinical practice.

Pharmacomechanical coupling has two mechanisms of action. Inhibitory or stimulatory transmitters can either alter membrane permeability by binding to membrane receptors or exert an effect through secondary messengers, a process referred to as signal transduction. Compared with electromechanical coupling the increase in intracellular Ca^{2+} is secondary to the release solely of intracellular ions from the sarcoplasmic reticulum. In smooth muscle the binding of acetylcholine to the muscarinic receptor activates phospholipase C (PLC), causing hydrolysis of phosphatidylinositol bisphosphate (PIP_2) into inositol trisphosphate ($InsP_3$) and diacylglycerol (DAG). Inositol trisphosphate elicits release of intracellular Ca^{2+} (levels rising from a baseline of 30–100 nM to 800 nM), which causes muscle contraction by promoting phosphorylation of the myosin light chain by myosin light chain kinase (MLCK). However, to activate this enzyme the Ca^{2+} must be bound to the protein calmodulin. Relaxation occurs by dephosphorylation of myosin via one of the many phosphatases, returning myosin to its inactive state. Reduction in intracellular Ca^{2+} or decreased sensitivity of the contractile proteins to it are other possible modes of relaxation. There is evidence to suggest that pathways involving cyclic AMP and cyclic GMP may be involved in reducing intracellular Ca^{2+} levels and uncoupling the force generation from myosin phosphorylation. In the bladder, β-adrenergic-stimulated bladder relaxation appears to be mediated by such a cyclic AMP-dependent pathway.

Classifications of incontinence

There have been several classifications of urinary incontinence but the advent of advanced physiological tests and a greater understanding of pathophysiology have allowed a more useful classification to evolve that has more relevance to planning therapeutic solutions. In its simplest terms any situation that causes the intravesical pressure temporarily to exceed intraurethral pressure will result in the passage of urine. Whether this rise is voluntary or involuntary distinguishes between voiding and incontinence. Thus incontinence may

Table 2.2 Causes of urinary incontinence (excluding congenital malformations and fistulae).

Overactive bladder
Idiopathic detrusor instability
Detrusor hyperreflexia
Reduced bladder compliance

Underactive sphincter
Sphincter impairment in men: mechanical disruption, scarring or neuropathy (usually following
    prostatic surgery or radical pelvic cancer surgery)
Female 'stress incontinence' due to urethral hypermobility or intrinsic sphincter deficiency
    (or both)

Underactive bladder
Neuropathies affecting bladder sensation or bladder contractility
Bladder outflow obstruction with overflow incontinence

be the result of abnormally high bladder pressure or abnormally low urethral pressure or both, and appropriate therapy simply aims to restore the normal pressure gradient that permits urine storage, if possible, without impairing the ability to void. A functional classification has been developed by the International Continence Society (ICS) that encompasses all forms of urinary incontinence (Table 2.2).

The aetiological factors responsible for faecal incontinence may vary considerably, from deterioration of cerebral function to intrinsic deficiencies of the anorectal control mechanisms, which are by far the most common causes. Patients may experience urge incontinence due to primary bowel pathology, such as Crohn's disease or ulcerative colitis, which results in the more rapid delivery of contents to the rectum. The patient's normal control mechanism is then unable to deal with this rapid arrival and incontinence ensues. However, in most cases of true incontinence there is a defect in anal/pelvic floor function and increased pressure within the rectum results in the passage of flatus, liquid or solid stool. This may result from morphological changes in the sphincter mechanism itself or the failure of innervation (Table 2.3).

Theoretically, the above classification is useful in explaining bladder and sphincteric dysfunction, although in practice patients frequently fall into more than one category. In particular, patients with neurological disease often have a combination of bladder and sphincteric dysfunction and therefore these conditions are discussed separately. The following section describes the aetiology of the common causes of urinary incontinence following the above classification as far as possible.

Table 2.3 Causes of anorectal incontinence (excluding congenital malformations and fistulae).

Colonic instability
Diarrhoea: whatever cause
Malabsorption: coeliac disease, blind loop syndrome, chronic pancreatitis, etc.
Laxative abuse: senna
Endocrine tumours: gastrinoma, VIPoma, carcinoid, etc.

Rectal instability
Reduced sensation: diabetes, childbirth, hysterectomy, pelvic trauma
Reduced capacity: radiation, trauma, inflammatory bowel disease especially Crohn's disease,
    tropical infections

Anal and pelvic floor instability
Neurological (motor or sensory): spina bifida, central disc prolapse, diabetic neuropathy,
    pudendal neuropathy, multiple sclerosis, trauma, rectal prolapse, chronic straining
Physical disruption (failure of EAS or IAS): vaginal delivery, fistula surgery, anal dilatation,
    sphincterotomy, haemorrhoidectomy

EAS, external anal sphincter; IAS, internal anal sphincter; VIP, vasoactive intestinal polypeptide.

Overactive bladder

DETRUSOR INSTABILITY

Detrusor instability refers to a urodynamic phenomenon. The ICS has defined the unstable bladder as one that is shown objectively to contract spontaneously during the filling or storage phase of cystometry while the patient is attempting to inhibit micturition. Previously a pressure limit of $15\ cmH_2O$ was set; however, no such limit now exists and an involuntary detrusor contraction at any pressure associated with symptoms of urge or leakage while the patient is attempting to inhibit micturition is recognized as instability. By definition, detrusor instability occurs in the patient with no identifiable neurological abnormality and the term 'detrusor hyperreflexia' refers to a similar urodynamic finding in patients with underlying neuropathy.

Incidence and epidemiology

It is difficult to assess accurately the true incidence and prevalence of detrusor instability because urinary incontinence is often underreported, is frequently treated without urodynamic assessment and conventional urodynamics may underestimate the incidence when compared with ambulatory studies (McInerney *et al.*, 1991). Studies have suggested that 7% of asymptomatic women over 65 years of age have evidence of detrusor instability (Diokno *et al.*, 1988). In the infant, instability could almost be considered physiological until the age when neurological maturation allows voluntary control of voiding. While urodynamic evaluation is usually normal in enuretic patients, the commonest urodynamic finding is detrusor instability (about 15%), the frequency of which increases to 97% in those with diurnal symptoms (Whiteside & Arnold, 1975).

Detrusor instability exists in about half of female patients presenting for evaluation of urinary incontinence. Hysterectomy and other pelvic surgery can potentially lead to peripheral nerve damage and have been implicated in the development of detrusor instability. Approximately two-thirds of men with bladder outlet obstruction have detrusor instability; however, it resolves in a similar number of patients when the outlet obstruction is dealt with (Abrams *et al.*, 1979).

Aetiology and pathophysiology

Bladder storage and voiding are under neural control and disruption of these pathways at any level affects bladder function. The aetiology of idiopathic detrusor instability is unknown. Infiltration of the spinal cord with local anaesthetic can abolish detrusor instability, indicating that it may represent a hyperexcitable micturition reflex. The Oxford group (Brading & Turner, 1994) have proposed a unified theory suggesting that instability arises because of a change in the properties of the smooth muscle of the detrusor which predispose it to unstable contractions and that this occurs secondary to a reduction in the functional motor innervation of the bladder. The findings in the obstructed pig model (many of which have been confirmed histologically in humans) of smooth muscle hypertrophy with reduced density of acetylcholinesterase-positive nerves and increased sensitivity to agonists such as carbachol all point to denervation supersensitivity. It has been proposed that the increased detrusor pressures in the obstructed bladder give rise to intramural ischaemia and subsequent damage to the intramural ganglia and hence denervation.

Underactive sphincter

Underactivity of the urethral sphincter commonly results in genuine stress incontinence, defined by the ICS as 'the involuntary loss of urine occurring when, in the absence of a detrusor contraction, the intravesical pressure exceeds the maximum urethral pressure'.

MEN

The commonest cause of sphincter failure in men is following prostatectomy, for several reasons. The operation may result in damage to the sphincter muscle itself or extravasation due to capsular perforation may result in pericapsular fibrosis with resultant nerve damage to the sphincter (Wein & Barrett, 1988). Residual apical prostatic tissue may interfere with sphincter closure, while the malignant gland may infiltrate the sphincter muscle, its nerve supply or both. The incidence of post-prostatectomy incontinence varies from about 1 to 5% depending on how one defines incontinence; however, the risk is higher for open prostatectomy and particularly after radical prostatectomy for carcinoma. Associated detrusor instability also increases the risk of post-prostatectomy incontinence.

WOMEN

An understanding of the normal urethral sphincter mechanism in women is crucial to comprehending the pathology of stress incontinence, yet it has been harder to reach international agreement on this subject than on the classification of detrusor activity. It is common to see female stress incontinence further subclassified as types I, II and III, although the ability to make this distinction depends entirely on the availability of videourodynamic testing. Type I stress incontinence is characterized by a closed bladder neck at rest that is situated above the inferior margin of the symphysis pubis; during stress there is leakage of urine but with less than 2 cm descent. Similarly in type II stress incontinence the bladder neck is closed at rest but may lie below the inferior margin of the symphysis pubis and demonstrates rotational descent characteristic of a cystocoele. Both these types are clinically associated with urethral hypermobility, usually following childbirth, and an associated pelvic floor neuropathy and subsequent endopelvic fascial defects. Type III stress incontinence is synonymous with intrinsic sphincter deficiency and demonstrates an open bladder neck at rest with no hypermobility. Type III incontinence may be associated with frank neuropathy or following previous anti-incontinence surgery or pelvic fractures. Obviously there may be an element of type III incontinence associated with types I and II.

Regardless of the classification used, it is clear that two main aetiological factors underlie the majority of cases of stress urinary incontinence in the female. Pelvic floor neuropathy (usually postobstetric) and changes in the type of collagen that contributes to the endopelvic fascia are the main factors, although in most cases it is multifactorial. Electrophysiological testing of the external anal sphincter shortly after delivery has revealed occult neurological damage in 80% of primigravida who deliver vaginally. Damage is related to

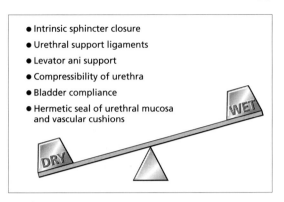

Fig. 2.21 The 'balance of continence' required to maintain female continence. If enough of the factors involved become impaired then stress leakage occurs, although it is unlikely that one defect alone is enough to account for such a problem.

parity, forceps delivery and prolonged second stage of labour (Snook *et al.*, 1984). This damage may persist and indeed become more marked with time and is associated with the development of faecal and stress urinary incontinence. Many of these women demonstrate perineal descent, which is a sign of pelvic floor weakness. Other factors, such as abnormal straining at defecation, may lead to a stretch-induced injury of the pudendal nerve. The extent to which each of these factors plays a role in the incontinence of any one individual varies. A useful concept to explain the multifactorial aetiology is the 'balance of continence' (Fig. 2.21).

Changes in the volume and type of collagen exist in women with genitourinary prolapse and in women with stress incontinence. The Bristol group have shown a reduction in the total collagen content of the vaginal wall in women with genitourinary prolapse associated with an increase in collagen turnover by a factor of four when assessed by matrix metalloproteinase activity (Jackson *et al.*, 1996). Similarly premenopausal nulliparous women with stress incontinence have significantly less collagen in their periurethral tissues and a decrease in the ratio of type I collagen (normally the predominant type) to type III collagen compared with continent controls (Keane *et al.*, 1997).

Urethral mucosal secretions create a surface tension within the urethra that helps to provide a watertight seal. Oestrogens maintain these secretions, as well as producing increased pulsation and lumen size of submucosal vascular 'cushions' that add to this effect (Raz *et al.*, 1972). Postmenopausal women may lose this rather subtle supplementary aid to continence.

Following previous bladder neck or urethral surgery, scar tissue often causes loss of elasticity and destruction of the urethral walls. The urethra is often short, but the bladder neck is usually well supported. However, normal sphincter closure cannot occur and proper pressure transmission is deficient. This is often referred to as 'pipe stem urethra', although this corresponds to type III stress incontinence.

Underactive bladder

The aetiology of reduced bladder contractility includes central neurological lesions affecting the conus medullaris and peripheral lesions affecting the cauda equina and the pelvic parasympathetic outflow. The autonomic neuropathy of diabetes is recognized as producing reduced bladder contractility; other causes include sacral shingles, pelvic fracture and radical intrapelvic surgery, such as Wertheim hysterectomy or abdominoperineal resection of the rectum. Overdistension of the bladder also results in non-contractility by producing a very peripheral submucosal neuropathy (Higson & Smith, 1981) and by overstretching of the smooth muscle itself. Non-contractility of the bladder may occur in isolation and may even be a normal finding in women; however, this is rarely associated with incontinence.

Patients with non-contractile bladders but with normal sphincter function may develop chronic retention of urine due to an inability to empty the bladder adequately. The same can occur as the result of bladder outflow obstruction. The bladder becomes progressively more distended and ultimately reaches the terminal part of its pressure–volume relationship, when terminal hypo-compliance occurs. The sphincter mechanism is unable to compensate for this and overflow incontinence is the result. This 'leak pressure' varies from one individual to the next and explains why some men have 'high-pressure' chronic retention and others have 'low-pressure' chronic retention. Where there is an efferent neuropathy affecting the sacral parasympathetic or somatic nerves, there will usually be associated sphincter weakness. In this situation, not only is there overflow incontinence but leakage also occurs with any rise in intra-abdominal pressure due to failure of the distal sphincter mechanism to augment its closure pressure appropriately. Nevertheless, there is not usually continuous leakage because residual smooth muscle tone of the distal urethral sphincter maintains a closure pressure adequate for continence at rest.

Incontinence in the elderly

The incidence of incontinence in the elderly hospitalized patient has been estimated to be about 40%. Although conventional diagnoses can usually be made, more than one functional disorder is often found (Table 2.4). Psychogenic responses to being in hospital, acute medical conditions, depression and drugs may all play a part. Loss of social awareness and normal inhibitions may complicate the issue, while immobility may simply make it impossible for a person to reach the toilet. With these extra complications, urodynamic diagnosis alone rarely provides an adequate basis for further

Table 2.4 Factors that may contribute to urinary incontinence in the elderly.

Reduced bladder capacity
Shorter times between voids
Detrusor instability
Inactivity or relative sensory deprivation leading to relative decreased bladder awareness
Bladder outlet obstruction with incomplete emptying and large residuals
Reduced strength of pelvic floor muscles
Increasing fascial weakness
Atrophic changes to urethra and trigone
Reduced mobility making toilet access difficult
Drugs (see Chapter 6)
Dementia

management. Indeed, invasive investigations may often be inappropriate in this age group.

Urethral instability

Urethral instability (defined as a spontaneous drop in maximal urethral pressure exceeding one-third of the resting pressure in the absence of detrusor overactivity) has been suggested as a cause of detrusor instability in approximately 40% of women (Wise *et al.*, 1993). Indeed these authors propose two subtypes of detrusor instability: those in whom the primary abnormality is a drop in urethral pressure and those in whom the initial event is an increase in detrusor pressure. It has been suggested that an α-adrenoceptor agonist may benefit those patients in whom the primary abnormality is a drop in urethral pressure.

Effects of common neurological disorders on bladder and bowel function (Fig. 2.22)

Cerebrovascular disease

The effect of a cerebrovascular accident depends on the site, size and location of the lesion. As previously mentioned, cerebral influences tend to have an inhibitory effect on voiding and therefore the end-result of a cerebrovascular accident is most commonly detrusor hyperreflexia with associated urinary incontinence, although retention is common in the early days. The clinical picture is influenced by immobility and mental confusion. Obviously any intervention must take into account both the urodynamic findings as well as the patient's general morbidity.

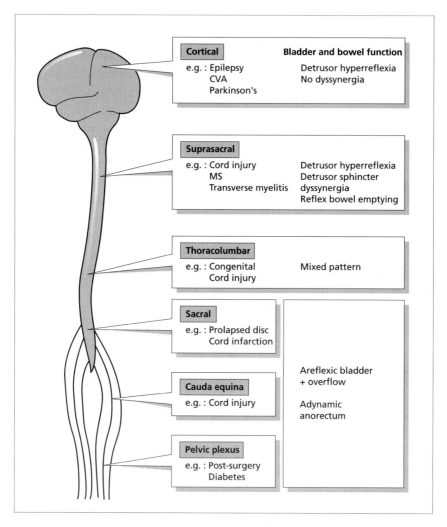

Fig. 2.22 The types of dysfunction of continence that can be expected to occur with lesions at various levels of the central nervous system. CVA, cerebral vascular accident; MS, multiple sclerosis.

Parkinson's disease and multiple system atrophy

Parkinson's disease is characterized by a resting tremor, 'cogwheel' rigidity and bradykinesia. Pathologically, it is distinguished by loss of the pigmented dopamine-rich neurones in the substantia nigra. In multiple system atrophy (MSA) there is a more generalized and diffuse loss of neurones and the prognosis is worse, hence stressing the importance of distinguishing between the two conditions. MSA is frequently confused clinically with Parkinson's disease, although there are several clinical symptoms and signs that help distinguish the two, including the presence of pyramidal or cerebellar features, autonomic failure and a poor response to L-dopa in MSA.

From a urological point of view, it is more common for urological symptoms to precede the onset of MSA than the onset of Parkinson's disease. Incontinence and erectile dysfunction are far more common in MSA, whereas irritative voiding symptoms are more common in Parkinson's disease. Sphincter electromyography is valuable in diagnosing MSA but is not commonly available and hence most clinicians need to pay particular heed to clinical findings. The importance in differentiating the two conditions is highlighted by the very high incontinence rates following prostatectomy in patients with MSA compared with those with Parkinson's disease (Chandiramani *et al.*, 1997). It has been suggested that the poor results reported following prostate surgery in Parkinson's disease may have been due to patients with MSA being misdiagnosed as having Parkinson's disease. Constipation is common in Parkinson's disease and may be aggravated by the anticholinergic drugs used to treat the associated detrusor hyperreflexia. The autonomic neuropathy in MSA may give rise to faecal incontinence secondary to altered bowel motility.

Spinal cord injury

Bladder dysfunction and renal tract disease remain an important cause of morbidity in the spinally injured patient, although thankfully the associated mortality rate has fallen due to improvements in patient care. A detailed discussion of spinal cord injury and its resultant disability is beyond the scope of this book. However, subsequent urological and anorectal function can in most cases be inferred from the level of the injury, although not always in a predictable manner. Men are far more commonly affected than women and the commonest cause is road traffic accidents. Regardless of the level of the injury, the initial trauma results in a period of what is referred to as spinal shock. This leads to flaccidity below the level of the injury and usually urinary retention. This areflexia lasts from days to months. Reflex activity first returns to the striated muscles of the pelvic floor, as can be detected by bulbo-cavernosus and anal skin reflexes. Urodynamic assessments both in the early phase of recovery and periodically, especially as neurological and urological symptoms change, are important in formulating subsequent management programmes.

Multiple sclerosis

Multiple sclerosis is a disorder of demyelination of the central nervous system that affects females twice as often as males and usually presents between the ages of 20 and 30 years. The lesions produced are known as plaques and in the spinal cord are more common in the cervical and suprasacral region, upper motor neurone-type lesions therefore being more common. It is probably an autoimmune condition and has an unpredictable course. Approximately 80% of patients have urological symptoms at some stage in the illness and in about 5% the sole presenting symptoms are urological. The common complaints are of frequency, urgency and urge incontinence, although some patients may present with obstructive-type symptoms or indeed in the acute phase with retention. There may be associated bowel dysfunction, either constipation or incontinence, and sexual dysfunction. Urological symptoms can be unreliable and therefore urodynamic investigation is the only way to reliably define the underlying abnormality; repeat testing is often necessary if the neurological findings change.

The most common finding is that of detrusor hyperreflexia, reflecting the preponderance of demyelination plaques in the suprasacral region; however, areflexia occurs in 5–10% of patients. Detrusor–sphincter dyssynergia is seen in about half of those patients with hyperreflexia, and these patients are considered to be at higher risk for upper tract damage.

Spina bifida

This refers to a group of developmental abnormalities of the spinal cord that vary enormously in the extent to which the patient is neurologically impaired. The spinal cord and vertebrae start to develop about day 18 of gestation and are completed by day 35, the canal closing in a caudal direction. The incidence of spina bifida is approximately 1 per 1000 live births in the general population, with the risk increasing significantly in a family with one previously affected child or in mothers with spina bifida. Supplementation of the diet with folate (400 µg daily) prior to conception reduces the incidence of neural tube defects by only 1 per 417 births, although in high-risk mothers high doses (5 mg daily) prevent the defect in 1 per 40 births.

The disability depends on the site and degree of the spinal abnormality. Most commonly the lower lumbar vertebrae are affected by a myelomeningocele (neural tissue protruding into a neural sac beyond the confines of the vertebral canal). Other abnormalities, such as meningocoele (the sac does not contain neural elements) or lipomyelomeningocele (the sac also contains fatty tissue), occur less frequently. About 85% of patients affected have an associated Arnold–Chiari malformation, in which the cerebellar tonsils herniate through the foramen magnum obstructing the free flow of cerebrospinal fluid and hence causing hydrocephalus, which normally requires shunting.

About 60% of patients have detrusor activity, reflecting sparing of the sacral segments; the remainder have areflexia. Similarly about 50% have intact innervation of the rhabdosphincter, with 25% having reduced function and 25% absent function. Those patients with leak pressures greater than 40 cmH$_2$O and dyssynergia are considered to be at higher risk for upper tract deterioration and warrant more intensive follow-up (McGuire *et al.*, 1981).

Cauda equina injury

The S2–S4 segments of the spinal cord lie at the level of the T12–L1 vertebral bodies. This portion of the cord is also known as the conus medullaris and the nerve roots that lie below this level are known as the cauda equina. The commonest cause of damage at this level is spinal cord injury at or below T12. Other common causes are central disc protrusion, root compression, spinal stenosis and primary or secondary malignant processes. Injury potentially impairs bladder, urethral and anal sphincteric function, in addition to erectile dysfunction, somatic paralysis and anaesthesia. Patients present with obstructive voiding symptoms or urinary retention and incontinence due to bladder and sphincter denervation, respectively. The classic neurological finding is of 'saddle' anaesthesia (i.e. perianal anaesthesia), reflecting S2–S3 nerve damage, and loss of bulbocavernosus and anocutaneous reflexes.

The predominant urodynamic finding is that of an areflexic bladder with or without sphincter weakness. Sphincter weakness is not always apparent because the dominant nucleus for the pelvic nerve may lie at a different level than that of the pudendal nerve. The diagnosis can be further confirmed with the bethanechol supersensitivity test. This is based on the phenomenon of supersensitivity, i.e. when an organ is denervated it becomes supersensitive to stimulatory transmitters. The administration of 5 mg of bethanechol chloride causes a positive response in detrusor pressure during cystometry. The effects of cauda equina damage on bowel function is more variable. A central disc prolapse can damage the entire sacral outflow, giving rise to a patulous anus with faecal incontinence with or without gross perineal descent.

Pelvic plexus injury

Due to its position this plexus or the nerves contributing to it are frequently injured in major pelvic surgery, such as abdominoperineal resection, low anterior resection and radical hysterectomy. Direct damage may occur to the nerves during dissection on the anterolateral aspect of the rectum, by traction on the rectum or, in the case of radical hysterectomy, by extensive dissection inferolateral to the cervix. Damage to the plexus affects parasympathetic, sympathetic and somatic fibres to the bladder and sphincter, and depending on the relative damage to each component the clinical picture varies.

Most commonly patients present with retention and are managed initially by catheter drainage. While the problem is transitory in the majority of patients, resolving over 3–6 months, approximately one-third of patients are left with long-term problems. After removal of the catheter the patient notices a poor flow and possibly urinary incontinence (Blaivas & Barbalias, 1983).

Urodynamic assessment reveals a hypocontractile detrusor with reduced compliance secondary to parasympathetic and β-adrenergic denervation, respectively. The α-adrenergic denervation of the bladder neck and sphincter mechanism gives rise to bladder neck incompetence and reduced urethral closing pressure. Unless there is associated pudendal nerve damage, faecal incontinence should not occur.

Diabetic neuropathy

Autonomic neuropathy giving rise to bladder dysfunction occurs in approximately 50% of diabetic patients. Its onset tends to be insidious and generally coexists with peripheral somatic neuropathy. Impaired bladder sensation is usually the first urological symptom, often with outflow symptoms and a sensation of incomplete emptying. The loss of the desire to void means that many patients void by the clock. Less commonly patients have urgency and urge incontinence with associated detrusor hyperreflexia, reflecting cortical or spinal tract involvement. Patients frequently have associated erectile dysfunction. Faecal incontinence may occur in up to 20% of diabetic patients secondary to pelvic floor somatic neuropathy, which can be exacerbated by recurrent diarrhoea as a result of the associated autonomic neuropathy (Rogers *et al.*, 1988).

3: Assessment of the Incontinent Patient

Lesley Irvine, Jo Laycock & John Beynon

Most patients with incontinence or functional disease are referred to individual specialists, continence advisors or possibly physiotherapists by their GPs. Following initial assessment there may be cross-referral for investigation or therapy to other members of this multidisciplinary team (Fig. 3.1). In an ideal world, members of this team should be located in the same clinic so that immediate interaction can occur, although in most hospitals this is not yet possible. Such a clinic employs the skills of the specialist continence advisor, specialist physiotherapist and relevant experienced clinicians backed by clerical support.

Layout should be designed to ensure adequate space for members of the team to function optimally, with appropriate facilities such as waiting and changing areas, toilets and investigation rooms. By implication, these facilities are ideally part of a purpose-designed and functional unit (see Appendix 1). This development in the out-patient management of incontinence ensures that the maximum cost–benefit is obtained for this area of healthcare. It should also reduce the need to recycle patients to each of these disciplines separately at different times with the inevitable problems of non-compliance.

Open access to this multidisciplinary team should already be possible, with patients self-referring or being referred directly to the continence advisor.

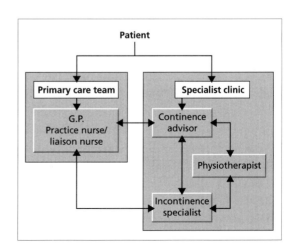

Fig. 3.1 The interaction of professionals involved in the running of a pelvic floor assessment clinic.

Integral to this sort of system is an appropriately trained staff on site, with a key liaison person and a telephone helpline for out-of-hours enquiries. Adequate time must be given to a consultation: up to 1 hour is usual for a specialist nurse continence advisor, although clinicians usually have to make do with less. Long consultations do not necessarily mean better compliance and if 'patient fatigue' is occurring then the consultation is shortened appropriately and a follow-up appointment offered reasonably quickly.

History in the incontinent patient

Incontinence is a symptom not a diagnosis. As in any medical condition, the initial diagnosis is suggested primarily by the clinical history reinforced by physical examination and followed, where relevant, by investigations. In taking the history, one must remember how the patient has been referred:

1   previously unassessed primary referral with the symptomatic diagnosis of incontinence;

2   secondary referral with a formal clinical diagnosis of which one symptom is established incontinence, e.g. a patient with multiple sclerosis and a presumed neurogenic bladder or a patient with rectal prolapse and faecal incontinence awaiting surgical repair;

3   secondary referral with a previous history of incontinence surgery that has failed and a request for further investigation and treatment.

In many ways the formal assessment is an integral part of the management and there often appears to be no clear dividing line between these two procedures.

Prior to the first appointment the patient is asked to complete an easy symptom questionnaire and a frequency–volume chart. The patient brings these documents to the clinic at the first attendance and these should be read through with the patient in order to clarify the history. Wherever possible the patient should be encouraged to give an account of the symptoms with as little interruption as possible from the assessor. Once this has been achieved, it is essential to explore the details of the history in depth in order to establish a working diagnosis. Taking a history is not just about recording responses to a series of predetermined questions; its purpose is to lead to a diagnosis. Thus, although questionnaires can be useful as an *aide-mémoire*, it is critical to probe the detail so that there is clarity not just a comprehensive list of ticked boxes. Beware that the relationship between symptoms of incontinence and the underlying functional disorder is often unclear and may be misleading.

By its very nature, incontinence of urine or faeces is socially embarrassing and eliciting a full history may be difficult. Symptoms may vary from slight leakage of flatus or mucus to passive incontinence of solid stool, either of which can be devastating in its effect. Patients may become confined to their homes and be afraid to venture out as they have to plan their routes with regard to the availability of toilet facilities. Assessment therefore needs to be directed not only to the form of incontinence but also to the effect on the overall quality of life. Does the patient need to wear pads? Are they aware of the urge to pass urine or faeces or the occurrence of incontinence that may indicate the existence of a sensory component to the incontinence?

In a large proportion of patients, urinary and anorectal symptoms may coexist and this may be indicative of pelvic floor failure and reflect a common aetiological background. There may also be the symptoms of gynaecological prolapse with these common functional symptoms. In our practice it is a fundamental philosophy that the pelvic floor is one entity with several closely related functions. Whether a patient is being seen by a specialist nurse, physiotherapist, gynaecologist, urologist or coloproctologist, the interelationship between urinary and bowel control and sexual function should never be forgotten. The questioning and examination must take this into account.

Learning point: Assessment of bladder and bowel function must include questioning about any sexual dysfunction

Pelvic malignancy is common and can manifest itself occasionally with symptoms of incontinence. It is particularly important to exclude this diagnosis by taking a good history and performing a general examination to exclude neoplasms of the anal canal, rectum, colon, vagina, cervix, uterus and bladder as well as the less common pelvic neoplasms.

Learning point: Exclude serious neoplastic disease within the pelvis

With these factors excluded one can then concentrate on the detailed history of symptoms and previous factors predisposing to the development of incontinence.

Urinary history

The following key questions need to be answered in making the initial assessment in all patients.

1 *How and when did the problem first start?* The length of the history gives little indication of the cause but association of onset (after childbirth, following a back injury) may be very important.

2 *What factors influence the incontinence?* Stress, urge and dribbling incontinence may have different causes.

3 *Does leakage occur without any warning?* If so, there is probably a sensory defect involved. Nocturnal enuresis sometimes occurs as the only problem but can be associated with daytime incontinence.

4   *Other urinary symptoms.* Frequency, urgency, dysuria, pain, infections, blood and bladder sensation are all important as they may give an indication of other bladder pathology.

5   *Type and amount of fluid intake.* Have patients restricted fluid and what effect did this have? Does the fluid intake include excessive caffeine?

6   *What assessment and treatment, if any, have been attempted previously?* For example, surgery or physiotherapy.

7   *What medication is being taken or has been used previously?*

8   *Problems with mobility and manual dexterity.* Mild urge incontinence becomes a serious problem if one is unable to reach the toilet because of immobility. Dexterity is vitally important if any form of assisted emptying is being considered.

9   *Pad usage, social interactions and psychosexual factors.* Offers both a qualitative and quantitative assessment of the impact of incontinence on day-to-day life.

10   *Obstetric and gynaecological history.* Information is required on parity, forceps delivery, large birthweight babies, prolonged delivery, episiotomy or tear and previous gynaecological procedures (vital if further surgery is planned).

11   *Do not forget the anorectal and sexual history.*

12   *General medical history.* Is incontinence the only symptom or is it part of an overall global disturbance of function?

Anorectal history

Patients need to be questioned on a variety of factors.

1   *Type of incontinence: solid, liquid, flatus?* This gives a clear idea of the treatment objectives, which are more varied for anorectal problems than for urinary incontinence.

2   *Impact of symptoms.* Does the patient wear a pad? Does it restrict their daily activities?

3   *Are they initially aware of the need to defecate?* If so, is the incontinence because of their inability to reach the toilet?

4   *Do they leak between normal bowel actions?*

5   *Other important questions.* These relate to possible aetiological factors.

    (a) Symptoms of obstructed defecation, such as straining at stool, incomplete evacuation, vaginal or rectal digitation to assist passage of stool, rectal bleeding, mucus discharge, feeling of perineal fullness.

    (b) Previous anal surgery: haemorrhoidectomy, sphincterotomy, fistula surgery.

    (c) Anoreceptive intercourse.

6   *Do not forget a urinary and sexual history.*

    Due to the multiplicity of symptoms it is useful to use a proforma to

Table 3.1 The history in the incontinent patient.

History	Urinary	Faecal
Duration and development	Descriptive	Descriptive
Type of incontinence	Stress, urge, constant dribble, no warning, nocturia, nocturnal enuresis	Solid, liquid, flatus, accidents, use of pads
Provocation	Cough, laugh, lifting, sneezing, sport, intercourse	Cough, laugh, lifting, sneezing, sport, intercourse
Other specific symptoms	Frequency, urgency, dysuria, pain, infections, blood, bladder sensation, voiding difficulty	Obstructed defaecation, incomplete evacuation, digitation, straining
Previous obstetric history	Parity, forceps delivery, large birthweight, prolonged delivery, episiotomy or tear	Parity, forceps delivery, large birthweight, prolonged delivery, episiotomy or tear
Fluid intake and diet	Descriptive	Descriptive
General medical history	Cerebrovascular accident, dementia, neoplasm, multiple sclerosis, neuropathies (diabetic/B_{12}), trauma, myelomeningocele	As urinary but also inflammatory bowel disease, infection, laxative abuse, overflow diarrhoea, intestinal fistula, radiotherapy
Previous surgery	Hysterectomy, anterior or posterior repair, bladder neck suspension or sling, endoscopic procedure	As urinary but also sphincter repair, colonic resection, prolapse repair, haemorrhoidectomy, sphincterotomy, anal stretch, fistulae in ano
Other therapy	Drugs/physiotherapy	Drugs/physiotherapy
Social/mobility	Descriptive	Descriptive

ensure that all factors are covered and a complete and comprehensive history is obtained (Table 3.1).

Scoring systems

Urinary scoring systems for incontinence have been developed and validated but are complex. Shorter more usable systems have been devised but as yet

Table 3.2 Cleveland Clinic scoring system for faecal incontinence.

Type of incontinence	Frequency				
	Never	Rarely*	Sometimes†	Usually‡	Always§
Solid	0	1	2	3	4
Liquid	0	1	2	3	4
Flatus	0	1	2	3	4
Requires pad	0	1	2	3	4
Alteration of lifestyle	0	1	2	3	4

Scores using this system vary between 0 (perfect continence) and 20 (complete incontinence).
*, Less than once per month.
†, Less than once per week, once or more per month.
‡, Less than once per day.
§, More than once per day.

have not been validated for clinical use. Various authors have developed scoring systems to evaluate the degree of faecal incontinence and these are undoubtedly useful in facilitating assessment and comparison of functional outcome following treatment. One commonly used system is that developed in the Cleveland Clinic (Florida) (Table 3.2).

General examination of the incontinent patient

It is paramount, for the reasons highlighted above, that the incontinent patient should be given a complete general examination and in most cases this should be performed by a clinician.

Learning point: Exclude neurological disease and pelvic malignancy. Consider specific urological, gynaecological and gastrointestinal disease

In particular, this examination should aim to exclude major neurological, endocrine (diabetes) and gastrointestinal causes for incontinence. A simplistic neurological examination should always include a sensory assessment of the sacral dermatomes (Fig. 3.2), the sacral reflexes and a general assessment of muscle tone and coordination. More detailed examination than this is unlikely to be worthwhile as the pelvic floor specialist rarely possesses the skills required to detect significant abnormalities. If a neurological defect is suspected then ask for a neurological consultation. A balanced judgement of the patient's mental state, insight and likely cooperation must be made. Intercurrent odour control, pad protection used, manual dexterity, mobility aids and, where relevant, information from the carer are noted at this point. The skin over

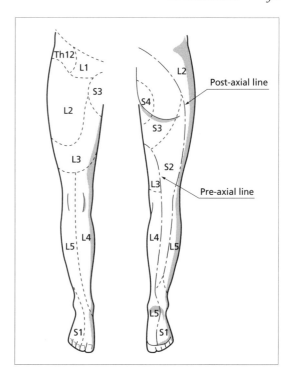

Fig. 3.2 The lumbosacral dermatomes.

the upper thighs and vulva should be inspected and if red, sore and excoriated, it may indicate severe incontinence, sensitive skin or possibly infrequent pad changes. A systematic pelvic examination should follow.

Systematic pelvic examination

The patient should be positioned supine in a good light, with head supported, knees bent and knees and feet apart. This places the hips in flexion and abduction; if the feet are together and the knees apart, the hips adopt a position of lateral (external) rotation, which can cause discomfort and fatigue of the hip muscles if the examination takes more than a few minutes. It is useful if the patient's left leg is supported (resting against a wall) and the right leg rests against the examiner, reducing muscle fatigue. By parting the labia, the vaginal introitus and the mucosa of the lower part of the vagina can be observed. This should appear pink and moist. In some postmenopausal women with oestrogen depletion, atrophic vaginitis may develop; this causes the vaginal mucosa to appear thin, red and sore. These symptoms are generally mirrored in the urethra, causing urethritis that results in irritative symptoms: frequency, nocturia, urgency and incontinence.

The patient is ask to cough vigorously and urinary incontinence can be observed if present. A bimanual examination is performed, with two fingers

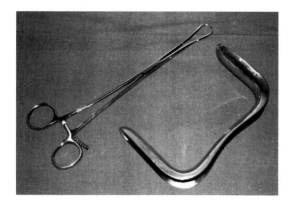

Fig. 3.3 The Sims speculum (right) is used to display the vaginal anatomy, while the vulsellum (left) is used to support the vaginal wall or to grasp the cervix and assess its mobility.

of the examiner's right hand in the vagina and the left hand on the abdomen to palpate the pelvic contents. In this examination the vaginal fingers are 'listening' and the abdominal hand is 'working'. The examination does not depend on the length of the examiner's fingers. The patient is also asked to squeeze as if resisting the flow of urine or stool in order to assess contraction of the pelvic floor muscles (see below). Palpation around all aspects of the vaginal walls and adjacent structures identifies localized pain or tenderness. This may be due to many factors and further investigations may be necessary. Pain elicited during a pelvic floor contraction should be identified, as this may inhibit muscle re-education.

The patient is then placed in the left lateral position. Three pieces of equipment are needed: (i) a Sims speculum (Fig. 3.3); (ii) a long-handled, single-toothed vulsellum or sponge forceps (Fig. 3.3); and (iii) a good light. The right leg is elevated actively or passively and the Sims speculum passed into the vagina following the contour of the posterior wall to the posterior fornix. Gentle traction then reveals the entire length of the anterior vaginal wall. The mobility of the bladder neck and presence of lateral sulci support are apparent when the subject strains downwards or coughs. If significant descent of the anterior wall is present this can be elevated by blunt pressure with the closed single-toothed vulsellum. Inability to control stress incontinence by this technique should be carefully noted and the accurate position of the bladder neck determined by other techniques. Support of any anterior wall prolapse allows visualization of the cervix, and this can be *carefully and partially* grasped by the vulsellum to allow distal displacement during straining to demonstrate the degree of uterine prolapse. Care should be taken to allow the Sims speculum to slide out of the vagina gently as the cervix is eased down in order to prevent inadvertent vault support. The vulsellum can be used to optimize inspection of the posterior fornix by lifting the cervix forwards or anteriorly. Posterior vaginal wall mobility is demonstrated by removing the Sims speculum and placing it so that it now holds back the anterior vaginal wall; again the closed blunt vulsellum is used to support any descent during straining. The left lateral position is also used for anal and proctoscopic examination. Bimanual examination of the perineal body and anterior sphincter complex, in addition to rectocele, is facilitated in this position.

Clinical assessment of the faecally incontinent patient

General examination is mandatory to exclude the other pathologies that may manifest as incontinence and which are documented above. Specific examination of the anorectum, which is normally conducted in the left lateral position, should concentrate on visual inspection, digital examination, proctoscopic examination and, if indicated, endoscopic examination.

The examiner should look for the presence of scars, gutter deformity, fistulae in ano, fissures, prolapsing piles and the presence of perianal excoriation (Fig. 3.4). Soiling may be grossly evident but it is always worth applying a moist white swab to the anal margin prior to digital examination to detect a small degree of soiling sufficient to initiate pruritic symptoms. At this stage the patient can be asked to strain against the closed anus and the amount of perineal descent assessed. Although instruments have been designed to quantify this descent, they are of little value clinically. The patient can be encouraged to push unrestrained and may prolapse piles or the rectum, although an indication of this is usually obtained first from the history. A fullthickness rectal prolapse may not be reproduced in the left lateral position, so in these circumstances the patient can be left to sit and strain on a commode for 20 min or so.

Prior to digital examination perianal sensation can be tested using a gauze swab. Digital examination is performed with the index finger of the right hand. Any ulceration or irregularity of the anal canal is noted, as well as the integrity of the sphincter complex and the anal tone, i.e. the tension the sphincter exerts around the examining finger at rest. By asking the patient to squeeze, as if arresting an urge to defecate, the function of the external sphincter can be estimated.

In the male the prostate should be evaluated for size and any suspicion of malignancy; in the female a rectocele should be palpated. Proctoscopic examination using either disposable or reusable instruments allows more detailed examination of the anal canal mucosa, haemorrhoids and fissure and detects anterior mucosal prolapse on withdrawal (Fig. 3.5). The rectum should be examined with a rigid sigmoidoscope to exclude malignancy and, if symptoms indicate it, flexible sigmoidoscopy, colonoscopy or barium enema need to be arranged subsequently.

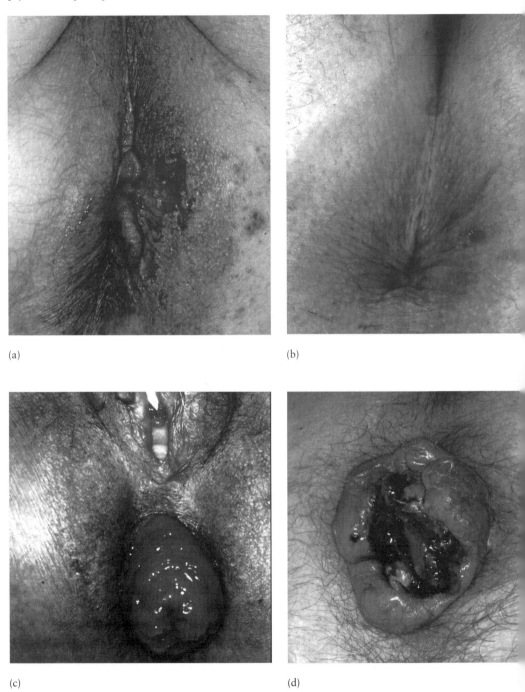

(a)

(b)

(c)

(d)

Fig. 3.4 (a) Anal excoriation; (b) external opening of fistula in ano; (c) full-thickness rectal prolapse; (d) thrombosed prolasped piles; (e, *opposite*) chronic fissure in ano and associated large piles.

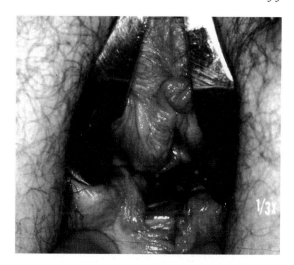

Fig. 3.4 *Continued.*   (e)

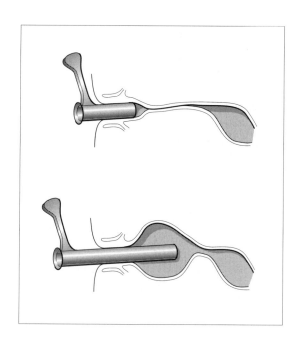

Fig. 3.5 The proctoscope
(above) allows examination of
the anal canal but not the
rectum. The sigmoidoscope
(below) is required to examine
the rectum adequately.

Standardized terminology of female organ prolapse and pelvic floor dysfunction

The aim of this system, formulated by the International Continence Society, is to produce an objective and reproducible description of vaginal wall prolapse. The system describes the position of the vaginal mucosa making no comment about the underlying structures, thus avoiding the terms 'cystocoele', 'urethrocoele', 'cystourethrocoele', 'enterocoele' and 'rectocoele'. It describes the maximal demonstrable prolapse in relation to the position of the hymenal ring. Measurements above the plane of the hymen are negative and those below are positive; the hymen is zero. There are six defined points in the vagina.

- Two points on the anterior wall:
  Aa: midline 3 cm proximal to external urethral meatus
  Ba: the lowest (most distal) point on the anterior wall above point Aa.
- Two points on the superior vaginal surface:
  C: the lowest (most distal or dependent) edge of the cervix or vaginal vault if the cervix is absent (hysterectomy)
  D: location of the posterior fornix (pouch of Douglas); this is omitted in the absence of the cervix.
- Two points on the posterior vaginal wall:
  Bp: the lowest position of any part of the posterior wall between point D and C and point Ap
  Ap: midline 3 cm proximal to the hymenal remnant on the posterior wall.
- Other landmarks:
  gh: genital hiatus (measured in cm) from the middle of the external urethral meatus to the posterior midline hymen
  pb: perineal body (measured in cm) from the posterior midline hymen to the mid anal opening and tvl: total vaginal length.

A scheme for the recording of findings is shown in Fig. 3.6. The recommended classification clusters groups of prolapse into five stages and then discusses ancillary techniques for describing organ prolapse, supplementary physical examination and imaging techniques. The basic concept has been described and although daunting at first impression is very straightforward. A significant shortcoming of the basic description is its failure to recognize the inadequacy or otherwise of the vaginal wall lateral sulci, which are vitally important in the understanding of bladder base and bladder neck support. This system is an excellent method for recording data on prolapse for research or comparison purposes, although it is somewhat exhaustive for everyday use. In most cases a simple line drawing of the lateral view and perineal view is adequate to record findings.

A simpler yet less comprehensive method is both quicker and easier to perform and record but runs the risk that significant findings will be over-

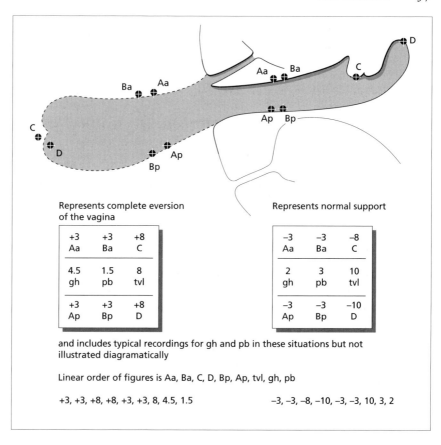

Fig. 3.6 Two notional examinations of the pelvis with the findings expressed numerically using the classification system formulated by the International Continence Society. On the left is a complete procidentia, while on the right is a normal pelvis. The findings can be displayed in either a grid or a linear fashion. Bump *et al.* 1996.

looked. An empty circle, representing the vagina, is drawn in the patient's medical records, the 'ring of continence', and any examination findings are drawn on this circle (Fig. 3.7). Physical examination alone does not determine the position of the bladder neck and the terms 'cystocoele', 'urethrocoele' or 'cystourethrocoele' can be misleading. Anterior vaginal wall defect, i.e. mild defect (1°), moderate defect (2°) and severe defect (3°), would be indicated as shown in Fig. 3.7a. Severe defect implies prolapse of the uterus or vaginal vault following total abdominal or vaginal hysterectomy. It is generally accepted that a 1° prolapse is not visible at the introitus on straining (but can be palpated or observed with a speculum), a 2° prolapse is visible at the introitus on straining and a 3° prolapse is outside the vagina. A posterior vaginal wall defect, generally indicative of a rectocele or enterocele, is represented on the ring of continence as shown in Fig. 3.7b; again, the same grading system is used. Full assessment of these posterior defects cannot be completed clinically and defecography is mandatory prior to considering

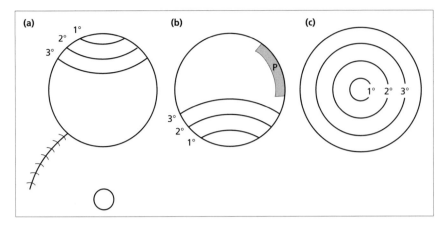

Fig. 3.7 The 'ring of continence'. This simple annotated diagram is quick and does not rely on artistic ability to convey its meaning. Abnormalities of (a) the anterior wall, (b) posterior wall and (c) vault are displayed, along with areas of pain (P) and any scarring. Previous scarring and the anus can also be represented as shown in (a).

any therapeutic manoeuvre. A uterine or vaginal vault descent is shown in Fig. 3.7c. A scar resulting from an episiotomy can be observed and recorded on the ring of continence (Fig. 3.7a). Observations should also be directed to the posterior fourchette and the length of the skin bridge between it and the anus.

Further assessment techniques

PELVIC FLOOR CONTRACTION

A good pelvic floor contraction can be observed in a number of ways: the anus retracts and the posterior vaginal wall is lifted in an anterior direction. Observation of 'bearing down' would indicate an incorrect (pelvic muscle) contraction, with the abdominal muscles straining. However, it is now accepted that the transversus abdominis works in synergy with the pelvic floor muscles and so some abdominal muscle activity can be expected, but certainly not straining. The deep muscles are palpated on the lateral walls of the vagina to a depth of 2–4 cm, whereas contraction of the superficial muscles is detected at the introitus. Many women demonstrate asymmetry of their pelvic floor muscles and this should be addressed, where possible, in the muscle strengthening programme. To enable a patient-specific exercise programme to be developed, the PERFECT assessment scheme is recommended and incorporated into the vaginal examination (Laycock, 1994).

PERFECT is a mnemonic to help all health professionals to assess the strength and endurance of the pelvic floor musculature and so prescribe an appropriate exercise regimen. *P* stands for power and is measured using a

Table 3.3 The modified Oxford grading system for pelvic muscle assessment.

0	Nil
1	Flicker
2	Weak
3	Moderate
4	Good
5	Strong

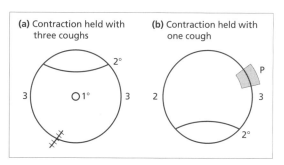

Fig. 3.8 Two notional patients with examination findings recorded prior to physiotherapy using the 'ring of continence': (a) patient with a grade 3 pelvic floor contraction demonstrating a 2° anterior wall defect, mild uterine descent and an episiotomy scar; (b) patient with a grade 2 contraction on the right and grade 3 contraction on the left, pain (P) at 2 o'clock and a moderate posterior wall defect.

modified Oxford scale (Table 3.3). The power (strength) of the contraction on the right and left may differ and can be shown on the ring of continence (Fig. 3.8). *E* stands for endurance and is the time (up to 10 s) for which a maximum contraction can be sustained. *R* stands for repetitions and is the number of maximum contractions, held for the specific time (endurance), that a patient can perform. *F* stands for the number of fast, maximum, 1-s contractions that the patient can perform. The remainder of the mnemonic (*E*, every; *C*, contraction; *T*, timed) reminds the examiner to identify the time and number of contractions that each patient can perform. The method of recording this assessment is shown below:

3/6/4//7

which represents a grade 3 contraction, held for 6 s, repeated four times and followed (after 1 min rest) by seven fast contractions. This method has demonstrated interobserver, intraobserver and test–retest reliability (Laycock, 1992) and is used extensively by physiotherapists in the UK. The system can be used not only for recording the status of the pelvic floor but also for tailoring a specific exercise regimen to the patient's needs (see Chapter 4).

Pelvic floor activity with cough

If the patient has stress incontinence with coughing, she is asked to contract the pelvic floor muscles and maintain the contraction while executing up to six coughs. This is recorded alongside the ring of continence.

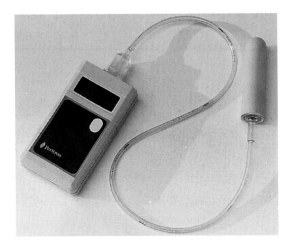

Fig. 3.9 The Peritron
perineometer with a digital
manometry display.

Accessory muscle activity

Recent studies have shown that the pelvic floor muscles work in synergy with
the transversus abdominis and multifidus spiniae (muscles of the lower back).
Consequently, concomitant activity of these muscles can be expected during
a maximum pelvic floor contraction. However, it is important to ensure that
a patient is not performing a Valsalva manoeuvre instead of the correct pelvic
floor contraction. Contraction of the glutei and hip adductors is also commonly seen when a patient performs a maximum pelvic floor contraction; we
feel that this should be minimized, but is admissible as long as the pelvic floor
is contracting adequately. This can only be detected on digital palpation, as
pressure perineometers may record transmitted abdominal pressure on the
vagina while electromyography (EMG) perineometers may record cross talk
from the abdominal, glutei or adductor muscles.

PERINEOMETERS

The Peritron (Fig. 3.9) is an electronic pressure-measuring device based on an
earlier design by Kegel in 1948. The vaginal probe, which is connected to a
manometer by plastic tubing and covered with a condom, is introduced into
the vagina. A pelvic floor contraction increases the pressure inside the probe
and this registers on the meter. Care should be taken to ensure that the correct pelvic floor muscle contraction is being recorded, as any increase in intra-
abdominal pressure may press the pelvic organs against the vaginal walls and
thus registers a false increase in pressure.

A simpler perineometer, the Periform, is shown in Fig. 3.10. This consists
of a vaginal probe (which can also be used for EMG biofeedback and electrical stimulation) and an indicator to measure angle of deflection. This

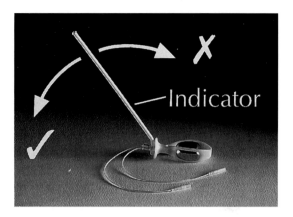

Fig. 3.10 The Periform
perineometer, complete with
indicator to show pelvic muscle
contraction.

device incorporates a modified Q-Tip technique and as the pelvic floor muscles contract, the indicator moves posteriorly. An inappropriate muscle action (e.g. bearing down) causes an anterior movement of the indicator, as does a cough. The strength of the contraction is measured by the angle of deflection, although this relationship can be complicated by vaginal wall laxity which itself can create a deflection.

URINE EXAMINATION

A dipstick examination of the urine usually detects the presence of protein, leucocytes, blood and glucose. If a dipstick test is normal and the patient's symptoms are not suggestive of infection, then there is really no need to send urine for microscopy as the chance of a positive result is remote. However, if the dipstick result is positive in any respect then urine should be sent for microscopy, culture and sensitivities.

BLADDER SCAN

It is important to know how efficiently the patient's bladder empties since, whatever the cause of incontinence, a large residual urine volume reduces functional bladder capacity and makes incontinent episodes more frequent. There is now a range of reasonably priced, hand-held, portable ultrasound scanners available that have been designed specifically for the purpose of measuring residual bladder volumes (Fig. 3.11). As part of the examination routine the patient should be asked to pass urine in private and a bladder scan immediately performed. A single measurement may, of course, be misleading if bladder emptying varies from one void to the next, so a series of scans on different occasions is sometimes worth while. The hand-held scanner is easy to use, requires very little training and avoids multiple referrals for pelvic

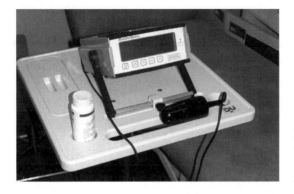

Fig. 3.11 A portable ultrasound bladder scanner is useful for measurement of residual urine volume.

ultrasound, which is quite unnecessary if the only question to be answered is whether the bladder empties. However, it should never be used in an attempt to scan other organs as its sensitivity is totally inadequate for this purpose.

UROFLOWMETRY

The urine flow rate is of fundamental importance in the assessment of patients with bladder outflow obstruction and a great deal has been written about the characteristics and relevance of each part of the flow trace. As an assessment of urinary incontinence it is of limited value, except in patients where bladder outflow obstruction is suspected. A prolonged flattened flow trace raises the suspicion of obstruction, although in the presence of incontinence this is almost always going to indicate a full urodynamic investigation (Fig. 3.12). Treatment of incontinence in the presence of obstruction or vice versa can lead to exacerbation of symptoms, so it is vital to be clear about the underlying dysfunction before any irreversible treatment is considered.

PAD TEST

The pad test is a useful way to quantify and confirm urine loss. Usually the patient is asked to empty the bladder and an absorbent pad is applied to the perineum. The patient is then asked to carry out a standard sequence of exercises over the course of an hour, including climbing stairs, handwashing, drinking, etc. At the end of an hour the pad is weighed and the patient passes urine again. The urine leakage (equivalent to the increase in pad weight) provides a representation of urine loss in relation to bladder volume for the hour. The test is a little unreliable because it is clearly dependent on the level of hydration and the enthusiasm with which the patient cooperates with the test. A variation is to collect pads over a full 24-hour period and measure both intake and output during this time. This gives a useful assessment of

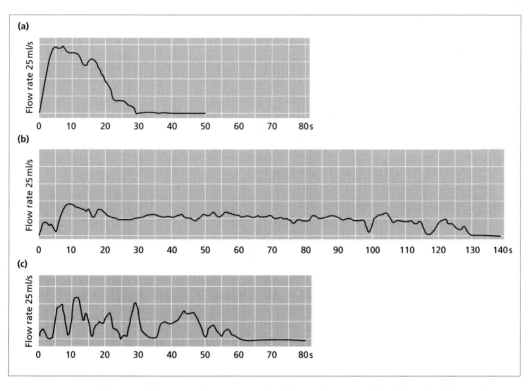

Fig. 3.12 Three urine flow rates showing (a) normal pattern, (b) prolonged and flattened pattern typical of obstruction and (c) intermittent flow typical of straining. Note that obstruction cannot be diagnosed confidently by uroflowmetry alone.

urine loss as a percentage of overall urine output. The chief value of the pad test is in a patient where there is real doubt about the severity of symptoms and whether they merit further therapy and also whenever one is looking for an objective measure of incontinence before and after treatment.

Correlation of findings with the clinical history and examination

The charts should be reviewed in the context of the history and examination findings. A great deal of important information can be derived from the charts (Figs 3.13–3.16). An assessment of the adequacy of fluid intake and total urine output is the first vital measure. Young women who complain bitterly of frequency and urgency and recurrent urinary infection often have very low volume output, which doubtless exacerbates the problem. Polyuria is obvious from the charts. The patient who passes small volumes throughout the day yet regularly voids over 400 ml in the mornings obviously does not have detrusor instability (more likely hypersensitivity), while detrusor instab-

	Monday	Tuesday	Wednesday	Thursday	Friday	Saturday	Sunday
Midnight							
1am							
2							
3							
4							
5							
6							
7	400	450		500			
8			350				
9							
10		250					
11	350						
Noon			300	250			
1pm		200					
2							
3							
4	450			350			
5							
6			250	150			
7		500					
8	300						
9							
10	200	350	450	400			
11			300				
Totals	1700	1750	1650	1650			

Fig. 3.13 A frequency–volume chart with a fairly normal pattern of voided volumes and timings.

	Monday		Tuesday		Wednesday		Thursday		Friday	Saturday	Sunday
Midnight											
1am	150		100		100		75				
2											
3	100		120		150		100				
4											
5	100				100						
6	75		120	W			150	W			
7	125	W	50		75		50				
8	130		75		75	W	75				
9	50		100		50						
10							100				
11	120		120		150						
Noon	50						130				
1pm			150		130						
2	100										
3			100		140		150				
4	150		75				50				
5					100	W	75				
6	120		120		75						
7							100	W			
8	130	W	150	W	100		100				
9	75		100				100				
10			50		150		50				
11	100		50		75						
Totals	1575		1480		1470		1305				

Fig. 3.14 A frequency–volume chart typical of detrusor instability. Note the consistently small volumes, the frequency and the leakage.

	Monday	Tuesday	Wednesday	Thursday	Friday	Saturday	Sunday
Midnight		50		20			
1am							
2							
3							
4							
5							
6	350		250	300			
7	50	300	50	50			
8	30	75	50	50			
9	40	75	120	50			
10	75	30	100	100			
11	120	100	75	100			
Noon	50	120	75	75			
1pm	40	30	20	20			
2	75	100	100	100			
3	120	120	100	75			
4	100	35	75	50			
5	110	75	100	100			
6	30	100	120	120			
7	100	50	75	50			
8	75	50	100	30			
9	75	100	30	100			
10	20	50	100	100			
11	75	50	50	30			
Totals	1535	1460	1590	1500			

Fig. 3.15 A frequency–volume chart typical of a habitually hypersensitive bladder. The volumes are remarkably small at times but the patient has slept well, passes good volumes in the morning and is not wet.

	Monday	Tuesday	Wednesday	Thursday	Friday	Saturday	Sunday
Midnight							
1am							
2							
3							
4							
5							
6	150						
7		200	250	250			
8							
9							
10	100						
11				100			
Noon							
1pm		200					
2							
3							
4	250		350				
5							
6				150			
7							
8							
9		150					
10	100						
11			200	100			
Totals	600	550	800	600			

Fig. 3.16 A frequency–volume chart of a young woman complaining of recurrent urine infections. Note the very small total urine output, indicative of an inadequate fluid intake. There is no need to record the intake as well.

ility is usually characterized by frequent small volumes both by day and by night. The charts provide a useful focus for the patient, who can use them both for gaining insight into her own problem and for monitoring progress with any treatment. Thus, whatever the underlying problem, there is value in the patient getting into the habit of charting.

By this stage the assessor usually has some idea of the pattern of urinary or faecal incontinence and the likely underlying cause. One must be aware, however, that the clinical impression can be wrong and symptoms may give little guide to the underlying pathophysiology. Attention should now be directed to whether further investigation is necessary and initial conservative therapy is almost always initiated within the same visit. Quite where assessment ends and conservative therapy begins is a somewhat artificial distinction and the two usually go hand in hand. However, for the sake of clarity of presentation, the techniques of conservative therapy are presented in Chapter 4.

Summary

Whatever the organization of incontinence services and whoever is seeing the patient at their first visit, it is important that the traditional clinical pathway of history, examination and special investigations is followed. This safeguards the patient who has concurrent or underlying serious disease, ensures that the patient's pelvic functions are considered as part of a whole and increases the likelihood that an accurate diagnosis is made at the outset. The division of chapters in this book into 'assessment' and 'conservative therapy' is somewhat artificial since the two usually come together in one session. At the end of the first consultation the patient should have had:
• an initial history taken, interpretation of the charts and symptom questionnaires;
• a mid-stream urine specimen and any relevant blood tests organized;
• assessment of the pelvic floor musculature and examination of the vulva, perineum and anus;
• a vaginal examination and/or rectal examination;
• relevant simple investigations;
• first-line management and treatment in line with Chapter 4;
• advice about follow-up;
• information sent to referring doctor, GP or colleague.
    The criteria for further investigation include the following:
• diagnosis not established;
• known multiple pathology;
• failure of conservative treatment;
• if surgery is contemplated;
• failure of previous incontinence surgery.

4: General Principles of Conservative Treatment

Jo Laycock, Lesley Irvine & Simon Emery

An initial conservative approach should be regarded as mandatory in the management of most patients with urinary or faecal incontinence no matter how tempting it may be to proceed straight to surgery. Between 30 and 70% will benefit and many prefer to live with persistent minimal symptoms rather than take the risks associated with a 'more successful' surgical solution. First-line management is usually provided by the specialist continence advisor, who should have the therapy skills and the complete repertoire of aids, devices, pads, protective clothing and literature immediately available. Many patients will never require surgical intervention, with its attendant risks, if the measures described in this chapter are applied with intelligence and diligence. Patients need to know about all the aspects of care that empower them in the control and management of a condition which may never be completely cured despite their clinicians' best endeavours. The continence advisor's office is a resource centre to be used by patients and specialists at any time. The cupboards may contain that long-forgotten pessary that exactly meets the needs of a difficult case. Lists of self-help groups and contact numbers of resource centres in other parts of the country are greatly valued by patients who are trying to come to terms with their condition or are afraid to venture far.

However, conservative treatment is not always successful and it is important to recognize this without undue delay. If a patient with instability is not making some progress after 2–3 months then persistence with bladder drill will benefit no one. Referral pathways need to be clear and group discussion, by clinicians, of difficult management problems is particularly helpful. If conservative management fails the patient is referred so that surgery by the appropriate gynaecologist, urologist or colorectal surgeon can be considered. The techniques described in this chapter remain relevant to almost all patients, as surgery rarely results in the restoration of long-term normality.

First-line conservative management

There are several essential practical measures that must be addressed in the first line of management:

1 fluid intake and types of fluid;
2 dietary requirements;

3 aspects of daily living;
4 toiletting guidance;
5 products and appliances;
6 collection devices, i.e. sheaths;
7 skin care, hygiene and odour removal;
8 psychological factors;
9 urethral plugs.

Fluid intake and output

The patient must clearly understand that measurement of fluid output is essential for ensuring a satisfactory outcome. An adequate measuring tool is required – plastic jugs are obtainable from all hardware stores. The optimum 24-hour fluid output is 1500–1800 ml. The assessor ensures that this output is achieved and questions, when relevant, why more or less fluid is being taken over 24 hours. Note that many patients perceive falsely that increasing fluid intake will make the incontinence worse.

Fluids containing three groups of substances may exacerbate urinary incontinence by both central and peripheral mechanisms: (i) caffeine-containing fluids, e.g. tea, coffee, colas, lager; (ii) sedatives, e.g. alcohol; and (iii) irritants, e.g. citric/carbonated drinks. Consideration must be given to discontinuing or reducing the input of such fluids.

Dietary requirements

Constipation may exacerbate urinary incontinence either by a volume effect or by promoting further pelvic floor damage through repetitive straining at stool. Encouragement must be given to increasing the intake of food with a high-fibre content, e.g. cereals, pulses, vegetables and fruit, together with an adequate fluid intake. There are numerous causes of constipation, some of which may be aided by manipulation of diet. If there is a change of bowel habit, underlying causes (e.g. neoplasia) should be excluded before concentrating on symptoms alone. In 50–70 year olds presenting with constipation, rectal bleeding or change in habit, there may be up to a 20% chance of significant neoplasia (10% polyp, 10% malignancy).

Constipation requires increased fluid intake and appropriate modification of diet, both to avoid exacerbating urinary incontinence and to overcome concomitant faecal overflow. Conversely, those with persistent loose faecal motions, as in structural bowel disorders or irritable bowel syndrome, may need to avoid exacerbating foods and/or use loperamide. Remember that if constipation is present, it may be caused or exacerbated by both analgesics and tricyclic antidepressants. Attention should therefore be given to rationalize such medications. Although these appear to be simple remedies, they are frequently overlooked and remain essential principles for management of incontinence.

Aspects of daily living

As equally important as fluid intake and diet is appropriate advice concerning the optimum arrangements for daily living. Adequate mobility within the house, good visual aids, manual dexterity, adjustment of clothing and access to laundry facilities and incontinence products are crucial for positive continence management. Sympathetic attention and advice are required when dealing with personal hygiene, especially in patients with physical disabilities, impaired dexterity and joint disorders. The characteristics of the toilet with regard to seating, height and support and access to the toilet and bath may require input from the social services. The team must also consider the problems experienced in the workplace, such as access to sufficiently private facilities (e.g. disabled toilets). A commode may be required downstairs if there is no downstairs toilet or upstairs by the bed in order to simplify bowel/bladder function. The local social services and primary care teams should be made aware of the problems.

Toiletting guidance

Based on the charted information, the continence advisor devises a programme of toiletting for the patient who may not have urgency or frequency but has an inability to recognize the need to void, mobility problems or apathy which results in inappropriate toiletting ('leaving it too late'). Advice about the national key scheme is given and a card provided to facilitate queue jumping when toiletting is urgent.

Products and appliances

These may be used in the short term for acute incontinence or be needed regularly and long term in cases where incontinence cannot be cured but can be helped. The continence advisor oversees their use. Products take the following forms.
• Perineal protection, i.e. pads/pants (Fig. 4.1). The patient and carer need to know from where supplies may be obtained.
• Bedding protection (Fig. 4.2): information is available about this from the clinic. The patient and carer need to know from where supplies may be obtained.
• Clothing adjustments: the clinic has a wide range of information available.

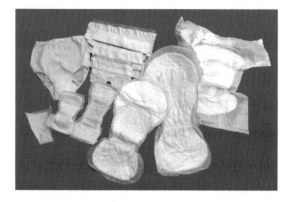

Fig. 4.1 A range of pads and pants that are available.

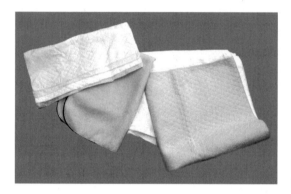

Fig. 4.2 A range of bedding protection.

Collection devices: sheaths

Several types of penile sheath are available that drain into a leg bag attached to either the thigh or calf. Some have self-adhesive strips and retaining band to minimize the risk of detachment (Fig. 4.3). In patients who have a retractile penis or inadequate penile length to retain a sheath, implantation of a simple malleable penile prosthesis or a penile-lengthening procedure will sometimes solve the problem. More antiquated forms of pressure appliance are still occasionally used in more elderly or immobile patients. There is still no adequate equivalent to penile sheaths for women.

Skin care, hygiene and removal of odours

Advice on skin care and topical medications for excoriated skin may be needed, because incontinent patients frequently have severe skin irritation and maceration with secondary bacterial and fungal infection. Advice on

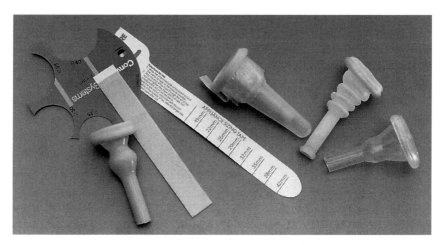

Fig. 4.3 The self-adhesive types of urosheath, together with the adhesive strips that can be applied to the penis in order to secure a non-adhesive sheath.

Table 4.1 Examples of useful creams for skin protection.

Conotrane
Kylie skin guard
Sudocrem
Metanium

Table 4.2 Examples of odour neutralizers and their manufacturers.

Products	Manufacturer
Day Drop (liquid)	Loxley
X-O (spray)	MMG (Europe) Ltd
Neutradol (liquid/spray)	M.S. George Ltd
NaturCare (spray)	Alphamed Ltd

washing, bathing and skin protection (Table 4.1) is given by the continence advisor. Deodorants/neutralizers may be an essential part of management, particularly in faecal incontinence which has a more immediate and obvious odour however adequate the hygiene. The continence advisor will advise about such products and from where they may be obtained. They are carried by the patient to neutralize odours when they attend to their toilet (Table 4.2).

Psychological and psychiatric factors

Any form of incontinence is both distressing and degrading. Much effort has to be made by the team to support the patient mentally and physically. In addition the team must instil the belief that the incontinence can definitely be

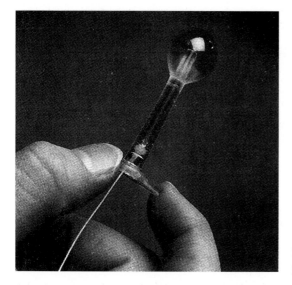

Fig. 4.4 The Reliance urethral plug.

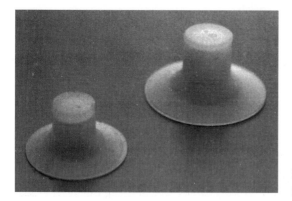

Fig. 4.5 The Femassist urethral plug.

helped by one method or another, and the patient must have confidence in him- or herself and in the support offered. Overdependence of the patient on the team or an individual should be avoided by not allowing 'recycling' or 'revisiting' to occur where no further therapeutic outcome is achievable. Re-referral is always an option. Remember that incontinence may be a symptom of an underlying anxiety/neurosis or a manifestation of a psychotic illness.

Urethral plugs

A wide variety of plugs has been marketed. These are worth considering but are not usually appropriate for long-term use. Two devices, the Reliance and the Femassist, are illustrated in Figs 4.4 and 4.5.

Active conservative management

Bladder or bowel drill and pelvic floor exercises are the mainstay of conservative therapy and are appropriate for patients with incontinence from any cause. Other management therapies, i.e. vaginal cones or weights, biofeedback, electrical stimulation, self-catheterization and long-term catheterization, are discussed later in this section.

Bladder drill

Bladder drill is used where there is a need to extend the time between the sensation of voiding and actual voiding, with the aim also of achieving increased bladder capacity and decreased frequency. Nocturia often improves spontaneously with improvement in daytime urgency and frequency. Bladder drill requires ongoing support and the patient must be well motivated and advised that persistence will be rewarded. The drill may be effective very quickly or take 3–4 months to achieve significant improvement. This behavioural training is usually performed and practised at home. Patients who fail to make progress at home may do better if the training is carried out in hospital, where they can be supervised more closely by experienced staff and followed up as outpatients.

The drill can be focused on times or voided volumes, and clear step-by-step targets are set. Motivation is of fundamental importance and the patient must be able to accurately complete a frequency volume chart. Increasing the voiding interval by as little as 15 min between each void is the usual starting point. This is maintained for 1 or 2 days before the interval is widened again. The patient steadily learns to control his or her urgency in this way. The small increments are needed to prevent discouragement and it is vital to provide continuous psychological support. Occasionally anticholinergic drugs are used in conjunction with bladder drill but this is not recommended as it undermines the principle of this extremely powerful behaviourist approach. Once a normal voiding pattern has been relearned care must be taken to avoid gradual regression. The long-term results of bladder drill have proved to be durable and compare favourably with any other treatment for detrusor instability.

Bowel drill

The principles underlying urinary drill may be applied to patients with faecal urgency by encouraging greater spacing between defaecations or by devising an individualized toileting programme. For example, patients with neurological disease can be encouraged to use an enema every third day in order to achieve complete emptying and they often remain clean during the intervening period.

Pelvic floor exercises

Voluntary contraction of the levator ani muscle generally involves synchronous contraction of the external urethral sphincter and the external anal sphincter. It is easier to explain to patients that they should tighten the pelvic floor muscles 'as if stopping wind escaping from the back passage and urine escaping from the bladder', rather than separate the different components of the continence mechanism. These exercises imply frequent contraction and relaxation of the pelvic floor muscles. However, simply tightening and relaxing a muscle will not necessarily strengthen it and so the four principles of muscle training should be applied.

PRINCIPLES OF MUSCLE TRAINING

Overload

To produce gains in strength or endurance, a muscle or muscle group should be overloaded, i.e. made to work beyond its normal activity level. This is easily demonstrated in athletic training schedules where runners, for example, are pushed to run further and faster in order to improve their performance. The same applies to pelvic floor training, so it is essential to carry out the PERFECT assessment (see Chapter 3) in order to identify the level of training required to satisfy this principle.

Specificity

This implies the need to train a patient to perform pelvic floor contractions specific to their needs and specific to the muscle's composition. Pelvic floor muscle exercises for urge incontinence involve learning to perform a long maximum contraction in an effort to inhibit the overactive detrusor. Specific exercises are performed for the slow-twitch muscle fibres (endurance exercises) and fast-twitch muscle fibres (power and speed exercises). Patients often present with a mixture of stress and urge incontinence, so appropriate exercise programmes should be devised. Pelvic floor exercises should be practised lying, sitting and, most importantly, standing.

Maintenance and reversibility

Pelvic floor exercises should continue as a lifelong habit, because if a trained muscle is not exercised it will, in time, simply revert to its pretrained state with a recurrence of symptoms. However, once an improvement is achieved, a less energetic regimen can be used. Exercising the pelvic floor maximally twice daily, e.g. while brushing the teeth, may well be sufficient to maintain the improvement in symptoms.

Once a patient-specific exercise programme has been devised, it takes 3–6 months to 'train' the muscles, i.e. increase their strength and endurance. However, some patients become 'dry' after only 1 week of therapy. These patients have 'found' their muscles (not strengthened them) and are using them at the appropriate time. For example, all patients should be instructed to tighten their pelvic floor muscles before and during any activity (coughing, bending, lifting, etc.) that normally makes them wet; this may be all that some patients require to become continent.

PROTOCOL FOR PELVIC FLOOR EXERCISES

The protocol used for any individual depends on the PERFECT assessment (see Chapter 3). Patients graded 0 or 1 on the modified Oxford scale are *not* suitable for pelvic floor exercises and need biofeedback and/or electrical stimulation. Patients graded 2, 3, 4 or 5 should be given a specific regimen that satisfies all the above principles of muscle training. An algorithm is shown in Fig. 4.6.

In principle, one is trying to improve performance by increasing strength, endurance, the number of possible repetitions or all of these. In addition to the PERFECT exercise regimen, long (up to 3 min) submaximal contractions should be practised during daily activities and short submaximal contractions can be performed in time to music for 2 or 3 min. For maintenance, one or two sessions of the specific regimen should be practised daily for life. Clear literature needs to be given to the patient for home reading (see Appendix 2).

Pelvic floor exercises are the mainstay of pelvic floor re-education, and both the referring doctor and the therapist must emphasize their importance. There is a tendency for us to stick to the treatments that we know; thus surgeons keep faith with surgery and the operations familiar to them and often fail to consider non-invasive therapies as a realistic option. The success of pelvic floor re-education is well documented. While this approach is highly dependent on the dedication and enthusiasm of the therapist and the commitment of the patient, any good incontinence unit should have a very close working relationship with the therapists and encourage this level of professionalism to develop.

POST-PROSTATECTOMY INCONTINENCE

Incontinence after prostatectomy should be evaluated using a pelvic floor PERFECT assessment of the puborectalis and anal sphincter complex. The pelvic floor exercises for stress and urge incontinence described above are

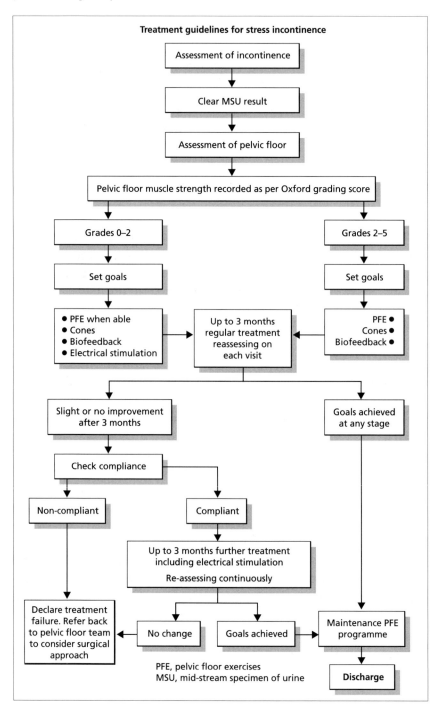

Fig. 4.6 Algorithm for conservative treatment of stress incontinence.

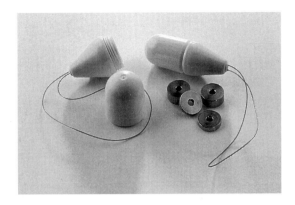

Fig. 4.7 Weighted vaginal cones used for pelvic floor retraining.

applicable to treating this condition. In some cases, it may take over 6 months of regular daily exercises to effect a change in symptoms. Pelvic floor exercises used in the treatment of faecal incontinence aim to increase both the resting tone and voluntary contractility of the puborectalis and external anal sphincter; again endurance and strength should be specifically targeted.

VAGINAL CONES OR WEIGHTS

Various types are available. Most cones are of similar size, with variable weights making up a set; an alternative is a hollow mould into which weights can be added (Fig. 4.7). These devices are useful adjuncts to a pelvic floor training programme and can be easily used after expert guidance. The lightest is inserted into the vagina and the patient encouraged to walk about or undertake normal activities. The cone will slip out if the muscles of the pelvic floor are not contracted. Sustained contraction is needed and the weight can be used for 10 min or more at each session. Progressively heavier weights are used as pelvic floor strength improves.

Cones can be used by most women, although some who never use tampons find them unacceptable and others with moderate to severe vaginal prolapse or a deficient perineum are unable to retain the cone when standing. The biofeedback aspect of cones can be particularly helpful in well-motivated patients. After a prolonged episode of exercise, patients develop aching muscles and may find their incontinence worse at these times of fatigue. Many report that they are able to hold heavier weights in the mornings and have more difficulty premenstrually.

Biofeedback

Biofeedback is a method of registering a state or a change in a body system that would not otherwise be detected; in the case of pelvic floor re-education,

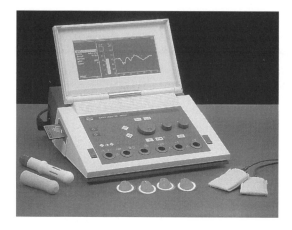

Fig. 4.8 Physiotherapy equipment incorporating biofeedback (manometric or electromyographic) and neuromuscular electrical stimulation.

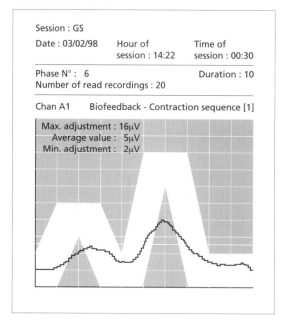

Fig. 4.9 Tracing of biofeedback session in which a patient has been asked to 'follow the blue line' (appears here as thick white band) with pelvic floor contractions.

it relies on any technique that will show a patient the extent of the effort of contracting the pelvic floor muscles. Biofeedback comprises a variety of treatment modalities, such as (i) verbal encouragement during digital pelvic floor muscle palpation; (ii) using a modified Q-Tip technique (Periform) (see Fig. 3.10); and (iii) sophisticated computerized recording equipment, with information on muscle contractility displayed on a colour monitor (Fig. 4.8). The latter uses a screen display (Fig. 4.9) to turn pelvic floor exercises into a game. The subject is told to contract their muscles so that the trace follows the blue 'track' (white track on figure). There is no doubt that patients respond to all types of biofeedback and put more effort into their treatment sessions.

Biofeedback equipment is available as a portable home unit or a clinic-based system; these hospital units provide more detailed information and generally have the added advantage of being able to print the results of the exercise session. This is a powerful tool for reporting on progress and further encourages the patient to produce a greater effort while performing his/her exercises, which in turn produces a greater training effect. Three techniques are described for biofeedback:

1   modified Q-Tip technique using the Periform indicator (see Chapter 3);
2   pressure (manometry) using the perineometers described in Chapter 3;
3   Electromyography (EMG) using the monitoring equipment described in Chapter 5.

There is debate about the necessity to completely isolate pelvic floor contraction from contraction of the abdominal and gluteal muscles during pelvic floor exercises. One group believes that better results (reduction in incontinence symptoms) are achieved when isolated contractions are performed; others believe that as the transversus abdominis works in synergy with the pelvic floor muscles one might expect co-contraction. Two-channel biofeedback equipment allows EMG monitoring of the abdominal muscles during pelvic floor training and helps the patient and therapist to check the activity in both muscle groups.

Exercise regimens using biofeedback to monitor effort and encourage greater performance should be done in all positions, especially standing, and use of the PERFECT scheme is recommended. EMG biofeedback has the extra advantage of detecting EMG activity from very weak muscles and so is an important step in the early stages of rehabilitation. All techniques described for manometric biofeedback can be applied to EMG biofeedback. Any electrode used for electrical stimulation can be used for EMG biofeedback, and some of these are shown in Chapter 5.

Electrical stimulation

Electrical stimulation is widely used in physiotherapy to strengthen and re-educate muscles, so it is the treatment of choice for patients with very weak pelvic floor muscles or for those unable to perform a voluntary contraction (this includes all patients graded 0, 1 or 2 on the modified Oxford scale). Studies have confirmed the beneficial effects of electrical stimulation for patients with detrusor instability and also for those with retention. This is thought to be due to the normalizing effect of electrical stimulation on micturition reflexes. There is a great variety of devices on the market (Figs 4.8 & 4.10) claiming benefit from one particular waveform or another, although very few randomized controlled trials using clearly comparable protocols have been published.

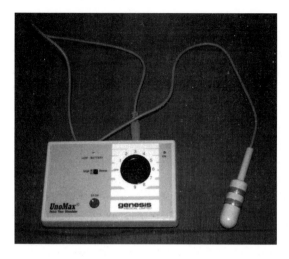

Fig. 4.10 A simple commercially available electrical stimulator for home use by patients.

TREATMENT

The following optimum parameters are recommended for the treatment of lower urinary tract dysfunction.
• Current intensity: maximum that the patient can tolerate. Always allow the patient to control the intensity. When purchasing equipment, especially battery devices, ensure that the generator can deliver 80 mA.
• Waveform: biphasic. Due to the high energy levels, interferential therapy is not generally recommended for treatment in the pelvis.
• Frequency: 35 Hz for stress incontinence, 10 Hz for urge incontinence.
• Pulse width: 0.25 ms for stress incontinence, 0.5 ms for urge incontinence.
• Duty cycle: off time equal to, or greater than, on time (measured in seconds), e.g. 5 s on and 10 s off for a weak muscle, 5 s on and 5 s off for a stronger muscle.
• Electrodes: route of lowest impedance recommended; therefore the vaginal/anal route is preferred.
• Treatment time: 20 min daily until symptoms improve.
Daily out-patient treatment is not practical, so home stimulation devices have been used in the majority of recent research studies.

When treating stress incontinence, a frequency of 35 Hz, applied via a vaginal electrode, is aimed at producing a tetanic contraction of the pelvic floor muscles and the external urethral sphincter. The patient is instructed to 'join in' with the current, so that cortical awareness is improved; thus the patient learns how to use the muscles voluntarily. Using the Periform, the result of the electrically stimulated muscle contraction is seen by posterior deflection of the indicator. As the muscles get stronger, the active assisted contraction causes a greater deflection that is held for longer. Progression to active voluntary contraction, associated with an Oxford scale grade 3, indicates that the stimulation can be discontinued and the patient continues with exercises alone. This illustrates the need for regular muscle assessment and that prescription of therapy, i.e. number of treatments, is inappropriate. Some patients may require only two treatments: once they have 'found' their muscles, stimulation is no longer needed as they can exercise without the device. Patients with very weak muscles may need many treatments. Most clinical research has used daily treatment for 30–50 days. A tetanic contraction of the pelvic floor muscles can be achieved with frequencies greater than 35 Hz and many home units are set at 50 Hz. This frequency is more likely to cause fatigue, so longer rest periods in the duty cycle are recommended. If this is not possible, a shorter treatment time should be used. The first treatment should be limited to 5 min in order to ensure that there are no adverse effects. Treatment time should then be gradually increased.

Treatment for urge incontinence follows similar guidelines, with the patient taking maximum intensity at a frequency of 10 Hz. As 10 Hz is a less fatiguing frequency, a duty cycle of 10 s on and 3 s off is adequate. Electrical stimulation at the parameters descibed has been shown to reflexly inhibit parasympathetic outflow to the bladder and activate the sympathetic inhibitory reflexes (Lindstrom, 1983). The treatment of urge incontinence should also include pelvic floor exercises and bladder training with or without medication.

The use of transcutaneous electrical nerve stimulation (TENS) for the treatment of urge incontinence has been demonstrated, with electrodes placed on the dermatomes of S2–S4. TENS units are less costly than muscle stimulation devices and some patients prefer this method to using internal electrodes. As with all therapies, treatment should be continued until improvement is reported, which may take as long as 4 months although a much quicker response is usual. Some patients may need to repeat the treatment from time to time, so the most cost-effective modality should be selected.

Clean intermittent self-catheterization

The management of most patients with poorly emptying bladders has been revolutionized by the use of clean intermittent self-catheterization (CISC). Any situation in which the bladder fails to empty may benefit, whatever the underlying cause. Failure of emptying often leads to overflow incontinence or reduces the functional capacity of a hyperreflexic bladder, thus increasing the frequency of incontinent voids. Thus, regular self-emptying of the system can reduce the likelihood of leakage and may also reduce the incidence of urinary infection compared with an indwelling catheter because of the completeness of bladder emptying and absence of foreign bodies.

Age and intercurrent disease are no bar to learning this technique, although severely impaired dexterity, e.g. multiple sclerosis or stroke, adduction hip deformity and urethral stenosis, may prevent its use. Most patients are reluctant to try it but conviction and persuasion on the part of staff usually overcome this psychological barrier. When CISC is taught in hospital an aseptic technique is used and catheters are only used once. At home, where only the patient's commensal organisms are present, a clean technique is employed and catheters can be reused for up to 1 week. A precoated catheter is the one of choice as its low friction minimizes urethral trauma; however, these can only be used once. The technique is simple to teach but adequate time must be devoted to careful explanation. Encouragement and support are needed at first as many patients are afraid of causing harm. Some practitioners use a mirror to help the female patient find her urethral meatus, although it is usually possible to locate the orifice by palpation alone.

The frequency of CISC is determined by the amount of residual urine (keep below 450 ml) and the patient's lifestyle. All patients should be given written details of prescription requirements, advised to drink freely (at least 1800 ml) and provided with adequate follow-up, including a local helpline number if possible.

Long-term catheterization

This is a last resort, as even with diligent catheter care and regular changes most patients eventually run into trouble with catheter blockage, recurrent infection and by-passing. Patients with a neuropathic bladder may develop urethral erosion and/or expulsion of the catheter caused by high-pressure bladder contractions. The erosion problems can be overcome by permanent suprapubic catheterization but the other problems remain. When leakage occurs around a catheter it is a common misconception that insertion of a larger catheter or bigger balloon will 'plug the hole'. It may for a while but the problems of erosion and expulsion will ultimately be aggravated because the larger catheter is a greater irritant than the smaller one. A better solution is to use a smaller catheter with a smaller balloon. Appendix 3 presents a summary of a protocol for choosing the most appropriate catheter.

Some patients with a permanent indwelling catheter find it easier to use a valve during the day rather than a leg bag. Catheter valves (Fig. 4.11) may be used when the patient is mentally alert, has a normal bladder capacity and is reasonably dextrous. A bag can be attached directly to the valve for night drainage.

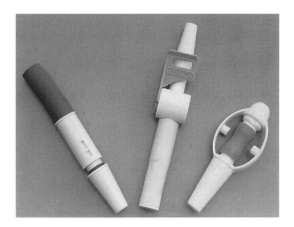

Fig. 4.11 Catheter valves used by patients with indwelling catheters to avoid the use of leg bags.

Synopses of conservative management of specific conditions associated with urinary incontinence

Remember that some of these conditions may coexist to different degrees within the same patient; collectively they form the bulk of clinical problems seen.

Urinary tract infection

The organism causing a urinary tract infection should be identified and isolated microbiologically. Appropriate treatment should be instigated and a satisfactory resolution ensured. Remember to keep in mind any underlying structural urological problems.

Childhood/adult nocturnal enuresis

Childhood enuresis is beyond the scope of this book. The core principles are described below.
- Ensure that any underlying structural abnormality has been dealt with, e.g. urinary tract infection, urethral valve, epilepsy, alcoholism.
- Provide star or picture charting, reward system and, for children aged 7 years and over, enuresis alarms; these are useful when the child is mature enough neurophysiologically and mentally for this behaviourist approach to succeed.
- Provide support for the mother/carer, with advice about fluid intake, and moral support for a potentially dysfunctional family situation.
- Use of appropriate products and appliances.
- Deamino-D-arginine vasopressin (DDAVP) tablets/spray 0.2–0.4 mg nocte (dosage independent of age and titrated to achieve results).

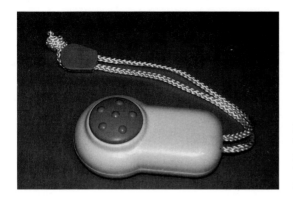

Fig. 4.12 Pressure-sensitive vibrator used by patients with multiple sclerosis to assist with bladder emptying (the Queen's Square bladder stimulator).

Overflow incontinence

Bladder outflow obstruction, either from mechanical obstruction or a neurological cause such as multiple sclerosis, Parkinson's disease or diabetic neuropathy, often leads to overdistension with overflow incontinence once the bladder's limit of compliance exceeds urethral closure pressure. If possible, treatment is focused on relieving the obstruction in order to improve emptying. Thus prostatectomy may be appropriate for benign prostatic hypertrophy (BPH), while CISC may be the most effective therapy for a patient with multiple sclerosis. The frequency of catheterization is determined by the need to keep residual volumes below 400 ml.

Where there is detrusor sphincter dyssynergia and detrusor instability, common in patients with multiple sclerosis, a regimen of CISC and an anticholinergic drug, with or without bladder drill, may be effective. Recent work (Dasgupta 1997) suggests that using a powerful pressure-sensitive vibrator applied to the suprapubic region improves bladder emptying in some patients with multiple sclerosis (Fig. 4.12; see also Chapter 6). Electrical stimulation at 10 Hz may have a similar effect. Self-care is encouraged wherever possible. Where CISC is not possible, e.g. patient with poor manual dexterity, management can be with an indwelling catheter. A suprapubic catheter may be needed where there is severe lower limb spasticity (adductor spasm), gross kyphoscoliosis or any condition rendering the urethra inaccessible. Voiding difficulties following abdominal and pelvic surgery can be resolved with a period of CISC.

Atrophic vaginitis and urethritis

This is diagnosed by history and examination of the vagina and perineum. It is associated with urgency, urethral irritation, reduced sphincter integrity and a tendency to stress incontinence. Oestrogen as a topical cream or vaginal tablets nocte for 2 weeks followed by one or two applications a week for 3 months are usually helpful. Long-term hormone replacement therapy should be considered.

Urethral stricture

Patients with urethral strictures may require regular dilatation of the stricture (by a urologist) in order to prevent overflow incontinence.

Synopses of conservative management of specific types of faecal incontinence

Management of hard faeces with or without overflow incontinence

Careful clarification regarding consistency, volume and appearance of stools, any laxative use and how the patient normally controls their bowels must be established. Infrequent defecators need to be encouraged to empty a soft stool more regularly; those who strain to pass a hard stool need faecal softeners. Patients who are faecally impacted need their rectum and left colon emptying by using suppositories, enemas or manual evacuation before an adequate pattern can be established with softeners or stimulants. Sometimes this may be required on a regular basis. Medication includes one or a combination of two preparations (Table 4.3). The aim is to achieve a daily, soft formed stool that requires no straining to pass.

Table 4.3 Useful preparations to encourage normal defecation.	Osmotic agents, e.g. lactulose Bulking agents, e.g. Fybogel, Isogel, Normacol Faecal softeners, e.g. Dioctyl, Movicol Bowel stimulants, e.g. senna, bisacodyl, picosulphate Combined stimulant and bulking, e.g. Manevac Rectal suppositories, e.g. glycerine, bisacodyl Bowel enemas, e.g. phosphate, Microlax

Management of liquid faeces

Loperamide hydrochloride and codeine phosphate are usually very helpful. Pads and advice about clothing, personal hygiene and odour control should be given. Small involuntary faecal leakages may be prevented by use of an anal plug device in carefully selected patients.

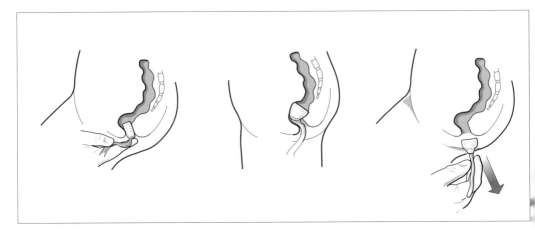

Fig. 4.13 Principle of the anal plug. The plug, once inserted, expands to improve the hermetic seal. It is easily removed by pulling on the attached 'tail'.

ANAL PLUG

Theoretically this method of controlling anorectal incontinence is attractive but has never really stirred the imagination of clinicians involved in the management of this problem. Original reports of this technique from Oxford were cautiously optimistic, although there were problems with design and manufacturing investment was not forthcoming at that time. Our own group has recently explored this idea further, with a new design (Fig. 4.13), but as yet we have no objective data concerning its value in the management of end-stage anorectal incontinence. Our belief is that while the anal plug is unlikely to control faecal incontinence, it may have a role in reducing the leakage of liquid, mucus and flatus in those patients who achieve a less than perfect result after sphincter reconstruction. Furthermore, many patients have leakage of mucus after antegrade colonic enemas or permanent colostomies because of continued sphincter failure or diversion proctitis (see Chapter 6). The anal plug may have a role to play in these situations.

Colonic irrigation

Colonic irrigation may have a part to play in the management of incontinence. By emptying the large bowel the patient has the confidence that they will not leak in an embarrassing fashion. Irrigation can broadly be accomplished in two ways, either perianally or through a specially constructed stoma or prosthesis, i.e. antegrade. The irrigation may be performed about once every 2–3 days (though it can be as often as twice a day) and can easily be managed by the patient themselves using isotonic fluids to prevent electrolyte disturbance.

5: Specialist Investigations

Malcolm Lucas, Simon Emery & John Beynon

In Chapter 3 the indications for considering specialized investigations were discussed in the context of a primary clinical assessment. This chapter presents a detailed description of all the special tests in common clinical use for the investigation of incontinence, whether of urine or of faeces. Some other tests, for instance neurophysiology, are described in less detail where it is felt that they belong largely in a research context, and this is clearly stated. If you have never seen some of these tests then go and observe them in your hospital or in another, whether or not they fall within the usual remit of your speciality. Not only will this broaden your appreciation of all pelvic floor abnormalities but it will also help to forge the links that are so vital to multidisciplinary working, the chief philosophy of this book. Ultimately, this can only benefit your patients.

Cystoscopy

Endoscopic examination of the bladder and urethra is often performed in the assessment of incontinence. The flexible cystoscope has made this a simple procedure that no longer requires a general anaesthetic. Although rigid cystoscopy is certainly possible in women without anaesthesia, the flexible scope provides a more complete examination including a good view of the anterior bladder wall. This area should never be omitted from bladder examination as it may be the site of the only abnormality and is the classic location for both Hunner's ulcer (interstitial cystitis) and adenocarcinoma of the bladder. Non-urologists may be unfamiliar with flexible cystoscopy but any specialist having an interest in bladder dysfunction should be able to examine the bladder competently and should learn this technique. However, bladder appearances rarely add to our understanding of the cause of leakage. The internal appearance of the bladder, bladder neck, prostate or sphincter tells little of their function. The importance of cystoscopy is in the exclusion of other bladder pathology (see Plates 1 to 5, opposite p. 148). Figure 5.1 shows an example of how the findings of cystoscopy can be recorded.

Any patient with blood in the urine should undergo cystoscopy regardless of whether there is associated infection or whether the haematuria has resolved. The same rule should apply for patients aged over 55 years with

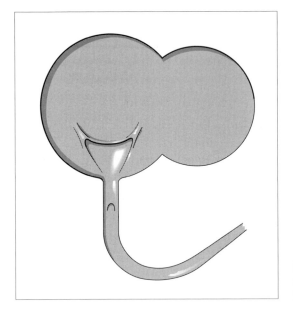

Fig. 5.1 Diagram commonly used for recording cystoscopy findings in a male patient.

dipstick or microscopic haematuria. Patients in whom the symptoms of frequency and urgency have failed readily to resolve with medication and especially those with bladder pain should have cystoscopy to check for inflammatory bladder disease such as interstitial cystitis, stones and carcinoma *in situ*. Abnormal-looking mucosa should be biopsied. This can be done using a flexible biopsy forceps passed through the operating channel of a flexible cystoscope; alternatively, the patient is brought back another day for cold cup biopsy using the rigid cystoscope under general anaesthesia. The bladder should not be biopsied unless you have the capability to stop bleeding with a diathermy probe. Beware, however, that while biopsy causes little discomfort, diathermy of the bladder wall through the flexible cystoscope is painful and must be done accurately and quickly.

Examination under anaesthesia

Patients who have previously had extensive pelvic surgery or radiotherapy, whether for incontinence or not, and those patients who cannot cooperate fully with pelvic examination because of either pain or embarrassment should have their endoscopic assessment under general anaesthesia so that a thorough examination can be performed. Only then can the degree of vaginal mobility and compliance and the full extent of any prolapse be adequately assessed.

Urodynamics

Prior to the advent of urodynamics the study of incontinence received scant attention from the medical profession and treatment was largely empirical. The development of electronics, reliable transducers and cheap recording equipment in the late 1960s moved the study of bladder function from smoked drums in the physiology laboratory to routine use in the clinic, and a clearer understanding of bladder function and dysfunction grew. The addition of synchronous radiological imaging in the 1970s increased this understanding and the treatment of incontinence began to be based on principles of pathophysiology. The International Continence Society (ICS) was inaugurated in Exeter in 1971 and the work of standardization of terminology began, upon which most of our current practice and communication about urodynamics and incontinence are based.

What is it?

Urodynamics is the physiological measurement of bladder pressure, sensation capacity and compliance during the cycle of filling and voiding. In its simplest form, bladder pressure is measured while the bladder fills and this can be done with a simple fluid-filled manometry line inserted through the urethra with the bladder being filled by gravity or natural filling. Changes in pressure can be observed by the rise and fall of the column of fluid in the manometer. Thus, at the very least, urodynamics allows the measurement of a filling cystometrogram and the demonstration of detrusor instability/overactivity under variable physiological conditions. Figures 5.2 and 5.3 illustrate methods of varying complexity used to measure urodynamics.

In the late 1990s, urodynamics is a study in which both bladder and rectal pressure are measured simultaneously and a third pressure, detrusor pressure, is electronically derived by the equipment by subtracting rectal from bladder pressure (Fig. 5.4). The bladder is usually filled with fluid artificially, by gravity or with a peristaltic pump. The bladder is filled until the patient has an intense desire to pass urine, at which stage they are encouraged to void to completion while pressure monitoring continues, thus completing a full cycle. During this process we attempt to provoke and observe an episode of incontinence so that the mechanism of incontinence becomes apparent. Analogue pressure data can now be displayed alongside X-ray images on the computer screen, with a facility for recording digital images one by one or even in rapid-fire sequences that mimic a video recording. However, such software is expensive and many clinicians still prefer to use videotape. In either case, the name has stuck and videourodynamics (VUD)

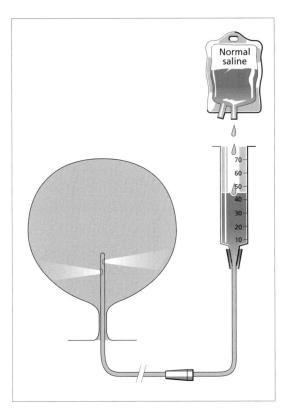

Fig. 5.2 Schematic diagram showing urodynamics in its simplest form, a single-channel fluid-filled manometer in the bladder. Changes in bladder pressure are detected by a rising column of fluid in the tube.

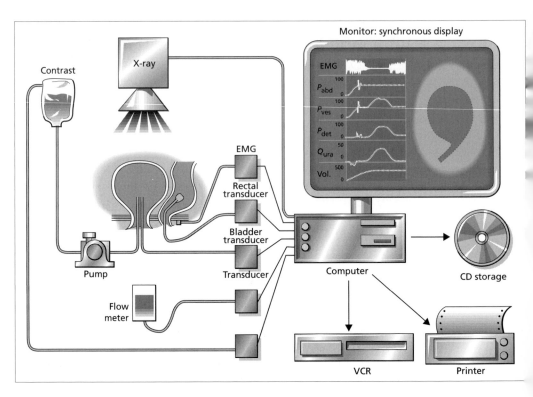

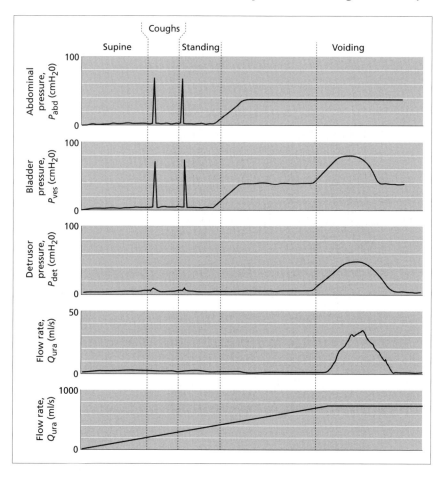

Fig. 5.4 Basic urodynamic tracing showing abdominal pressure (P_{abd}), bladder pressure (P_{ves}), subtracted detrusor pressure (P_{det}) and flow rate (Q_{ura}) during a normal filling and voiding cycle.

means the ability to synchronously image the bladder during urodynamics (Fig. 5.5).

When to do urodynamics

The measurement of urodynamics is often ordered as a knee-jerk response to certain clinical situations without much thought being given to the reason for the request. However, the test is invasive, carries a risk of infection and is not

Fig. 5.3 (*opposite*) Modern videourodynamics with bladder and rectal pressure monitoring, bladder filling via a peristaltic pump, and synchronous computer display of subtracted pressures and radiographic images. The recordings can be viewed on-screen, printed to hard copy or archived on to videotape or optical magnetic disc.

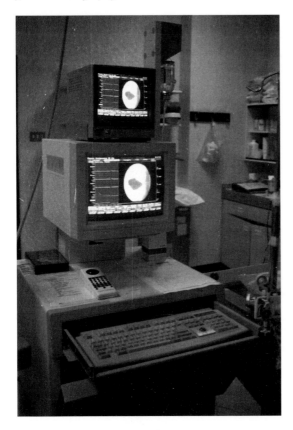

Fig. 5.5 The computer system during videourodynamics: the pressure displays are on the left of the screen, with a synchronous X-ray image on the right.

always diagnostic. Abnormalities such as detrusor instability may be seen in up to 69% of asymptomatic patients, while it may be missed in others who are undoubtedly suffering from the problem. The test is unphysiological in the sense that filling rates are abnormally fast, the catheters act as foreign bodies lying within the lower urinary tract and thus alter voiding dynamics, and the immobility imposed by the test conditions inhibits attempts to reproduce normal activity. It is helpful therefore to have a clear concept of the indications for urodynamics (Table 5.1).

With the exception of the conditions listed in Table 5.1, empirical therapy for incontinence is perfectly reasonable as a first approach and can be based simply on symptomatology. However, once such an approach has failed then a full urodynamic evaluation is usually required, and the following are indications for peforming such an evaluation: (i) to distinguish between stress incontinence and detrusor instability; (ii) neuropathic patients with incontinence where renal function is not impaired; (iii) post-prostatectomy incontinence; (iv) younger men with voiding difficulties; and (v) any patient in whom one needs to know whether detrusor instability could account for

Table 5.1 Absolute indications for urodynamics.

Indication	Reason
Prior to any corrective surgery to the bladder neck or reconstructive bladder surgery for incontinence	To confirm the diagnosis and appropriateness of planned surgery. Also because there is a significant failure rate from all interventions so a baseline investigation may be essential for assessing the reasons for failure
To investigate recurrent incontinence where surgery has failed	An accurate diagnosis is vital before any further definitive treatment is given. It may be important medicolegally
In neuropathic patients in whom there is real or threatened impairment of renal function	Renal impairment is usually secondary to bladder dysfunction in these patients. Accurate urodynamic evaluation will reveal the pattern of bladder dysfunction that needs to be treated to correct renal function
In all spinal cord-injured patients once the neurological status has stabilized	Bladder function cannot always be accurately predicted from the neurological lesion. By definition, therefore, these patients have threatened renal impairment until there is urodynamic evidence to the contrary

their symptoms or where incontinence cannot be explained and has failed to respond to empirical therapy.

How is it done?

Urodynamic evaluation is best performed in a room dedicated to the purpose. The room should afford privacy and be well heated (Fig. 5.6). There is a compromise to be made between privacy (where investigator and patient would ideally be in separate rooms, with all the monitoring equipment linked at a distance) and interaction (where the patient and investigator are together in the room and able to communicate). The choice may depend on the type of clinical practice that you have; complex neuropathic and reconstructive problems require a greater degree of interaction in their assessment and the addition of X-ray screening usually implies the use of a dedicated screening room adapted for urodynamics rather than the other way around (Fig. 5.7). None the less, an effort should be made to minimize the patient's feelings of exposure and embarrassment. The test usually takes between 20 and 40 min depending on the complexity of the problem. Busy clinics will be able to process six patients in a half-day session. However, this leaves little time for

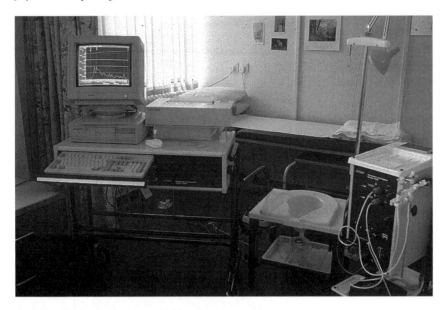

Fig. 5.6 Arrangement for simple urodynamics testing, with recording apparatus close to the couch and the room curtained off at one end.

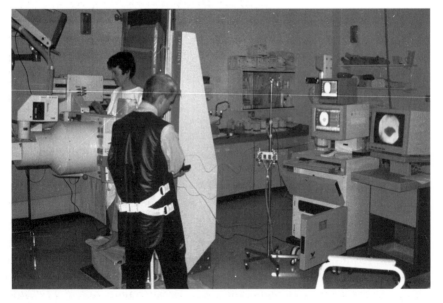

Fig. 5.7 Arrangement for videourodynamics. This female patient is in the standing position for provocation of stress incontinence.

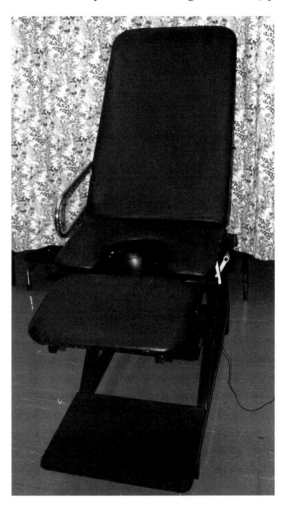

Fig. 5.8 The urodynamics couch has a cut away to facilitate voiding study.

interaction, which we feel is a vital part of the study and we rarely attempt more than four patients per session.

An examination couch is a bare essential, allowing the patient to be catheterized in the supine position, and there should be enough room for the patient to stand during the investigation. An X-ray screening table fulfils these requirements. Purpose-built couches for urodynamics are available that allow the patient to lie or sit and to void through a hole in the couch directly to the flow meter (Fig. 5.8). A C-arm image intensifier can be used with one of these couches but these systems tend to discourage examination in the standing position.

The patient is asked to attend with a full bladder. At the start of the study a free flow is obtained without any catheters, partly to see the unimpeded flow pattern but mainly to ensure that the bladder is working from its normal

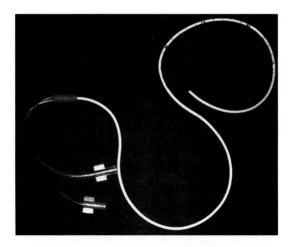

Fig. 5.9 Double-lumen catheter used for urodynamics.

baseline residual volume. This should, of course, be zero. Some investigators empty the bladder by catheterization at this stage in order to measure the residual volume accurately. However, this can create artefactual filling characteristics, especially in some neuropathic patients. It is much better to start filling on top of the residual volume, thus demonstrating the functional bladder capacity and reflecting what usually happens for that patient. If an accurate assessment of residual volume is necessary then a simple bladder scan will suffice or the bladder can be emptied by catheter at the end of the test.

The bladder is catheterized urethrally. Two catheter lumina are required, one for filling and the other for pressure measurement. A separate line is also inserted into the rectum or the vagina for measurement of intra-abdominal pressure. The ideal system is easy, safe and comfortable to insert, allows filling at any rate, provides accurate and sensitive pressure recording and yet does not interfere in any way with the dynamics of voiding. Such a system does not exist, since good recording requires rigidity in the tubing while comfort requires the opposite and so a compromise has to be struck. The best laboratories will be aware of several techniques and use them as appropriate in particular clinical problems. For instance, the frightened adolescent with myelomeningocele is best investigated by performing preliminary cystoscopy, when a suprapubic urodynamics catheter is inserted that allows the test to be performed the following day. The younger man with equivocal voiding is best studied with rapid filling and removal of the filling line so as to interfere as little as possible with the urethral cross-section during the voiding study.

Double-lumen catheters (6 French gauge) are available for the bladder line (Fig. 5.9). Alternatively, two separate fine-bore tubes (maximum 3 French gauge) can be used; their total cross-section is smaller than a single 6 French gauge tube and so they interfere less with voiding dynamics, although they

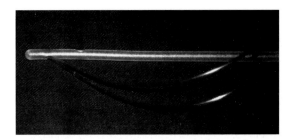

Fig. 5.10 Two small-diameter tubes 'hitched' into a Nelaton catheter, which is used to insert them into the bladder in men.

still alter flow characteristics by flattening the maximum flow. These are 'hitched' into the side hole of a larger 14 French gauge Nelaton catheter, which is used to insert them into the bladder (Fig. 5.10). Once they have been inserted, pulling sharply backwards on the small tubes disengages them from the larger one, which is then completely removed. The technique is easy to master and allows some very cheap catheters to be created that perform well. However, we have recently been converted to the convenience and reliability of patented double-lumen catheters and feel that the minimal additional cost is more than justified. Their disadvantage is that they are more prone to kinking within the empty bladder, leading to a dampened bladder pressure with pump artefact until the bladder is full enough to allow the catheter to straighten (usually at about 50 ml). Some investigators use a large-bore filling catheter and remove it once the bladder is full, leaving only a fine-bore pressure line for the voiding phase of the study which thus minimizes flow artefact. While this allows a quicker fill it eliminates the ability to perform a second filling cycle, which is an invaluable adjunctive technique; occasionally the pressure line will accidentally fall out at the crucial moment of commencing voiding, rendering this part of the test useless. All lines must be secured to the penis or the inner thigh with a piece of Micropore tape. In order to avoid the catheters falling out during a forceful urinary stream they are best secured as close as possible to the urethral meatus; however, in females, if rigid tubes are held firmly to the thigh this can result in a 'splinting' open of the meatus with possible effects on continence and voiding (Fig. 5.11). Finally, suprapubic catheters can also be used. The easiest way to do this is to pass a 10 or 12 French gauge suprapubic cannula (Bard, Porges, Sherwood) into the bladder suprapubically and then slip a double-lumen urodynamics catheter through it. The cannula is removed and the urodynamics catheter is left taped to the abdominal wall, allowing separate filling and pressure measurement. This gives much better results than the previous technique that used a Y-piece connector and a damping chamber on the filling line to eliminate filling artefact.

Catheter-tip strain gauge transducers have been available for several years. They are manufactured with up to three transducers with end or side mountings that allow a range of studies, from simple cystometry to static

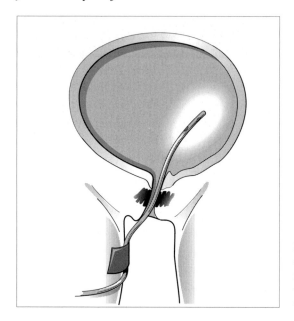

Fig. 5.11 If a rigid tube is
secured too close to the meatus
in a female, it distorts the
urethra and interferes with the
urodynamic study.

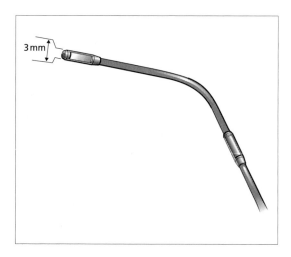

3 mm

Fig. 5.12 Catheter-tip and side-
mounted transducer. This can
be used for simultaneous
measurement of two pressures,
e.g. bladder and urethral
pressures.

urethral profilometry, to be performed (Fig. 5.12). They should be calibrated
to atmospheric pressure before insertion into the bladder. They are expensive
and require sterilization after every case but are easier to use than fluid-filled
tubes. Some laboratories may feel their use is worth while, particularly if
ambulatory studies are also regularly performed; if the cost is spread over a
couple of years they are no more expensive than disposable tubing. Pressure
catheters are usually connected to Statham-type strain gauge transducers,
which are very reliable and can be mounted on a stand, level with the

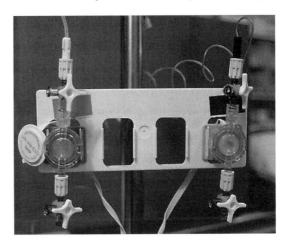

Fig. 5.13 Statham-type transducers mounted on a stand alongside the patient.

symphysis pubis (Fig. 5.13), or strapped to the upper thigh. The lines and transducer chambers are filled carefully with sterile water or saline while gently tapping to exclude any air bubbles, which dampen pressure signals. The transducers are 'zeroed' to atmospheric pressure before recording.

Pressure recording is started and the bladder filled with saline or radio-paque contrast medium, either by gravity or using a peristaltic pump. For urodynamic tests it is usual to fill the bladder artificially as it speeds up the whole cycle. The equipment should be calibrated to the specific gravity of the filling fluid, since the filling volume is calculated from a weight transducer that assumes the specific gravity of the fluid used. Carbon dioxide is used in some laboratories, especially in the USA. It is easier, less messy and much faster to use than saline or contrast and appeals particularly to 'office' urologists. It is effective as a way to detect or exclude detrusor instability but is more prone to artefact and does not allow for screening, nor can it be used to assess the voiding cycle. However, artificial filling is non-physiological and the increasing use of ambulatory monitoring, in which filling is natural over a few hours, has revealed fundamental differences in the filling cystometrogram which suggest that hypocompliance and some instability may simply be an artefactual finding caused by rapid filling. Medium filling rates (10–100 ml/min) are usual. Slow rates are used largely for neuropathic patients (see below) while rapid rates are used usually only on a second fill. The filling rate should always be recorded in the urodynamics report. The total bladder pressure (P_{ves}), abdominal pressure (P_{abd}) and subtracted detrusor pressure (P_{det}) are recorded simultaneously on a pen-and-ink recorder or, more usually nowadays, a computer software package displays the pressure changes on a monitor.

The bladder is filled until the patient is anxious to pass urine. He/she is asked to state when they feel a first desire to void (FDV) and subsequently a

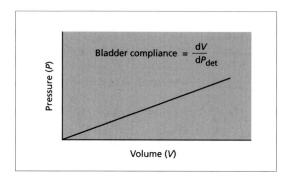

Fig. 5.14 Relationship between pressure and volume, which gives a measure of bladder compliance. The trace shown illustrates severe hypocompliance.

strong or urgent desire, or any pain. Attempts are made at intervals to provoke urine leakage or unstable activity. Events must be marked on the trace, if only by scribbling with a pen, although most modern systems have event markers. The bladder capacity at FDV and strong/urgent desire are measured. Maximum cystometric capacity is the volume at which the patient is no longer able to delay voiding and filling should be stopped at this point. In practice, filling is usually stopped at 500 ml when one full bottle of saline or contrast has been used. Functional capacity is the maximum capacity minus the residual volume. End-fill detrusor pressure and bladder compliance (change in volume divided by change in detrusor pressure, dV/dP_{det} in ml/cmH_2O) can be measured (Fig. 5.14).

The test is usually started in the supine position, although the most important part is with the subject in the standing position when incontinence is more likely to be seen. Some investigators perform separate supine and standing fills; we simply stand the patient halfway through filling. Incontinence is often seen during the filling phase and these events should be recorded on the trace or on VUD, with either video recording or digital image storage so that the precise relationship of anatomical and physiological events can be reviewed later (see Figs 5.12 & 5.14). One useful interactive tool is to include an audiochannel into the videotape recording so that a running commentary can record important events. This may be particularly useful in units where the tests are being done by a technician.

Detrusor instability that occurs during filling shows as a rapid rise in detrusor pressure accompanied by an urgent desire to void and possibly by incontinence (Fig. 5.15). If filling is stopped, a detrusor contraction usually settles down within seconds. Hypocompliance, on the other hand, is a gradual rise in the baseline detrusor pressure throughout or towards the end of filling that does not usually decline once the filling is stopped. Two patterns are typically seen: in neuropathic patients the hypocompliant pressure rise usually tends to occur steadily throughout filling, while in the 'stiff' bladder

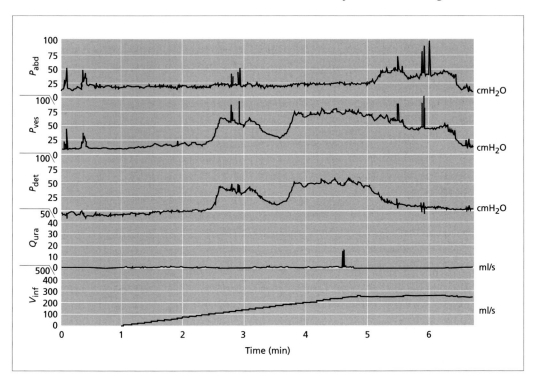

Fig. 5.15 A urodynamic trace showing detrusor instability.

the rise tends to be in the terminal phase of filling (Figs 5.16 & 5.17). The filling study is done lying and standing in either one or two fills, although if instability is not evident it should be provoked. Coughing, jumping up and down, washing hands in cold water and running the taps all help in this respect. Telling a joke often works, although it is remarkable how the presence of urethral and rectal catheters can limit one's sense of humour and we have been accused in this situation of not taking the patient's problem seriously enough.

Once the patient is anxious to pass urine he/she should be allowed to do so. Older systems tended to require a change of recording mode (filling to voiding) at this point but the better modern systems allow all parameters to be recorded at once and there is no longer a need for this somewhat inconvenient interruption in recording. The patient is asked to void either sitting on the commode over the flow meter or by voiding directly into the funnel (Figs 5.18–5.20). During VUD this is difficult if the camera is directly in front of the patient and a flow tube has to be attached to the patient's leg or between the thighs that will direct the urine flow to the funnel, which stands just to one side of the table. This all creates a highly artificial environment

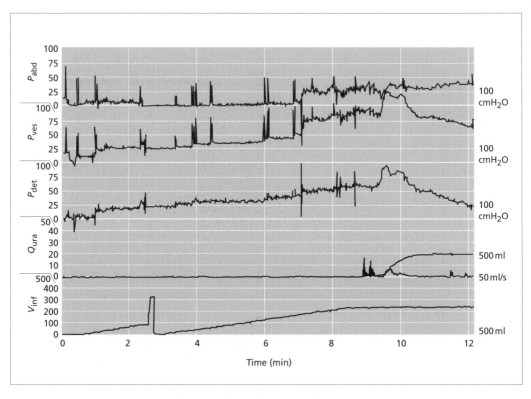

Fig. 5.16 A urodynamic trace showing hypocompliance throughout filling in a patient with spina bifida.

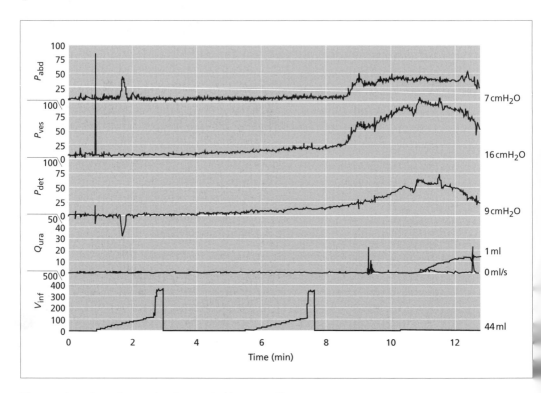

Fig. 5.17 A urodynamic trace showing terminal hypocompliance.

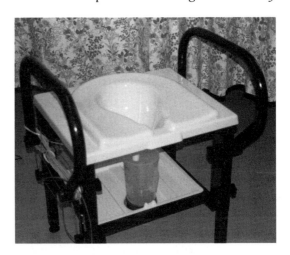

Fig. 5.18 Commode used for voiding studies with flow meter positioned below.

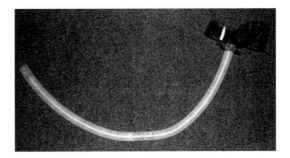

Fig. 5.19 Voiding tube used for women. The moulded plastic funnel is held between the thighs, whilst the flexible tube is directed into the flow meter.

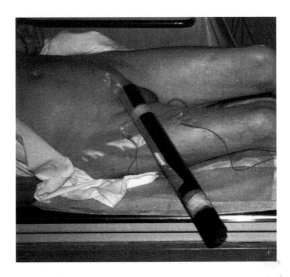

Fig. 5.20 Voiding tube used for men fixed to the thigh. This can be pointed directly into the flow meter in the standing position or in recumbency for non-ambulant patients.

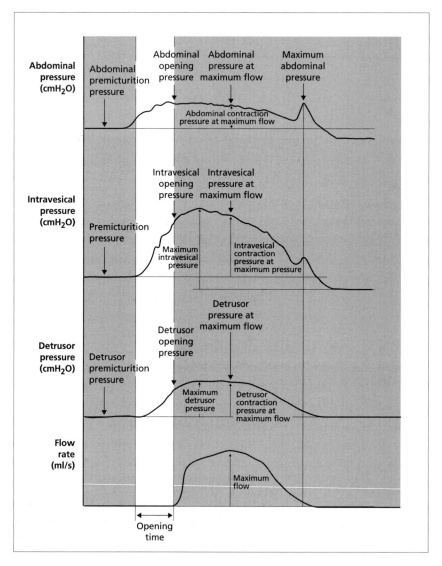

Fig. 5.21 Relationships between pressure and flow throughout a normal voiding study. Based on Abrams P. *et al.* (1998), with permission.

for voiding, often exacerbated by the presence of an enraptured audience. It is hardly surprising that many patients find it impossible to void in these circumstances and thought should be given in each laboratory as to how this psychological 'pressure' can best be alleviated, otherwise the voiding studies will be uniformly disappointing in their diagnostic yield. Maximum flow rate (Q_{max}), average flow rate (Q_{ave}) and voiding time are usually recorded (Fig. 5.21). In the investigation of bladder outflow obstruction the relationship between voiding pressure and flow rate is very important,

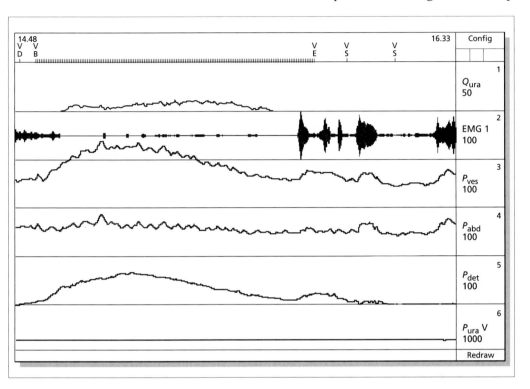

Fig. 5.22 Urodynamics study showing filling and voiding in a man with lower urinary tract symptoms.

obstruction being characterized by high voiding pressures with low flow rates. Nomograms have been produced and many of the modern computerized systems automatically superimpose these on the pressure flow plot for a given patient in order to assist with the urodynamic diagnosis of obstruction (Figs 5.22 & 5.23). While this subject is beyond the scope of this book, a confident diagnosis of obstruction may be important in incontinent men with detrusor instability since in these patients little will be achieved in the control of the instability until the underlying obstruction has been removed.

Halfway through the free urine flow the patient should be asked to stop the flow as quickly as possible; this is known as a stop test. It is regarded as positive if the patient can interrupt voiding with a pelvic floor contraction within 5 seconds or so. It is normal in the stop test for the detrusor pressure to rise momentarily and then decline quickly (within a couple of seconds), presumably in response to a spinally mediated inhibitory reflex. In patients with detrusor instability this is less likely to occur and one may see a rise in the isovolumetric pressure (P_{iso}) sustained for several seconds (Fig. 5.24). Indeed these patients may find it impossible to stop the flow.

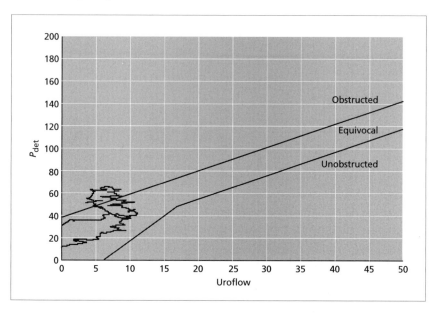

Fig. 5.23 The same pressure–flow study as seen in Fig. 5.22 displayed on the Abrams Griffiths nomogram, showing the trace lying within the equivocal (i.e. not definitely obstructed) part of the graph.

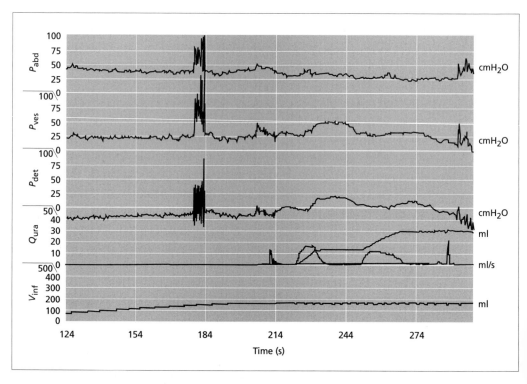

Fig. 5.24 Urodynamic trace showing a stop test in which P_{iso} rises significantly.

The test results are recorded on a proforma, an example of which is shown in Appendix 4 (a and b). If there is any suspicion that the first filling and voiding cycle has not answered the clinical questions posed then a second fill should be performed. This might require a faster or a slower filling rate and, perhaps, more careful screening of a particular event, such as a cough or the first unstable contraction. It is usually worth the extra time and the second fill may confirm your existing impressions or clarify an area of doubt. This is one reason why the best results are usually obtained by the individual who has to make the clinical decisions rather than a highly trained technician, who may not appreciate the nuances of the clinical problem.

Table 5.2 lists the problems commonly encountered during the performance of a urodynamics study and describes solutions to these problems.

Special tests of urethral function

One limitation of conventional urodynamics is that the test gives little information about urethral function. Urethral pressures can be measured in two ways: by leak point measurement and urethral pressure profilometry. The beauty of leak point pressures is that their measurement requires no additional equipment to that already used for cystometry. There is a poor correlation with the findings of urethral pressure profilometry but since we know that maximum urethral closure pressures do not correlate well with symptoms of stress incontinence this probably emphasizes that urethral pressure profilometry is an outmoded and unreliable investigation. It is described here for completeness only.

The detrusor leak point pressure is a measurement that was developed in neuropathic patients for the evaluation of risk to the upper urinary tract. It is the subtracted detrusor pressure at which urethral leakage occurs and reflects the competence of a neuropathic sphincter mechanism. McGuire *et al.* (1981) showed that provided the leak point pressure is < 40 cmH$_2$O then the upper tracts are safe, even if the total bladder pressure exceeds this level. From this measurement was derived the method of assessing abdominal Valsalva leak point pressure (VLPP). The patient is asked to perform a Valsalva manoeuvre with a comfortably full bladder. A good way is to ask the subject to blow into the chamber of a 10-ml syringe with steadily increasing force and observe for leakage, either with direct observation or on synchronous screening. The total abdominal pressure at which leakage occurs is recorded. The normal urethra does not leak even with a very high abdominal pressure. Patients with VLPP of < 65 cmH$_2$O are thought to have intrinsic sphincter weakness, while those who leak at pressures > 100 cmH$_2$O usually have a purely hypermobile bladder neck. This makes the technique particularly useful for patients with stress incontinence and may help in making the choice of operation for this problem.

Table 5.2 Troubleshooting with urodynamics.

Problem	Cause	Avoidance	Solution
Catheters will not pass through urethra	Urethral stricture	Flexible cystoscopy is advisable in most men before performing urodynamics	May require urethrotomy
	False passage Sphincter spasm	Use plenty of lignocaine gel: milk into posterior urethra and leave for several minutes before trying again very gently	Suprapubic lines can be used
Lines fall out during test	Inadequately secured lines or strong bladder contraction	Rectal lines best secured to natal cleft. Bladder lines secured in several places. Explain each step to patients and encourage them to move slowly and carefully	Rectal line can usually be simply reinserted even in standing position. It is better to replace the bladder line completely as it is probably contaminated. If you do not do this the entire test will have to be repeated another day
No pressure response	Kinked tubing (especially in the bladder)		Ease the bladder line back slightly and reflush. Sometimes it does not work properly until there is some fluid in the bladder
	Blocked tubing		Change the tube
	Air bubbles		Careful flushing, making sure there are no air locks in syringe. Tap the transducer gently to release bubbles
	Defective transducer/connections		Check and service or replace defective kit
Unequal subtraction	Obesity The bladder and rectal lines are basically different systems (different tubing diameter, length and rigidity) and respond at different rates		Careful flushing. Set height of transducers carefully to symphysis pubis. If this fails then cheat by zeroing the pressure channels after closing the system to air
Artefact in pressure traces	Pump artefact due to pump line touching filling line Double-lumen tubes, if kinked, will give pump artefact Movement artefact	Separate the filling and manometry lines by fixing with different tape	
Bladder spasm	Gross instability/reflexia		Stop filling and take a break. Do a second and third fill slowly

Continued.

Table 5.2 (*cont'd*)

Problem	Cause	Avoidance	Solution
Gross leakage will not allow any bladder filling	This can occur in any patient with gross incontinence but the study will not then give information about the potential bladder capacity and compliance after surgery		In men, a penile clamp will help the bladder to fill more. Alternatively the bladder-filling line can be a Foley catheter with the balloon inflated and pulled down against the bladder neck to prevent leakage
The patient does not leak	Either the test is not sufficiently provocative/physiological or the catheters are masking the leakage		Do a second or third fill and remove all of the catheters. Then try again to provoke leakge. Mild sphincter weakness incontinence may then become apparent. Failing this, proceed to ambulatory monitoring
Patient feels faint on standing up	Usually men		Lie the patient down immediately. Try again after a few minutes and keep him pushing up and down with calf muscles. Abandon if necessary and do ambulatory test instead
There is a large residual urine volume and the bladder cannot be seen			Use 50 ml of high-density contrast injected directly through filling line. Then roll patient from side to side to mix in the bladder. A good image will then be obtained

The static urethral pressure profile (UPP) was described by Brown and Wickham, 1969. A perfusion catheter or microtip transducer is inserted into the urethra as far as the bladder and the catheter gradually withdrawn using a mechanical puller at a steady rate of 1 mm/s. The recording equipment thus prints a pressure 'profile' that represents the distribution of pressure along the length of the urethra. Vesical pressure (P_{ves}), maximum urethral pressure (P_{ura}), maximum urethral closure pressure ($UCP_{max} = P_{ura} - P_{ves}$) and functional urethral length are all measured (Fig. 5.25). Though low pressures may be associated with poor results from surgery, women with low UCP_{max} may be dry while others with high UCP_{max} may have stress incontinence; this renders the test of little practical value in patient management (Wan *et al.*

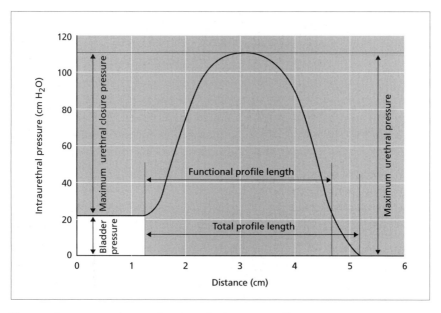

Fig. 5.25 Components of a normal static urethral pressure profile.

1993). The stress UPP records bladder pressure and maximum urethral pressure synchronously during stress with a full bladder. It is a complicated way of demonstrating hypermobility of the bladder neck and of no practical use.

The dynamic UPP is a technique that was developed for investigation of the neuropathic patient. As for the stress UPP the tranducers are positioned to record bladder and maximum urethral pressures but the bladder is also filled in order to allow a cycle of filling and voiding to be studied. The main purpose of this technique is to detect detrusor sphincter dyssynergia in the spinal cord-injured patient, but it is unreliable because of difficulties in determining the position of the catheter in relation to the bladder outlet and yields high false-positive and false-negative rates.

The urethral electrical conductance test is simply a way of confirming the existence of stress incontinence. A catheter is mounted with two electrodes and the conductance between these is constantly measured. One electrode is positioned in the bladder, while the other sits in the distal urethra. With a full bladder the patient is asked to cough and a sudden increase in the conductance indicates that urine has escaped into the urethra, resulting in better conduction between the two electrodes. The test is little used and actually demonstrates bladder neck incompetence, which is known to be present in 40% of asymptomatic females. The fluid bridge test is similarly flawed. Watching the urethra during straining is a much simpler, though undignified, way to identify stress incontinence.

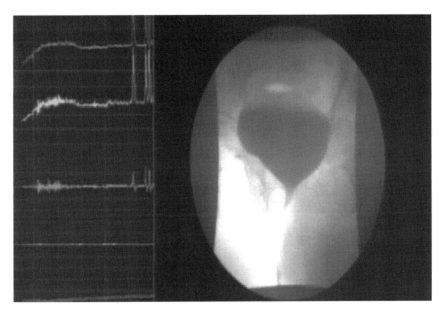

Fig. 5.26 Videourodynamic display showing type I stress incontinence. There is mild descent of the bladder neck alone.

Videourodynamics

VUD allows the synchronous screening of the bladder and urethra during a complete filing and voiding cycle. Although much of this information can be obtained from simple urodynamics and a lateral cystogram, or even a micturating cystourethrogram, it is the combination of synchronous events in one recording that allows a more complete picture and a subtlety of diagnosis that is not possible by any other means. Synchronous ultrasound recording fulfils the same requirements and allows screening to continue throughout the study. It provides good images in the sagittal plane that show the bladder neck and urethra, particularly in relation to the pubic symphysis in women, but it does not allow evaluation of bladder shape or vesicoureteric reflux, both of which are important in the assessment of neuropathic patients. We have used it for a period but abandoned it because of our discomfort with the images and some evidence that the presence of a large probe in the rectum or vagina interferes with the normal function of the urethrosphincteric complexes. The development of perineal probes or smaller intraluminal probes may help this problem.

VUD allows imaging of the bladder base and bladder neck anatomy during filling, stress and voiding and any incontinent episode. This helps in the distinction of urethral hypermobility from intrinsic sphincter weakness and from bladder base prolapse (Figs 5.26–5.29). It also reveals the dynamics of

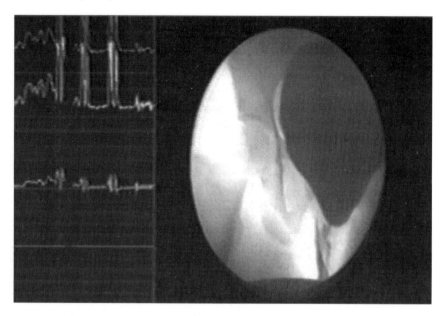

Fig. 5.27 Videourodynamic display showing type II stress incontinence. The bladder base prolapses as well as the bladder neck. Clinically, there is loss of lateral support and demonstrable anterior vaginal wall descent.

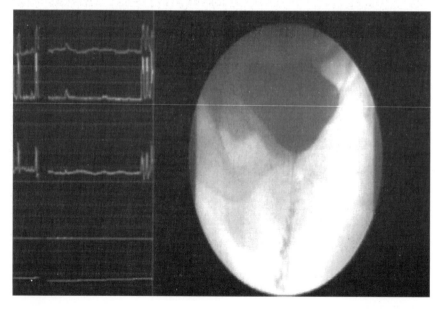

Fig. 5.28 Videourodynamic display showing type III stress incontinence in a woman who had previous bladder neck surgery. The bladder neck remained static during cough despite gross leakage.

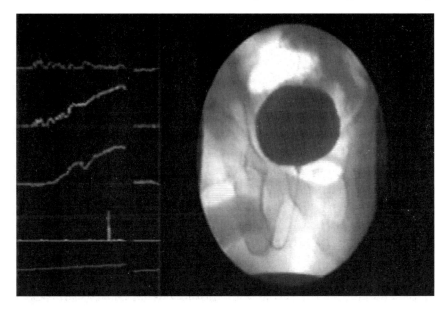

Fig. 5.29 Videourodynamic display showing urge incontinence due to detrusor instability.

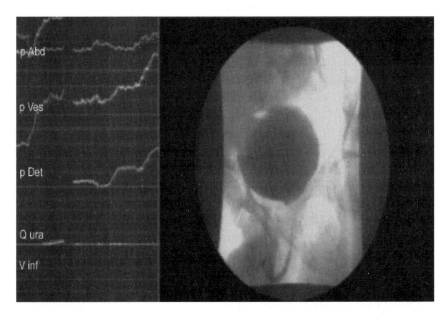

Fig. 5.30 Videourodynamic display showing bladder diverticulum in a man with obstructed voiding. Note the high voiding pressure and poor flow, with little opening of the posterior urethra.

bladder diverticula (Fig. 5.30) and sacculation in the obstructed or neuropathic bladder; the appearance of the bladder neck and posterior urethra during voiding (Fig. 5.31), where urodynamic parameters of obstruction may be equivocal; and reveals the presence, severity and behaviour of vesicoureteric reflux in the neuropathic patient (Fig. 5.32).

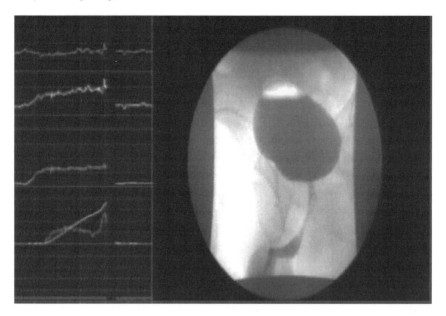

Fig. 5.31 Videourodynamic display showing a normal male void.

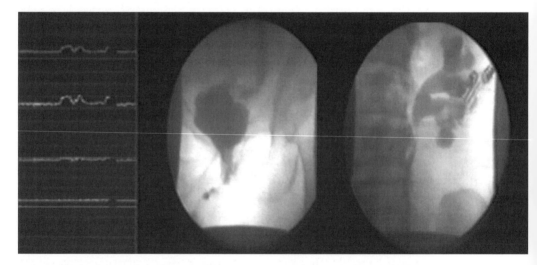

Fig. 5.32 Videourodynamic display showing a paraplegic with hyperreflexic cystometrogram and grade 4 left vesicoureteric reflux.

The basic requirements in terms of facilities are the same as for simple cystometry but X-ray screening is also required. There are three types of image intensifier. The mobile C-arm is versatile and can be used outside the X-ray department, although any room used requires the safety features of a theatre or X-ray room (wall and floor lining and reinforcement). The C-arm is rarely powerful enough to provide satisfactory full lateral images and the quality of still images obtained is usually poor. However, its major advantage is that it can be used to screen the patient during voiding in a sitting position. Screening tables come with either an over-couch or an under-couch tube. The over-couch tube is easier to use as it is less bulky and does not get in the way of flow meters, although the X-ray scatter (reflection from the patient) is worse. The under-couch tube has a cumbersome camera system that is placed so close to the patient that access to the patient is awkward and flow meters cannot be positioned and have to be placed remotely alongside the patient. However, the under-couch tube is safer for the investigator who, for these tests, has to be in the room with the patient in order to obtain the best results. Screening tables do not allow screening of voiding in a sitting position because there simply is not room.

Screening during VUD requires another compromise to be made. We want to see as much of what is happening to the bladder as possible but must minimize the X-ray screening time. Well-coordinated screening and video recording are essential and this can best be done by one person who controls both screening and recording. The urodynamic investigator therefore needs to have received basic training in radiation protection and control. In our experience this leads to shorter screening times that rarely exceed 1 min per patient. 'Freeze frame' is helpful for teaching since the obvious abnormality seen by an experienced tester may require prolonged examination to become apparent to the novice. Digital image recording, particularly with modern high-capacity computers, may well replace video recording in time and offer the additional convenience of faster access for review. Video recording is remote controlled and the 'on-screen' display of pressures and X-ray image is stored on videotape. Recording is usually in 'snippets' of important events so as to save tape. Synchronous control of X-ray screening, computer keyboard, video remote and digital image capture while trying to focus on the patient's clinical problem requires practice and should not be left to the inexperienced.

Ambulatory urodynamics

Ambulatory urodynamic monitoring was introduced for two reasons. Firstly, it was appreciated that conventional studies are unphysiological in that the filling rate is abnormally fast. Secondly, there is a significant number of patients in whom conventional studies fail to clarify the diagnosis because the symptoms of which the patient complained fail to occur during the test. Ambulatory ECG and oesophageal pH monitoring have been used for years, but the availability of computer chips with large memories has made the digitalization of physiological recording possible and for hours of recording to be made on one chip within an easily portable recording box (Fig. 5.33).

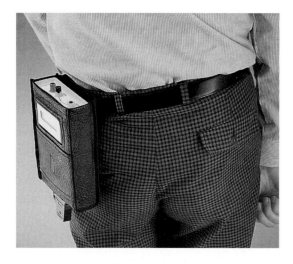

Fig. 5.33 Patient wearing recording box for ambulatory monitoring.

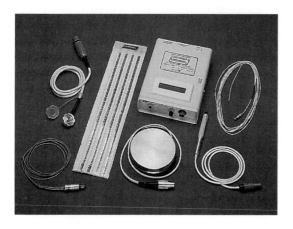

Fig. 5.34 The Uroloss pad together with recording box and transducers used for ambulatory monitoring. Reproduced with kind permission of Lectromed UK Ltd, Letchworth, Hertfordshire.

The patient is catheterized with microtip transducers that have been calibrated to atmospheric pressure and which minimize the movement artefact. The transducers feed directly into a compact recording unit that the patient wears on a strap over the shoulder or around the waist. A sampling rate is usually set and this determines the length of recording. Slow sampling rates allow longer recording periods. While a sampling rate of 1/min might suffice for a pH recording, changes in pressure are faster and require a sampling rate of at least 1/s. Typically, the sampling rate is 2–5/s and recording lasts for 3 hours.

Urine loss can be detected by the use of a special pad, of which there are two types. One type contains a series of metallic strips laid between layers of absorbent nappy material and the system detects sudden changes in electrical impedance between the strips (Fig. 5.34). Alternatively, some pads

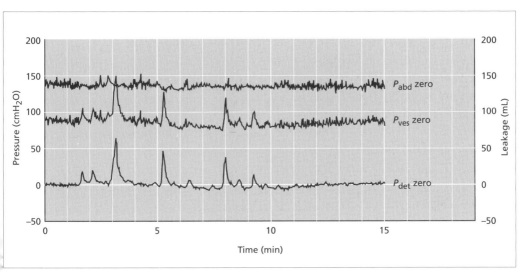

Fig. 5.35 Section of ambulatory urodynamics trace showing detrusor instability that had been undetected on conventional videourodynamics. From *British Journal of Urology* (1996) 77, 333–8, Blackwell Science.

contain a thermocouple device that detects the sudden increase in temperature of urine leakage. Total loss of urine is measured at the end by weighing the pad.

The unit is fitted with an event marker, which allows the patient to mark the trace whenever a significant event occurs. The patient is sent for a predetermined sequence of exercises that includes such things as climbing stairs, taking a drink, going for a walk in the cold wind and so forth. This programme is tailored to fit the patient's symptoms. Ambulatory recording allows several cycles of filling and voiding to be completed within the recording period. The patient is told to keep a simple diary during the study so that, as well as pressing event markers, a record is made of the time a drink was taken, the time stairs were climbed, etc. On return to the department after the predetermined period the unit is disconnected and the digital data downloaded to the software of an accompanying personal computer (often the one used as the basis for conventional urodynamic studies). This software allows trace analysis with focusing on events.

DIFFERENCES FROM CONVENTIONAL STUDIES

Ambulatory monitoring detects unstable contractions not apparent during conventional filling (Fig. 5.35). Unfortunately, these are also seen in asymptomatic subjects and this raises questions about the significance of the finding. However, reproducible recordings of instability associated with

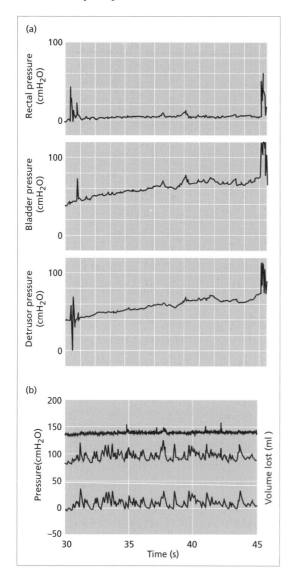

Fig. 5.36 Traces of conventional (a) and ambulatory (b) urodynamics showing the difference in the appearance of hypocompliance. From *Journal of Urology* (1992) 148, 1477–8, American Urological Association.

a sense of urgency or incontinence indicated by the event markers would be good evidence of instability and would justify further invasive treatment. Stress incontinence is nicely demonstrated because it occurs in the absence of detrusor contraction and this is a valuable finding where it has proved impossible to demonstrate leakage on conventional studies. Hypocompliance is a finding of conventional studies that cannot be reproduced by ambulatory testing. Instead repeated, regular, phasic contractions are seen that rise to a pressure equivalent to that seen in the hypocompliant trace (Fig. 5.36). This finding has made the interpretation of ambulatory studies in neuropathic patients particularly difficult.

Ambulatory studies are time-consuming and expensive of manpower since considerable time has to be spent preparing the patient and explaining the purpose and procedure. The investigator has to be available throughout the study in case a problem develops. Thus it is rarely possible to study more than two or three patients in a day. The analysis is all done retrospectively, which is a different philosophy to conventional studies where patient–investigator interaction is essential. The software and hardware are expensive, which means that the effective cost per investigation far exceeds that of conventional studies. For these reasons ambulatory studies will probably not replace conventional monitoring, although they have become a vital part of the urodynamic armamentarium of any department dealing with complex cases on a regular basis.

Equipment

The purchase of urodynamic equipment is a major capital outlay for a hospital and the choice should be made with care. Choice of equipment depends on the case composition in the area, the expertise and experience of the investigators, the availability of X-ray facilities, back-up by local medical physicists and, of course, the budget. If there are likely to be large numbers of spinally injured patients, neuropathic patients and a large reconstructive surgical practice, then full screening facilities with VUD are essential. However, a busy general unit in which most tests are done simply to exclude or confirm the presence of instability would be wasting money to buy more than a basic system for simple cystometry.

Most equipment now on the market is based on the personal computer. To some extent this has made urodynamics more complicated and certainly more expensive. Software packages have minor variations in configuration but these can usually be learned easily. There is much emphasis on programs that 'interpret' the recording; however, these must be viewed with scepticism since they depend on the quality of analogue data entered, which are subject to a great many artefactual errors. There is still much to be said for an old fashioned pen-and-ink trace laid out across the floor.

Always arrange for a demonstration in your hospital and always with real patients. Prepare a 'wish list' of the features that you seek in your ideal system and press relentlessly to see these in operation. Ideally, you should operate the system yourself. After-sales service is crucially important and all companies will tell you how excellent they are in this respect. Find out where the system is already operating and contact them to find out just how it performs in real life. Decide whether you want an after-sales service contract or whether your medical physics department can do the job. It is remarkable how a company can lose interest in you if they do not hold a service contract.

Who should do it?

Clinics have used different approaches to this. Many medical physicists and specialist nurses have been trained to perform urodynamics to a very high standard. Some would argue that the trained laboratory technician or nurse performs tests with greater obsessiveness and attention to detail than most doctors. However, our belief is that urodynamics should be an interactive process between investigator and patient, where physiological readings are coupled with observation of the patient experiencing the symptoms and, in particular, an attempt is made to answer specific clinical questions. This is best done by the clinician who has to make the management decisions about the patient. While this individual is probably a costly resource, it is likely that his/her presence increases the usefulness of the test and reduces the need for repeat testing or misleading reporting. We categorize patients prior to urodynamics so that consultant-led sessions focus on the more complex problems, e.g. neuropathic patients or surgical failures.

Interpretation of results: specific clinical situations

FEMALE INCONTINENCE

The prime reason for performing urodynamics on incontinent women is to detect the presence of detrusor instability; if it is not readily apparent it should be provoked. VUD allows an assessment of the functional defect associated with leakage. With coughing, the bladder neck should remain fixed in relation to the pubic symphysis and the bladder base likewise. Downward movement of the bladder neck on coughing is referred to as descent or hypermobility of the bladder neck (type I genuine stress incontinence (GSI)). There may also be descent of the bladder base posterior to the bladder neck, either independent of the bladder neck or all moving as one (type II GSI) (see Figs 5.26–5.28). When GSI occurs without any movement of the bladder neck it implies intrinsic sphincter weakness (type III GSI). Undoubtedly there is always an element of intrinsic weakness in patients with stress incontinence with or without hypermobility. We know this because there are many women with very mobile bladder necks and often marked prolapse who have no incontinence at all. The distinction is important if one is trying to decide between an operation to provide renewed support or one to simply increase urethral resistance (i.e. an obstructive procedure), and this decision can only really be made with synchronous screening.

The voiding study is important for two reasons. Firstly, a normal emptying phase means that postoperative voiding problems are less likely to occur. Secondly, it may help to identify a group of women in whom there is no measurable rise in bladder pressure yet who are able to void with a normal flow. These are the patients more likely to need intermittent self-catheterization after any attempt to augment urethral closure. Any patient in whom the bladder appears unstable during filling and yet who cannot initiate detrusor contraction for voiding may have a suprasacral neuropathy such as disseminated sclerosis.

Only about 50% of women show a rise in bladder pressure during voiding despite emptying the bladder well. You should remember that this does not necessarily mean that the bladder is not contracting. A contraction against an outlet resistance causes a pressure rise but if urethral resistance is negligible very little pressure rise may be recorded. This is why it is important to do a stop test, since in the latter group the sudden introduction of obstruction to flow causes a brief rise in pressure, showing that the detrusor is in fact contracting.

If the patient has experienced failure of previous surgery for GSI then the bladder neck is observed during filling. Bladder neck incompetence with minor filling of the posterior urethra may be the reason for a persistent urge syndrome and might be easily resolved with a local injection of silicone gel or collagen.

POST-PROSTATECTOMY INCONTINENCE

It is essential to identify detrusor instability in these patients and so the study should include provocation. If present then it is the detrusor instability that needs to be treated primarily. The real question being asked is whether the patient might benefit from insertion of an artificial urinary sphincter (AUS).

The patient should be standing, if possible. Sphincter weakness incontinence can only be shown with VUD, where contrast fluid will be seen leaking through the distal sphincter region with vigorous coughing (Fig. 5.37). Remember, as with women, that if no leakage is observed on the first fill despite provocation, then a second fill and removal of all catheters may reveal a leak that was masked by the presence of the urethral catheter. If sphincter weakness incontinence is present then bladder compliance and capacity should be assessed. These must be normal if an AUS is to be inserted; if not, they should be corrected at the same time. With gross sphincter weakness incontinence it may be necessary to obstruct the bladder outlet so that this assessment can be made; use either a penile clamp or predict the problem and for the filling study use a Foley catheter, which can be pulled down against the bladder neck to prevent leakage.

The voiding study is also important here. There must be no outlet obstruction if an AUS is to be inserted, since any future attempts to deal surgically with the obstruction will be compromised by the sphincter cuff or vice

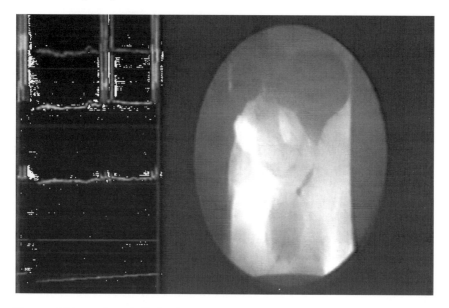

Fig. 5.37 Videourodynamic display showing a patient with post-prostatectomy incontinence secondary to sphincter weakness.

versa. For this reason these patients must have cystoscopy in addition to their urodynamic evaluation.

NEUROPATHIC BLADDER DYSFUNCTION

Assessment of the neuropathic bladder is probably the most interesting application of urodynamics and the area where the findings are important not only for the control of incontinence but also preservation of renal function. This is specialized work and for a detailed discussion of the neuropathic bladder the reader is directed to the recommended further reading in the Bibliography. We recommend that simple cystometry is an inadequate assessment for the neuropathic patient. The behaviour of the bladder neck and of the vesicoureteric junctions is important and can only be assessed with synchronous screening.

Collecting the urine flow may present a problem, especially in non-ambulant patients. A collection tube can be fitted to men that directs the flow towards the flow meter. Non-ambulant women are best studied in a sitting position over the flow meter and with lateral C-arm screening or ultrasound screening, although these are not available in most departments.

Intrinsic rectal activity is often seen in the neuropathic patient during the filling study (Fig. 5.38). It is therefore important always to view the detrusor trace in the light of the other two pressure traces and with what was happening

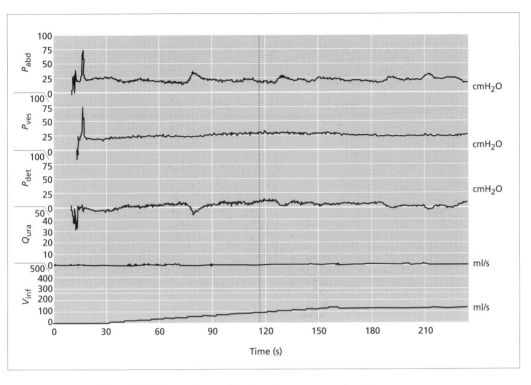

Fig. 5.38 Urodynamic trace showing spontaneous rectal activity.

to the patient at the time. In the severe tetraplegic patient it is easier not to use a rectal line at all, since the abdominal movements are so minimal that they induce little or no pressure change and intrinsic rectal activity serves only to complicate the picture.

Traditionally, the bladder is filled slowly in neuropathic patients. Undoubtedly, rapid or even medium fill rates can induce artefactual hypo-compliance and reflex bladder contractions that are not seen at more physiological rates. However, the finding during ambulatory monitoring (natural filling) that hypocompliance does not exist but is replaced by repeated short-lived phasic contractions implies that much of what we see in a cystometrogram is artefactual anyway. None the less, slow filling is the standard recommended by the ICS and should be used as routine in these patients. There is sometimes concern that the presence of a urethral catheter may interfere with the usual urodynamic behaviour of the bladder. This effect can be minimized by the use of suprapubic filling, as described earlier in this chapter.

There are always two questions to be answered in neuropathic patients: what is the reason for, and pattern of, the incontinence and what is the risk

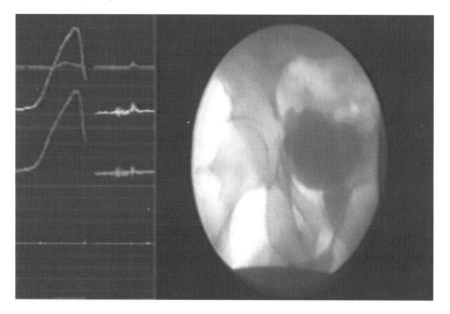

Fig. 5.39 Videourodynamic display of a patient with T6 syringomyelia showing high-pressure hyperreflexia and detrusor sphincter dyssynergia with no bladder emptying. This was a recumbent study and one would expect the situation to be worse when the patient is ambulant in his wheelchair. This is a high-risk bladder.

posed by the bladder to the upper urinary tracts? Abnormal compliance, high-pressure contractions, detrusor/sphincter and bladder neck dyssynergia, poor detrusor contractility with impaired emptying and vesicoureteric reflux may all represent a risk to the upper tracts and should therefore be carefully investigated (Figs 5.39 & 5.40). The bladder of a supine paraplegic may behave differently when he or she is mobile or is in a wheelchair. Thus provocation (e.g. with suprapubic tapping) may be essential in order to recreate as far as possible the normal situation for that patient. A second fill is usually worth while and in cord-injured patients is essential since the first fill is often quite different from subsequent fills, which reach a 'steady state' of repeated filling and voiding and show the same parameters on each cycle.

Any urodynamic department studying patients with spinal cord injury must be aware of the importance of preventing autonomic dysreflexia. This potentially dangerous phenomenon occurs in patients with cord injuries above the level of T6. It is characterized by a rapid rise in blood pressure, sometimes to dangerous levels, severe headache and profuse sweating. It is caused by perineal or bladder stimulation leading to a mass reflex response of the sympathetic nervous system with arterial vasoconstriction; however, the normal baroreceptor response producing vasodilatation is prevented because of the dissociation of the sympathetic system by the cord injury. Congenital cerebral aneurysms have been known to burst in these circumstances, with

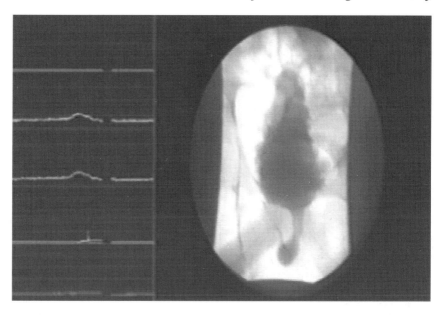

Fig. 5.40 Videourodynamic display of a T6 paraplegic showing a 'fir tree' bladder typical of longstanding severe hyperreflexia. However, he had a sphincterotomy and the pressures are now low with effective emptying of the bladder, which is consequently a low risk to the upper tracts.

catastrophic results. Autonomic dysreflexia can be avoided by giving a spinal anaesthetic, although this destroys the normal bladder reflexes. For urodynamics it can be prevented by oral nifedipine or glyceryl trinitrate before starting the test and by using an extremely gentle catheterization technique and slow filling with monitoring of blood pressure. An attack should be treated by immediately tipping the table to raise the head, stopping filling and emptying the bladder, sublingual administration of glyceryl trinitrate or intravenous injection of any vasodilator. Chlorpromazine and phentolamine have been recommended in this situation.

OTHER SPECIAL SITUATIONS

Post-reconstruction urodynamics

Beware of overfilling the reconstructed bladder as there is a risk of rupture.

Artificial urinary sphincter failure (see Chapter 6)

When an AUS fails, VUD is essential in order to elucidate the cause of failure (Fig. 5.41). Plain X-ray films are taken in two oblique positions to show the location of the AUS components and reveal any kinks (now unlikely with

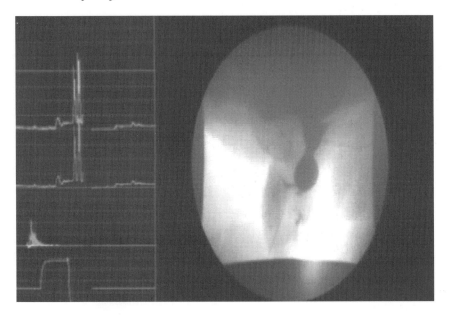

Fig. 5.41 Videourodynamic display of a leaking artificial urinary sphincter placed around the bulbar urethra. Videourodynamics with leak point pressure assessment is vital in these patients.

improved manufacture) and the presence of air bubbles in, or of contrast fluid outside, the system implying the presence of a leak. Care is taken on catheterization. The cuff is emptied by pumping prior to catheterization and then allowed to refill before the start of bladder filling. During the filling study a leak point pressure is measured. This may be slightly misleading as the catheters tend to improve the water seal of the cuff. Alternatively, the urethra can be filled retrogradely using the twin-lumen catheter and the pressure recorded at which contrast can be seen to leak retrogradely into the bladder. It is not a good idea to use a suprapubic tube for patients with an AUS because of the risk of infection or of damage to the tubing.

Patients with no rectum

In patients who have undergone abdominoperineal resection of the rectum, urodynamic studies are commonly needed in order to determine whether they are obstructed or have bladder failure from pelvic nerve damage. The rectal line can be inserted into the colostomy and this gives reasonable results provided that it is inside the abdomen; however, it very often sits within the subcutaneous tissues, where it is unhelpful. Alternatively a single pressure line (the bladder) can be used. In this case it is wise to refill the bladder two or three times to eliminate confusing artefact.

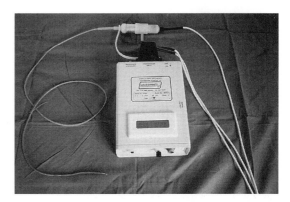

Fig. 5.42 Microtip transducer used for anorectal manometry attached to ambulatory monitoring box.

Anorectal function tests

Further investigation of anorectal disorders should be contemplated in any incontinent patient in the following circumstances:

1 any faecal incontinence;

2 associated rectal prolapse;

3 constipation, where the patient wants to pass a stool but has to strain or is unable to do so naturally.

There are various methods available to assess the functional capabilities of the anorectum, particularly those functions necessary to maintain continence. These tests are described below.

Anorectal manometry

Initial techniques used single-channel or multichannel recorders with a wide variety of pressure-determining devices, including balloons, microballoons, open tip catheters and perfused catheters. All have had their advocates and all rely on the estimation of static pressures rather than dynamic measurement during defaecation (i.e. with the patient usually in the left lateral position). As the techniques and the equipment varied so did the normal ranges and estimates, making comparisons of data difficult. More recently a wide variety of microtransducers have been developed with multichannel recorders which, because of their smaller size, are suitable for ambulatory and static assessments (Fig. 5.42). Variable numbers of channels can be recorded and subsequently downloaded to a personal computer. Not only are pressure measurements possible but also recordings of mass electromyography (EMG) and multifibre EMG, which can be assessed synchronously. These systems provide a highly accurate and reproducible method of assessment.

The basic estimations necessary are (i) resting pressure, reflecting internal anal sphincter (IAS) activity; (ii) maximal squeeze pressure, reflecting external anal sphincter (EAS) function and innervation; and (iii) anal canal length.

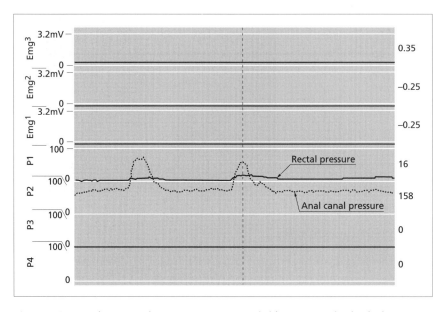

Fig. 5.43 Anorectal resting and squeeze pressures recorded from a normal individual.

RESTING PRESSURE

Both the EAS and IAS are responsible for maintaining resting pressure. Intraluminal pressures can be measured by a pull-through technique using microtransducers or any of the techniques described above. The pressure increases gradually from proximal to distal, the highest value being found 1–2 cm from the anal verge. Resting pressure varies according to gender and age, with women and older patients having a lower pressure (Figs 5.43 & 5.44). Resting pressure also varies circumferentially in the anal canal, with the resting pressure posteriorly being highest proximally and lowest near the anal verge. In contrast, resting pressure anteriorly is highest near the anal verge and lowest proximally. Therefore the pressure is distributed radially in an unequal fashion and gender variations have also been noted.

The contributions that the individual muscles make to the resting pressure is difficult to estimate, although studies have suggested that the IAS contributes about 85% of the resting tone. There is also a contribution to this pressure from the anal cushions, which tend to close the anal canal at rest. In addition to these static pressures there is a dynamic component to resting pressures, with slow waves and ultraslow waves clearly observed in the pressure recordings.

The normal range of resting pressure is 30–100 cmH$_2$O. For slow waves, the normal range of amplitude is 5–25 cmH$_2$O and frequency is 10–20/min.

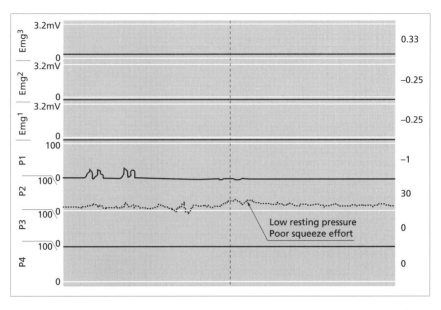

Fig. 5.44 Anorectal resting and attempted squeeze pressures from a faecally incontinent subject showing low pressures.

For ultra-slow waves, the normal range of amplitude is 30–100 cmH$_2$O and frequency is < 3/min.

SQUEEZE PRESSURE

This pressure is produced by the combined contraction of the EAS and puborectalis and reaches levels approximately twice that of the resting pressure (see Figs 5.43 & 5.44). There is a decline in the pressure over a period of 3 min, with maximum pressure lasting for < 1 min because of fatigue. As with the resting pressure, squeeze pressure is unequally distributed because the puborectalis provides force directed anteriorly in the proximal anal canal and squeeze pressures are therefore higher posteriorly and lowest anteriorly. The pressures in the middle of the anal canal are radially equal, while in the lower anal canal the pressure is highest anteriorly and lowest posteriorly. The function of the squeeze pressure is to prevent the leakage of contents at socially unacceptable times, with the rectum accommodating because of the rise in outlet resistance.

ANAL CANAL LENGTH

The length of the anal canal varies according to gender, with women having shorter anal canals. The length is easily measured using a pull-through technique that measures the high-pressure zone, which on average is 4 cm. The normal anal canal length ranges from 2.0 to 5.5 cm; the mean in women is 3.7 cm and in men is 4.6 cm.

Anorectal sensation

The two most important sensory functions of the anorectum are detection of rectal fullness and discrimination between solid, liquid and gas. Disorders may occur as a separate entity or, more commonly, as a combined sensory–motor disorder that is much more difficult to treat successfully. Three simple methods can be used to assess sensory function.

1   The anorectal inhibitory reflex tests the function of the sensory-rich area in the upper part of the anal canal and the subsequent sensory and motor pathways that lead to EAS contraction.

2   Rectal filling and compliance: filling a rectal balloon in a standard fashion allows crude estimates of rectal distensibility to be made, as well as allowing the calculation of compliance.

3   Mucosal electrosensitivity evaluates mucosal sensitivity by means of electrical stimulation.

RECTOANAL INHIBITORY REFLEX

As stool fills the rectum and causes distension, it comes into contact with the anorectal junction because of slight relaxation of the proximal portion of the anal canal. This initiates a reflex at the level of the spinal cord that results in relaxation of the IAS and an immediate feeling of call to stool. This reflex process has been termed the anorectal inhibitory reflex; if there is a deficient EAS or interruption of the neural pathways to the EAS then incontinence results. The reflex is present in patients who have had rectal excision with a coloanal anastomosis and this supports the theory that the reflex is dependent on pelvic wall stretch receptors and is spinally mediated. The physiological function of this reflex is not fully understood, although some workers have speculated that it is related to sensory function in the anorectum, referred to as sampling. This hypothesis postulates that solid, liquid and flatus can be differentiated in this part of the proximal anal canal and that the patient can respond accordingly, either deferring the call to stool or releasing flatus if socially convenient.

The test is easily performed by inflating a balloon in the rectum (Fig. 5.45), with a manometry catheter being placed in the high-pressure zone of the anal canal. As the volume in the balloon is increased, the point is reached where there is a rapid and profound decrease in resting pressure (Fig. 5.46). The reflex is present in all healthy people and is produced by a volume of 10 ml or less. The reflex is absent in patients with Hirschsprung's disease.

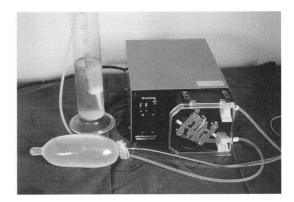

Fig 5.45 Inflation balloon used for measuring rectal sensation and for initiating the rectoanal inhibitory reflex.

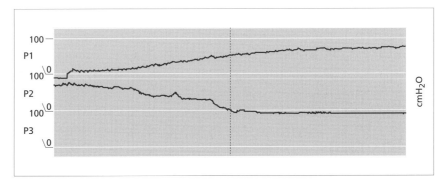

Fig. 5.46 The graph shows a normal rectoanal inhibitory reflex. The upper line indicates the increase in the rectal pressure associated with inflation with intrarectal balloons. The lower line records anal resting pressure. As the volume in the rectum increases, the pressure in the anal canal decreases eventually to zero. This is an illustration of a normal rectoanal inhibitory reflex.

RECTAL FILLING AND COMPLIANCE

Rectal sensation can be crudely tested by inserting a balloon and filling this with fluid. The volume at which the patient first becomes aware is termed the minimum perceived volume and some authors have noticed a difference in this volume between incontinent and normal patients. Continued inflation allows the determination of the maximum tolerated volume, when the desire to defaecate becomes overwhelming. The rectum distends passively but reaches a maximal tolerable volume at around 400 ml. Despite this, the pressure tends to remain low at around 20 cmH_2O. Calculating the change of volume and comparing it with the pressure gives an indication of the distensibility of the rectum, i.e. its compliance, which is normally around 17 ml/cmH_2O. However, in conditions that affect the distensibility of the rectum, such as Crohn's disease or ulcerative or radiation proctitis, the compliance is decreased. This results in the urgency associated with these conditions and potential incontinence if the sphincter mechanism is not sufficient to deal with the more urgent call to stool.

MUCOSAL ELECTROSENSITIVITY

Anal canal sensation can be tested by means of electrical stimulation. A metallic probe is inserted into the anal canal and an increasing current applied until the patient first becomes aware of the sensation. This method does give useful reliable data and has shown that sensation is decreased in patients with neuropathic incontinence. In addition, electrical sensitivity has been measured and raised thresholds found in patients with haemorrhoids; conversely, in fissure there is a lower threshold. Temperature sensation has also been investigated and shown to be altered in incontinent patients, although this has no practical use clinically.

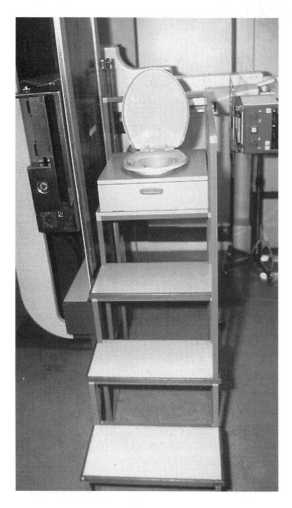

Fig. 5.47 Arrangement for defaecating proctography.

Defaecography

The pelvic floor and rectum can be assessed at rest and straining using defaecography. The patient is seated on a special commode constructed of any radiolucent material, although wood or Perspex are the most commonly used, and the evacuation is collected in a receptacle or bag placed underneath. A semi-solid radiopaque paste is introduced into the rectum until the patient experiences the need to defaecate. The patient then sits on the commode (Fig. 5.47) and lateral projections are obtained (Fig. 5.48).

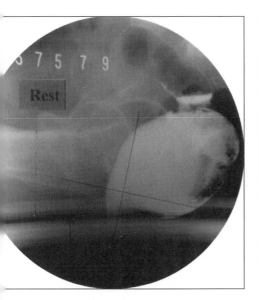
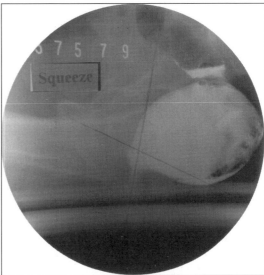
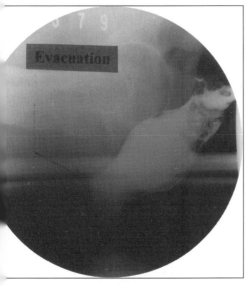
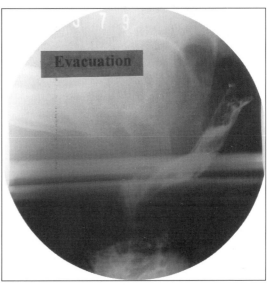

Fig. 5.48 Normal defaecating proctogram. Lateral projection.

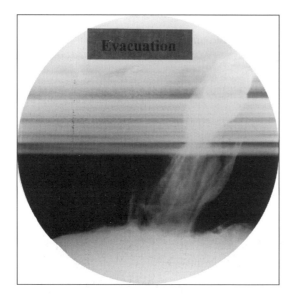

Fig. 5.49 Defaecating proctogram in a patient with intussusception.

Evacuation can be evaluated at rest, evacuation and after evacuation. Anteroposterior films can also be useful in order to clarify lateral appearances. Specific features and measurements can be made that allow more objective evaluation and those commonly determined include (i) anorectal angle, (ii) pelvic floor descent, (iii) anal canal length, (iv) presence or absence of rectocoele, (v) presence or absence of intussusception, (vi) trapping of paste and (vii) need for digitation or perineal/vaginal pressure in order to complete evacuation. Pelvic floor descent is recorded as the vertical distance below the line between the coccyx and the pubic bone. A correlation has been reported between the extent of descent and pudendal neuropathy. Defaecography is also used extensively in the assessment of disordered defaecation in order to evaluate intussusception, solitary rectal ulcer and rectocoele (Figs 5.49–5.51).

Anal endosonography

This technique has found increasing application over the last 5 years and has largely replaced EMG mapping for the morphological assessment of the anal sphincters. In most units, anal endosonography is performed using the Bruel and Kjaer ultrasound scanner in association with endoprobe type 1850 and involves the introduction of a rotating ultrasound transducer (7–10 MHz) into the anal canal. The transducer is covered by a plastic nose cone filled with gel that allows the transmission of the ultrasound signal. The individual layers of the anal canal can be clearly identified: the IAS produces a hypo-echoic image, the EAS has a mixed pattern but is mainly hyperechoic and

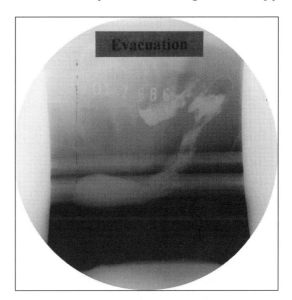

Fig. 5.50 Defaecating proctogram with rectocoele and trapping.

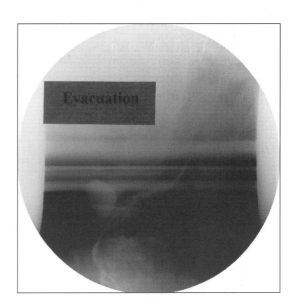

Fig. 5.51 Defaecating proctogram showing rectal prolapse.

the subepithelium and longitudinal muscle are both hyperechoic. However, the anatomy of the EAS differs according to the level in the anal canal, being circumferential superficially and diverging widely in the proximal canal. The IAS and EAS can be delineated and defects noted (Figs 5.52–5.55). Care is needed in the interpretation because, as mentioned above, the anatomy of the anal canal varies according to the distance from the anus.

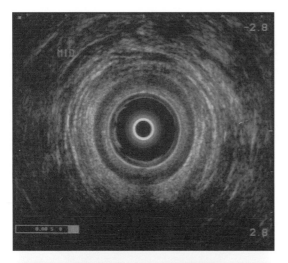

Fig. 5.52 Anal endosonography showing a normal external anal sphincter.

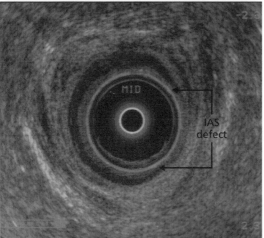

Fig. 5.53 Anal endosonography showing a defect of the internal anal sphincter (IAS) after sphincterotomy.

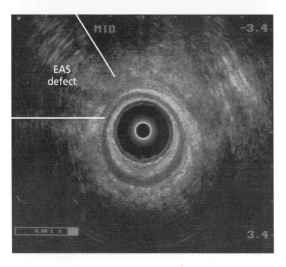

Fig. 5.54 Anal endosonography showing a defect of the external anal sphincter (EAS) after obstetric injury.

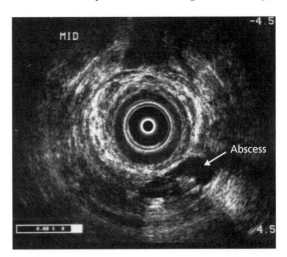

Fig. 5.55 Anal
endosonography showing a
fistula and abscess.

Colonic transit studies

Anorectal function differs fundamentally from bladder function because it is
dependent on the consistency and mode of delivery of its contents from the
upper parts of the gastrointestinal tract. The assessment of colonic transit is
essential before treating the constipated or incontinent patient, since in these
patients there can be overlapping functional problems. For example, in the
patient who is unable to evacuate the rectum and who also has disordered
proximal bowel transit, focusing only on the defecatory disorder will yield
disappointing results.

In order to assess transit most clinicians use a 'shapes' study, although
other workers have advocated isotope transit studies (Plates 6 and 7, opposite p. 148). The advantage of a shapes study is that it is relatively quick and
simple to perform. The patient is given 20 radiopaque shapes orally and plain
radiographs of the abdomen taken at days 3 and 5 (Figs 5.56 & 5.57). In
normal subjects 80% of the shapes are eliminated by day 5. It is obviously
important to ensure that patients do not take laxatives for 48 hours before
and also for the duration of the investigation.

Although this method gives a good indication of overall colonic transit,
it has limitations if colonic resection is being considered as a therapeutic
option. Ideally, if there is a segmental transit problem then resecting the
appropriate portion would be less radical and possibly more predictable
in terms of functional outcome. In order to achieve this, segmental transit
studies have been attempted with both multiple shapes studies and, more
recently, isotope transit studies, in which the patient is given a technetium-
labelled meal and transit is mapped by repeated scanning with a gamma
camera over the following few days. The evidence of isotope studies suggests

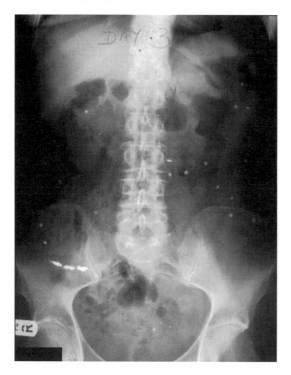

Fig. 5.56 Shapes transit study: radiograph taken on day 3.

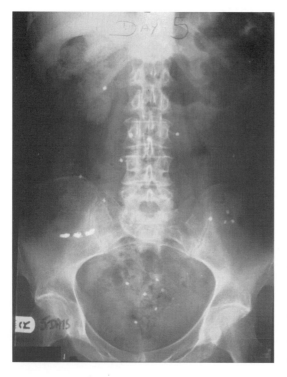

Fig. 5.57 Shapes transit study: radiograph taken on day 5. Although shapes have entered the rectum there are still some in the right colon. This is slow-transit constipation.

that this differentiation may be possible, while multiple shapes studies have found little application clinically.

Where does neurophysiology fit in?

While urodynamic investigations have increased our understanding of normal and disordered bladder function, these remain at best only functional studies of an end organ that require deductions to be made about underlying causation and neuropathology. Anorectal physiology and imaging is similarly limited, although anal endosonography offers a degree of understanding lacking in our assessment of the bladder outlet. Detailed neurohistochemistry and *in vitro* pharmacology of bladder and pelvic floor muscles have increased our understanding of bladder and anorectal function but the findings have to be extrapolated to the living person. However, clinical neurological examination, expertly performed, allows approximate localization of lesions though often fails to detect subtle functional abnormalities in neural pathways. The field of clinical neurophysiology theoretically provides the tools with which nerve function can be measured and quantified directly. Sadly, the potential benefits of clinical neurophysiology in clinical practice have been very disappointing and, despite a flurry of enthusiasm for the techniques in the 1980s, most working urodynamic and anorectal laboratories would only use neurophysiology in a research setting. Therefore, basic techniques are described for completeness. Essentially, clinical neurophysiology encompasses two fields of study: EMG and nerve conduction studies or electroneurography.

Electromyography

EMG is the study of the bioelectrical potentials generated by the depolarization of muscle and can establish whether the muscle under study is normal or shows evidence of denervation. In practical terms this means striated muscle, because of the technical difficulties of recording from smooth muscle. Electrodes are used to detect this depolarization which, after appropriate amplification, is displayed on an oscilloscope/monitor with a very fast frequency response or audibly through a loudspeaker. Integration of the EMG signal is an electronic trick that allows an increase in muscle activity to be displayed as a deflection from the baseline rather than as a complex repetitive series of deflections. This can be demonstrated audibly by a change in pitch of the sound.

Recruitment EMG is a technique commonly used during urodynamics to indicate contraction of the pelvic floor or urethral sphincter. Using either surface epithelial electrodes (Figs 5.58 & 5.59) or simple needle electrodes

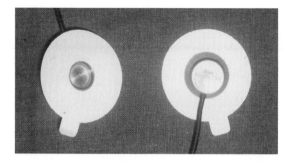

Fig. 5.58 Stick-on surface electrodes used for simple EMG recording.

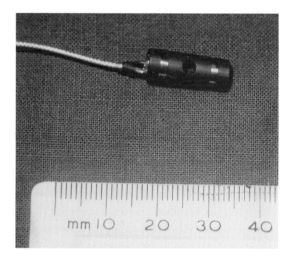

Fig. 5.59 A urethral electrode is mounted on to a urethral catheter either to stimulate the posterior urethra or to record surface EMG from within the urethral sphincter.

inserted directly into a muscle, compound action potentials are displayed. An increase in activity represents a mass muscle contraction (Fig. 5.60). This is sometimes referred to as kinesiological EMG. Separate components of the pelvic floor can be shown to behave independently if EMGs are recorded synchronously from different muscles. While the anal plug electrode has been commonly used in urodynamic practice as an indication of pelvic floor activity, this independent function means that anal plug recording may be an unreliable indicator of urethral sphincter activity (Snooks & Swash, 1986). Some urodynamic laboratories use recruitment EMG as an indicator of external sphincter activity, particularly in patients with spinal cord injury (Fig. 5.60). In the absence of video X-ray screening, EMG would be an essential adjunct to simple cystometry in these patients as the best alternative to demonstrate detrusor sphincter dyssynergia.

The functional unit of the EMG is the 'motor unit', i.e. a moter neurone and all the muscle fibres that it innervates (Fig. 5.61). Concentric needles are used to detect potentials from individual motor units by implanting directly into the muscle mass. These needles may be monopolar or bipolar, the latter

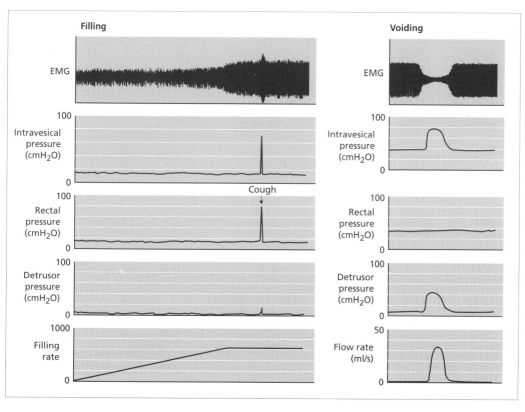

Fig. 5.60 Pelvic floor recruitment EMG during filling and voiding. Note that when the patient voids the resting EMG activity disappears.

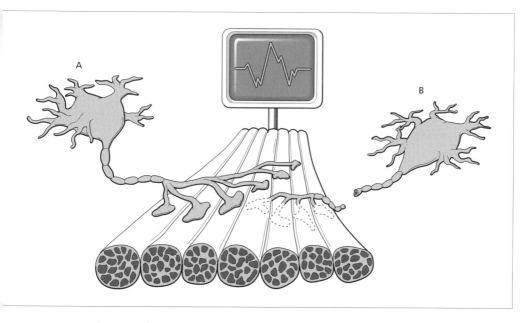

Fig. 5.61 Schematic diagram of the 'motor unit', which comprises the motor nerve cell and its axon, endplates and all the muscle fibres that it innervates. (A) shows a sprouting motor unit which is reinnervating fibres previously supplied by (B). From Siroky, M.B. (1984), with permission.

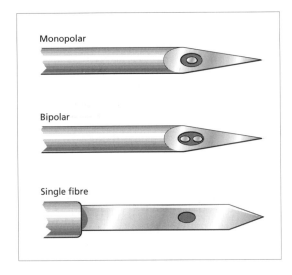

Monopolar

Bipolar

Single fibre

Fig. 5.62 Different types of needle used for EMG recording: unipolar and bipolar concentric needles and single-fibre needle (increasing specificity for volume of muscle captured by recordings).

being more specific to individual motor units because of a smaller recording surface area (Fig. 5.62). Single-fibre needle electrodes, with a still smaller recording surface, can be used to look at the activity of single muscle fibres as opposed to entire motor units. Pathological processes that affect the nerves supplying muscle groups produce characteristic changes in the motor unit potential recorded by these methods. Although normal skeletal muscle is silent at rest, the sphincters and pelvic floor often manifest several motor unit potentials per second even at rest. Potentials of increased amplitude and duration, 'fibrillation' and polyphasic potentials and positive sharp waves (Fig. 5.63) are characteristic signs of reinnervation of a motor unit and, by implication, prior denervation. Single-fibre EMG analysis also makes possible the quantitative assessment of motor endplate stability and fibre density by making 20 measurements within any muscle into which the needle is placed. It is also a measure of reinnervation but is much more difficult to perform and to interpret.

EMG of the anal sphincter, urethral sphincter or pelvic floor muscle (levator ani) can clearly be used to show that a muscle has been denervated and that neuropathy is at least a part of the patient's underlying aetiology. The measurements are made during squeeze and at rest. EMG has been used in the past for sphincter mapping prior to sphincter repair, although this has now been superseded by anal endosonography. The finding of denervation makes little difference to subsequent management decisions in urinary incontinence, which are largely based on an assessment of function, i.e. the balance of pressures, or on an attempt to restore or even overcompensate functional anatomy. However, knowledge of underlying neuropathy may be of prognostic significance and, occasionally, of medicolegal interest.

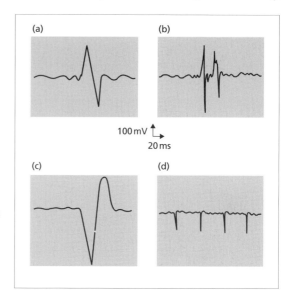

Fig. 5.63 Motor unit potentials showing (a) normal recordings, (b) polyphasic traces, (c) fibrillation potentials and (d) positive spike waves indicative of denervation.

Nerve conduction studies

Nerve conduction studies are used to test the integrity of neural pathways, either to establish a neurological diagnosis (e.g. multiple sclerosis) or to investigate whether the pathways thought to be relevant to urinary or faecal control are abnormal. It is most unusual to find abnormalities on neurophysiological testing in the absence of any clinical neurological signs. Nerve conduction studies involve the application of a stimulus and measurement of the latency between this stimulus and a nerve-mediated response at a distant site. The stimulus may be applied to a sensory field or directly to a named nerve; the response may be detected from a muscle (motor latency or reflex latencies) or from the central nervous system itself (evoked potentials). The stimulus can be electrical, which is painful, or magnetic using the magnetic induction coil over the cerebral cortex or the spinal column, which is painless. Modern computer technology has allowed the development of software that performs rapid analogue-to-digital transformation and averaging of multiple signals, time locked to a stimulus, with elimination of stimulus artefact to give accurate determination of minimum latency times. Latencies are usually expressed in milliseconds from the onset of the stimulus to the first deflection of the response (Fig. 5.64). These developments have facilitated the routine use of conduction studies in neurological and neurophysiological practice.

The pudendal nerve motor latency is the simplest nerve conduction study used in pelvic floor assessment. The examiner performs a rectal examination while wearing a specially designed finger cot on the index finger that is

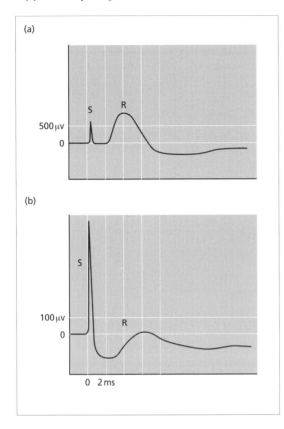

Fig. 5.64 Sacral reflex latency recording. (a) A single response in which it is hard to see any particular pattern. (b) An 'averaged' response from several hundred stimuli, in which the response is easy to see.

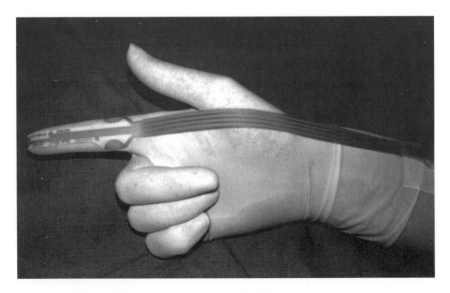

Fig 5.65 St Mark's/Kiff glove used for recording pudendal motor nerve latencies.

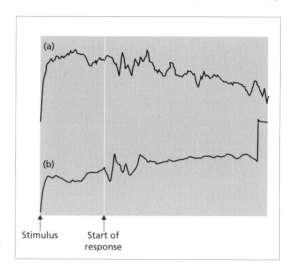

Stimulus   Start of
response

Fig. 5.66 Normal pudendoanal
motor nerve latency.

mounted with two surface electrodes (Fig. 5.65). One electrode sits within
the anal canal while the one at the tip of the finger can be applied laterally to
the pudendal nerve as it wraps around the iliac spine, close to the rectum. The
stimulus is applied to the pudendal nerve at this point and the latency to an
anal sphincter response is recorded (Fig. 5.66). A prolonged latency is taken
as evidence of neuropathy, though whether this is neuropraxia secondary to
nerve stretching associated with prolapse is unclear.

The sacral reflex latency (Fig. 5.67) gained popularity in the 1980s as
techniques were developed involving stimulation of either the dorsal nerve
of the penis or posterior urethra with recording from the anal sphincter, the
urethral sphincter and the bulbocavernosus muscle. Each combination of
stimulation and recording sites involves a subtly different neural pathway
and slightly different latency times. It was anticipated that it would be possible
to identify not only an occult neurological lesion but also to localize or even
lateralize this lesion by analysis of different responses. Many clinical studies
have been performed in different groups of patients with varying clinical
syndromes, including spinal cord injury, GSI and multiple sclerosis. Meagre
normal data are available owing largely to the fact that the tests are unpleasant and few normal volunteers can be encouraged to subject themselves to
these tests. Despite a high incidence of apparently occult neuropathy being
demonstrated in many different patient groups, the lack of clear correlations
and doubt about the reproducibility of the tests led to a rapid loss of interest.
Abnormal sacral reflex latencies are evidence of disorders of sacral reflex
activity. Whether this is due to a disruption of the microarchitecture of the
conus or whether it represents abnormal modulation of reflex activity from
higher centres is not known.

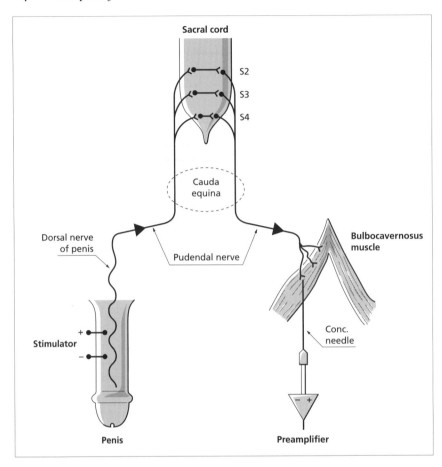

Fig. 5.67 The principle of sacral reflex latency.

An evoked potential is an action potential recorded from the central nervous system, usually in response to electrical stimulation of a peripheral sensory field or a named nerve. Such recordings formed the basis for mapping the cortical representation of sensory fields over the last 100 years. Cortical somatosensory evoked potentials (stimulation of a sensory field with recording over the cerebral cortex) following bladder and urethral stimulation and pudendal nerve stimulation result in characteristic waveforms (Fig. 5.68) that may be useful in assessing afferent conduction relevant to bladder function. Cortical somatosensory evoked potentials are recorded with electrodes similar to those used for EEG and are placed on the cranium over the cerebral cortex. The test is relatively easy to perform because impulses arising at the cerebral cortex recruit a large number of neurones so that the brain acts as a sort of biological amplifier. Evoked potentials can also be recorded from the spinal cord but this is technically difficult because of the relatively low signal

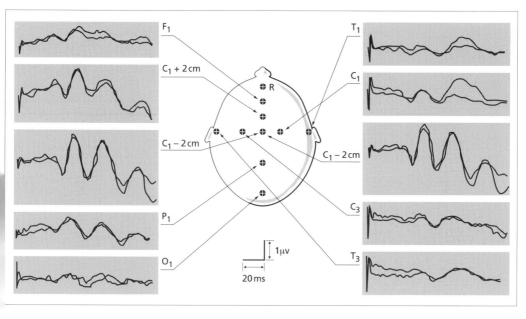

Fig. 5.68 Drawings taken from a series of recordings of cortical evoked potentials in response to stimulation of the pundendal nerve. It can be seen that a map of cortical representation can be drawn and abnormalities indentified by comparison with normal. From Hadelman (1982), with permission.

to noise ratio (little signal, lots of noise) and is therefore a highly specialized technique. This method has been used in some research laboratories in an attempt to localize lesions of the central nervous system to different levels of the spinal cord and to relate this to abnormalities in bladder function following spinal cord injury, although it has no value in routine assessment of the incontinent patient.

Sensory testing

Sensory thresholds have been measured from the urethral mucosa, the perianal skin and the anal canal. This is usually regarded as the minimum stimulus that can be felt by the patient or, alternatively, that will cause an evoked response. The measurements are heavily dependent on electrode characteristics and probably totally unreliable.

Summary

Despite the sophistication of the neurophysiological techniques described, they are still remarkably crude in terms of their ability to localize neurological lesions. Nevertheless it seems likely that the relationship between bladder dysfunction and neuropathy will be clarified as a result of the further development, understanding and application of these techniques in well-coordinated research. Sadly, or happily, depending on your viewpoint, they have little to offer in routine clinical practice and need not be considered in the establishment of a routine urodynamic department.

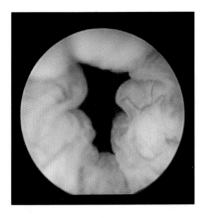

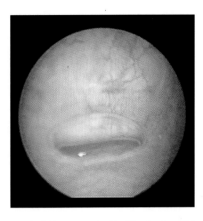

Plate 1 Normal bladder neck in a postmenopausal woman. (Kindly supplied by Christopher G. Eden, Consultant Urological Surgeon, The North Hampshire Hospital, Basingstoke.)

Plate 2 Air bubble seen in the bladder fundus. (Kindly supplied by Christopher G. Eden, Consultant Urological Surgeon, The North Hampshire Hospital, Basingstoke.)

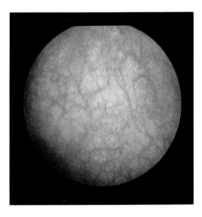

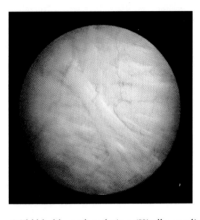

Plate 3 Typical inflamed appearance of interstitial cystitis with petechial haemorrhage, which is classically seen after release of the fluid from the first fill of the bladder; bladder filling induces pain that may break through light anaesthesia causing hyperventilation. (Kindly supplied by Christopher G. Eden, Consultant Urological Surgeon, The North Hampshire Hospital, Basingstoke.)

Plate 4 Mild bladder trabeculation. (Kindly supplied by Christopher G. Eden, Consultant Urological Surgeon, The North Hampshire Hospital, Basingstoke.)

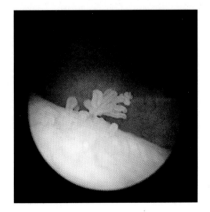

Plate 5 *Opposite.* Papillary bladder tumour. (Kindly supplied by Christopher G. Eden, Consultant Urological Surgeon, The North Hampshire Hospital, Basingstoke.)

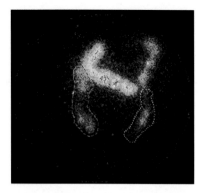

Plate 6 An isotope colonic transit study showing separate count areas for the ascending, transverse and descending segments of the colon.

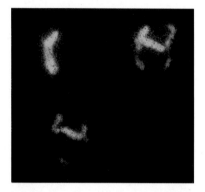

Plate 7 Isotope colonic transit study showing images at three points in time. There is no isotope entering the descending colon. This is described as right-sided delay.

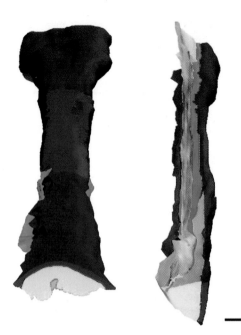

Plate 8 Computer-generated three-dimensional reconstructions of the female pig vesicourethral junction and urethra viewed from (a) a direct anterior perspective and (b) a right direct lateral perspective, 'clipped' so that the internal spatial relationships are visible. Wall components include: lamina propria (green), circular (magenta) and longitudinal (red) smooth muscle, circular (blue) and longitudinal (cyan) striated muscle and cavernous tissue (yellow). The distal urethra extends towards the bottom of the picture. Bar represents 1 cm.

(a)

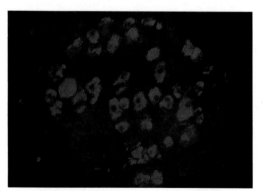

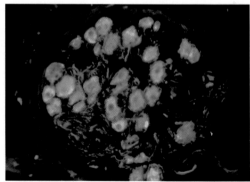

(b)

Plate 9 Ganglion cells in the proximal third of the female urethra (human). With double immunolabelling techniques, cell bodies with haemoxygenase II fluoresce red (a) and those with nitric oxide synthase immunoreactivity fluoresce green (b).

6: Specialist Treatment: Drugs and Surgery

Malcolm Lucas, Simon Emery & Nicholas Carr

Drugs

Despite a wealth of research on bladder smooth muscle pharmacology, there remains a relative dearth of useful drugs available to the clinician for the treatment of incontinence and extraordinarily little comparative data about their efficacy. The problem with the comparison of drug therapies for incontinence is that there is always a real placebo effect of about 30–40% that can be further enhanced by the enthusiasm of the physician. Since the best response with any drug used for treating incontinence is only 60%, any differences between drugs are likely to be small and require large-scale studies to demonstrate them. The fact that incontinence is an ill-defined subjective symptom rather than a measurable physiological parameter adds to this difficulty. Even if urodynamic parameters are employed in such studies, our lack of knowledge of the natural variability of these tests makes valid conclusions difficult, except perhaps in neuropathic patients, who are more predictable. Double-blind studies are largely impossible since most of the drugs mentioned below have side-effects when given in effective doses. Pharmacologically, the *in vitro* mode of action of most drugs is understood but the site of action *in vivo* is less certain (Tables 6.1 & 6.2).

Drugs that decrease bladder activity

Acetylcholine is released at postganglionic parasympathetic nerve terminals and acts on muscarinic receptor sites on detrusor smooth muscle to cause a propagated bladder contraction. Atropine and atropine-like drugs (anticholinergic or antimuscarinic drugs) depress bladder contractions of any aetiology by blocking binding at these receptors. However, *in vivo* there is a degree of resistance to atropine at these sites, presumably due to the action of other non-adrenergic non-cholinergic neurotransmitters. This may account for the clinical unpredictability of these drugs. There are four types of muscarinic receptor in the human body (M_1–M_4); M_3 receptors have been shown to predominate in the bladder although M_2 receptors are also present. Unfortunately M_3 receptors are also found in the salivary glands and the

149

Table 6.1 Drugs currently available on prescription in the UK that have an effect on bladder or urethral function and their relative usefulness for specific functional problems (modified from lecture given by Cordozo). The number of crosses indicate relative efficacy.

Generic name	Dose	Enuresis	Bladder outflow obstruction	Nocturia	Detrusor instability	Stress incontinence	Hyperreflexia	Sensory urgency
Propantheline	7.5–30 mg t.d.s. on empty stomach	+		+	+		+	
Imipramine	Usually 25–50 mg at night	++		++	+		+	
Oral oxybutynin	2.5 or 3–5 mg t.d.s.	+		+	++		++	
Tolterodine	1–2 mg b.d.	+		+	++		++	
Intravesical oxybutynin	5 mg in solution up to t.d.s.						++	
Flavoxate								+
α-Adrenoceptor antagonists	Vary with preparation		++					
Desmopressin		++		++				
Ceteprin								+
Potassium citrate						+		
α-Adrenoceptor agonists						+		
Oestrogens						+		+

Table 6.2 Drugs that may provoke or exacerbate urinary incontinence.

α-Adrenoceptor agonists
α-Adrenoceptor antagonists
Anticholinergics
Antipsychotics
Bromocriptine
Calcium blockers
Clonazepam
Diuretics
Ethanol
Lithium
Metoclopramide
Misoprostol
Phenytoin
Sedatives/hypnotics
Skeletal muscle relaxants: baclofen and dantrolene
Sympatholytics: methyldopa, reserpine, guanethidine

bowel and so dry mouth and constipation are usually associated with non-selective antimuscarinic drugs.

The mainstay of anticholinergic therapy for years has been oral propantheline bromide (15–60 mg t.d.s.) and it is still the cheapest drug in this group. Unfortunately, when given in effective doses it almost always causes the atropine-like side-effects of dry mouth, blurring of vision, constipation and abdominal distension.

Imipramine is a tricyclic antidepressant agent that, in doses of 25–75 mg b.d. or nocte only, has a strong inhibitory effect on bladder contractions. Although its systemic anticholinergic effects are marked, this is not its primary effect on the bladder. Instead, it appears that it has a local anaesthetic-like action in stabilizing the smooth muscle membrane. While its antidepressant action (used in higher doses) takes 2–4 weeks to occur, the effect on the bladder is immediate. Imipramine is particularly useful at night because of its longer half-life and is much used for primary enuresis. A combination of diurnal oxybutynin supplemented by imipramine at night is still an effective way to control detrusor instability throughout the day.

Antispasmodic drugs act at a site distal to the cholinergic receptor to relax the smooth muscle. Oxybutynin hydrochloride is mainly a potent smooth muscle relaxant but also has a strong anticholinergic effect and is said to have local anaesthetic effects. Given in doses of 2.5–5 mg t.d.s. it reaches therapeutic levels very rapidly and has a short half-life that make it easy to titrate dosage against symptoms (Fig. 6.1). Unfortunately, oxybutynin seems to have a more reliable effect on salivary secretions than on bladder contractions and so usually causes a dry mouth even in the absence of a therapeutic effect. It is widely used for detrusor instability in spinal cord injury and

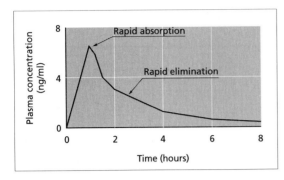

Fig. 6.1 Pharmacokinetic curve for oxybutynin. Note how quickly effective levels are obtained from a single oral dose; this is the rationale for its use on a p.r.n. basis.

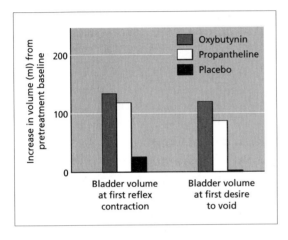

Fig. 6.2 Efficacy of propantheline, oxybutynin and placebo.

multiple sclerosis and must now be the commonest prescribed drug for incontinence. Like the anticholinergic drugs it induces atropine-like side-effects. There is some evidence to suggest that oxybutynin is more effective than propantheline although it probably has a similarly poor side-effect profile (Fig. 6.2) (Thuroff *et al.*, 1991).

There is much to be said for encouraging patients to use oxybutynin on an occasional basis. Patients know the behaviour of their own bladder and can usually predict when they are most likely to have trouble, for example when out for a walk or at a football match. Oxybutynin taken 30 min before such activity may provide adequate symptomatic control while the patient tolerates the side-effects in order to carry out the desired activity. At other times, particularly when the patient is at home, they will prefer to avoid the side-effects and go without the drug. In this way we have achieved a high rate of compliance and apparent efficacy with oxybutynin. The dry mouth of anticholinergic medication can be alleviated with boiled sweets.

Intravesical preparations of oxybutynin have been used successfully in patients with detrusor hyperreflexia due to neuropathy (Madersbacher &

Jilg, 1991; Madersbacher *et al.*, 1991; Weese *et al.*, 1993). This method of administration lends itself particularly to neuropathic patients who also have to self-catheterize in order to empty. High serum concentrations of oxybutynin are achieved, giving control of hyperreflexic contractions without the systemic side-effects of the oral preparation, which seem to be caused by hepatic metabolites that are avoided by intravesical instillation. Its efficacy in idiopathic instability is unknown as yet. Prescribing intravesical therapy has been on a named patient basis only and has involved preparation of the solution for instillation by the patient. However, an intravesical preparation is to be introduced to the market soon and patients who already self-catheterize may find this helpful.

Tolterodine is a new muscarinic blocker that lacks receptor selectivity but appears to have some specificity to the bladder and, reputedly, has eight times less affinity for parotid receptors than oxybutynin. There have been a number of published trials comparing tolterodine with placebo and with oxybutynin. These show that tolterodine 2 mg b.d. is effective in reducing urinary frequency and incontinent episodes and that it is as effective as oxybutynin without causing the same side-effect profile (although the difference in side-effects is not as dramatic as the pharmacological profile would suggest). The drug has been used in elderly patients without serious adverse events. Patients with hepatic or renal impairment should be treated with caution and lower doses used. It seems very likely therefore that tolterodine will rapidly establish a major place in the drug management of detrusor instability.

All antimuscarinic drugs must be avoided in patients with glaucoma. Oxybutynin should be used with care in patients with known cardiac dysrhythmia, although it appears that tolterodine may be safer in this respect. Since both of these conditions are common problems, this is a serious limiting factor in the use of drugs for detrusor instability. If one drug with an anticholinergic action fails to work when given in large enough doses, there is little point in trying another. However, if side-effects have prevented adequate doses being given, another drug in this group may be worth trying.

Calcium antagonists, e.g. nifedipine, have been shown to block the non-adrenergic non-cholinergic portion of the mammalian bladder response to electrical field stimulation by opposing the influx of calcium required to activate ATP-dependent muscle contraction. Terodiline is an anticholinergic drug that in higher doses also has a calcium antagonistic effect on mammalian bladder detrusor muscle *in vitro*. It is effective in the treatment of detrusor instability (Norton *et al.*, 1994) but, unfortunately, has now been withdrawn from the market because of anecdotal reports of sudden death in patients with cardiac dysrhythmias. Although calcium antagonists have been shown to stop contractions *in vitro*, clinical studies have not been done in patients with incontinence.

Other drugs used for 'irritable' symptoms

Although flavoxate hydrochloride (antispasmodic) is still widely prescribed in general practice and probably has a place in treating hypersensitive bladders, it is of little practical use for detrusor instability. Emepronium has also been used in the same way but there is little evidence to support its use for detrusor instability and it has been found to cause oesophageal strictures. Alkalinizing agents are widely prescribed in general practice for the symptoms of cystitis; these include potassium citrate, sodium citrate and sodium bicarbonate. It is worth measuring urinary pH before prescribing these drugs since the urine may not need alkalinization. Acidification can be achieved with ascorbic acid. Dicyclomine (antispasmodic) has been used sporadically but has not gained wide acceptance. The β-adrenoceptor agonists have been shown to have a dose-related relaxant effect on detrusor muscle *in vitro*, but although terbutaline has been tried no satisfactory clinical trials have been completed on this drug.

Drugs that increase outlet resistance

There may be value in pharmacological therapy that increases urethral sphincter tone. In theory, α-adrenoceptor stimulation or β-adrenoceptor blockade may be expected to have this effect. Only the oral sympathomimetic phenylpropanolamine has been shown to have any value and then only in mild genuine stress incontinence (GSI). Administration of oestrogens, either topically or in the form of hormone replacement therapy, should improve the surface tension of the opposing surfaces of the urethral mucosa by restoring normal urethral secretions, although the evidence of this working in practice is sparse. Women with urethral instability may benefit from an α-adrenoceptor agonist, which could be expected to increase smooth muscle tone in the distal sphincter mechanism. Pharmaceutical companies are developing specific α-adrenoceptor agonists with a view to marketing these drugs for patients with stress incontinence and clinical trials are underway. Their value in the control of stress incontinence is always likely to be limited given the importance of anatomical defects in these patients.

Drugs that improve emptying

Cholinergic drugs may improve bladder emptying by increasing the force of detrusor contraction. This may help to prevent overflow incontinence in patients with poor detrusor contractility due to either obstructive chronic retention or neuropathy. In practice, however, only those drugs that can be given parenterally are effective, e.g. bethanechol 5–10 mg subcutaneously and carbachol 0.2–0.5 mg subcutaneously. Oral bethanechol and distigmine bromide have been shown to be of little therapeutic value.

The α-adrenoceptor antagonists are a group of drugs that improve bladder emptying by selective blockade of α-adrenoceptors in the bladder neck and urethral sphincter mechanism. They are widely used in the treatment of bladder outflow obstruction due to benign prostatic hyperplasia and in this context have nothing to offer in the treatment of incontinence. However, we believe they may have a role in patients with multiple sclerosis, assisting with bladder emptying and thus allowing the bladder to fill from smaller volumes, diminishing the impact of hyperreflexic contractions. Thus, the drug might be used in conjunction with oxybutynin.

Desmopressin, a synthetic analogue of vasopressin, has been a great leap forward in the treatment of nocturnal enuresis (Meadow, 1988). Given as a nasal spray at night it reduces nocturnal urine production. Disadvantages are the rebound diuresis that occurs the following morning and our lack of knowledge about the long-term effects of manipulating pituitary function in this way, although emerging evidence suggests that its long-term use is safe. It is difficult to reconcile the philosophy of desmopressin with our usual advice in these patients to increase fluid intake.

The future

In view of the abundance of M_3 receptors in the bladder, selective M_3-receptor antagonists might be expected to control the overactive bladder and indeed there are drugs undergoing clinical trials that will doubtless reach the market in due course. These include darifenacin and vamicamide, which may prove to have better specificity for the bladder than existing drugs. A new agent, duloxetine, is currently undergoing phase II and phase III trials. It is reported to be a blocker of serotonin and noradrenaline reuptake, resulting in stabilization of the neuromuscular junction and decreased detrusor contractility. Potassium channel openers are a group of drugs that activate the ATP-sensitive potassium channels on the smooth muscle membrane, leading to hyperpolarization of the cell and inhibition of muscle contraction. One such early drug was cromakalim, which although controlling unstable contractions in the obstructed pig model (Foster, 1989) and human tissue (Nurse *et al.*, 1991) seems to be ineffective in controlling detrusor contractions in doses that do not reduce the blood pressure *in vivo*. Newer drugs (e.g. Zeneca ZD6169) are currently undergoing clinical trials and may prove to be more effective.

It is now realized that non-adrenergic non-cholinergic transmission at the neuromuscular junction is modulated partly by nitric oxide and that nitric oxide synthetase is widely distributed throughout the lower urinary tract and the central nervous system. The precise role of nitric oxide in the modulation of lower urinary tract function is still hotly debated but it seems likely that specific inhibitors or agonists of this molecule will have a role in the control of bladder dysfunction.

Surgery

When conservative treatment of incontinence has failed it is usual to consider surgical therapy. The expectation of patients is usually that an operation will restore them to normal bladder or bowel function. Although delightful when it occurs, such an outcome is actually rare and in reality what we usually achieve is to exchange one abnormality that the patient finds totally intolerable for another that is, hopefully, easier to live with. This is also often done in the context of progressive failure of the pelvic floor and hence the possibility that improvement in function may be only temporary. Our objective with all surgery for incontinence should be to restore the patient as closely as possible to normal function with the minimum short-term and long-term morbidity and for this improvement to be durable. However, we do our patients no service if we fail to explain the realities of surgical intervention carefully.

This section describes the variety of surgical approaches to urinary and faecal incontinence, some of which have proved disappointing yet may still have a place in our armamentarium, while others may be highly effective yet carry risks that might not always be justified. We have not attempted to review the management of individual neurological states because the principle of providing urodynamic solutions to urodynamic problems remains the same. The poorly emptying bladder of diabetes and cauda equina injury is dealt with in the same way. Similarly, the high-pressure bladder can be dealt with in the same way whether it is due to detrusor instability or congenital myelomeningocele. However, one must remember that the priorities of treatment are fundamentally different in many neuropathic patients where renal function is often in jeopardy and preservation of renal function must be the first priority. On occasions, this may mean sacrificing continence in the interests of protecting the kidneys (as with external male sphincterotomy). Additionally, it is vital to see the urodynamic problem in the context of the whole patient and their neurological disorder. Patients with progressive degenerative disease cannot be treated in the same way as congenital neuropathic patients who are planning for 30 years of improved function. For any one patient there will commonly be a range of options available. A discussion about how these choices should be made is presented at the end of the chapter.

Table 6.3 Risk analysis for patients with intractable detrusor instability (failed conservative and drug therapy). The figures are based loosely on published evidence but also personal experience and are therefore representative of real situations.

Choice	Chance of normality	Chance of being dry	Risk of early morbidity	Risk of late morbidity
No treatment	Zero	10% spontaneous resolution	Zero	Zero
Phenol injection	Zero	20–60% short-term success	1%	Impotence in men
Detrusor myectomy	Zero	60%	10%, especially wound infections, urine leak	CISC, 20% UTI, 10% Late failure, 50%
Clam cystoplasty	Zero	90%	20%: thromboembolic, cardiorespiratory, gastrointestinal, urine leak and infection	Voiding/CISC, 50% Infection, 25% Metabolic, 50% Bowel, 80% Mucus, 100% Malignancy, 2%
Ileal conduit	Zero	80% with bags and occasional accident	10%: as above	Infection, 25% Metabolic, 25% Bowel, 50% Mucus, 100% Malignancy, 1%

CISC, clean intermittent self-catheterization; UTI, urinary tract infection.

Surgery for urinary incontinence

SURGERY FOR THE UNSTABLE OR HYPERREFLEXIC BLADDER

Approximately 10% of patients who present with symptoms of detrusor overactivity fail to improve with conservative therapy or drugs and require some form of surgical therapy. The procedures available are based on two alternative principles of 'cure', denervation and augmentation, although some procedures may combine the two. The choice of therapy for individual patients with detrusor instability depends on careful discussion and assessment of the risks and benefits of each therapeutic approach. A typical conceptual framework for such a discussion is shown in Table 6.3.

Denervation

Patients with neurological lesions affecting the cauda equina or sacral spinal cord usually have either a poorly contractile or a non-contractile bladder. The rationale of bladder denervation procedures is to interrupt the sacral reflex upon which the propagation and continuation of a detrusor contraction depends. It is known that epidural and spinal anaesthesia and posterior root section (rhizotomy) obliterate detrusor contractions. The latter renders reflex detrusor contraction impossible, although direct stimulation of anterior sacral roots still results in powerful detrusor contraction. Thus, interruption of this reflex at some point seems a logical therapy for instability. However, it is hard to rationalize trying to produce peripheral denervation of the bladder with experimental evidence that the denervated bladder, both in animal models and humans, exhibits postjunctional supersensitivity, a hallmark of the unstable bladder.

Denervation has been performed at nearly all levels of the efferent limb from the spinal cord to the neuromuscular junction with varying degrees of success (Fig. 6.3). In general all denervation operations have acceptable early success rates (though they have never been compared with a control group) but long-term follow-up has always been disappointing. This may be partly a manifestation of the placebo effect and partly the 'opening up' of alternative neural pathways that allow new reflex detrusor contractions to occur. The disadvantages of all methods of denervation proximal to the bladder are the risk of impotence and the loss of sensation or volitional control of voiding. Manipulation of the sacral roots interferes with anorectal innervation and can result in difficulty with defaecation. Failure of bladder emptying is not a disaster especially with the advent of clean intermittent self-catheterization (CISC), although loss of vaginal sensation is an unwelcome additional handicap.

Phenol injection. This is the only method of denervation that we still use in our practice. The technique involves the use of a 30-cm long needle that can be passed through the deflecting mechanism of a standard cystoscope. The needle is inserted through the bladder mucosa halfway between the bladder neck and the ureteric orifice lateral to the trigone (Fig. 6.4). About 2 cm of the needle is inserted so that the tip lies just outside the bladder wall at the point where the perivesical pelvic plexus splays out to enter the bladder base (Fig. 6.3) and 10 ml of 5–6% aqueous phenol is injected on each side under endoscopic vision. There is little resistance to the injection provided the needle is in the right place. The technique is easy for any endoscopic urologist to learn and is safe provided that the phenol is not injected in the midline, when vesicovaginal fistula has been reported as a complication. Great care

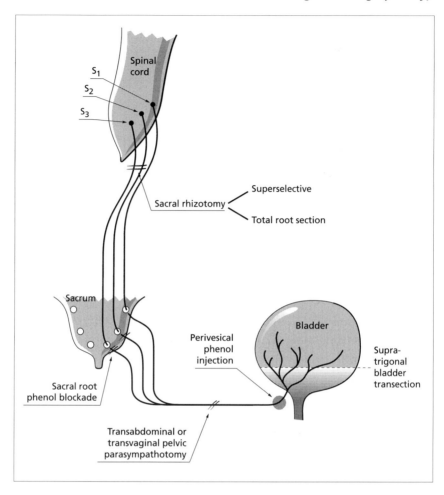

Fig. 6.3 The various neurological levels at which denervation, or decentralization, of the bladder has been performed.

must be taken to avoid any spraying of the solution and both surgeon and scrub nurse should wear protecive goggles.

There is some evidence that it is primarily the sensory fibres from the bladder that are damaged (Ewing *et al.*, 1983). The technique has fallen from favour because of poor long-term results (Chapple *et al.*, 1991), though Mundy (1993) reports a 68% success rate in women aged over 55 years. There is little morbidity associated with the procedure and occasional patients do have a dramatic and prolonged improvement in symptoms. For this reason we feel that phenol injection still has a valid place in the treatment of any patient with detrusor instability although it should not be used in sexually active men, who may be at risk of impotence.

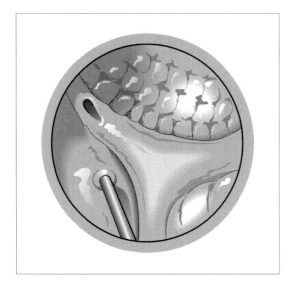

Fig. 6.4 Phenol injection, showing the needle as seen through a cystoscope. It is inserted halfway between the bladder neck and the ureteric orifice and passes outside the bladder wall to the perivesical nerve plexus.

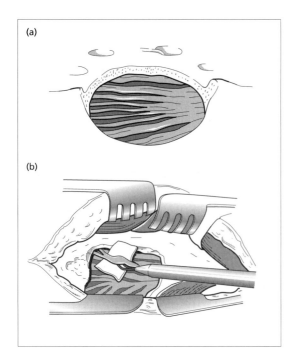

(a)

(b)

Fig. 6.5 Sacral neurectomy: (a) sacral laminectomy exposes the sacral roots; (b) a root is isolated and stimulated with a hooked electrode to see if it generates a bladder contraction.

Sacral rhizotomy. This is an operation performed by a neurosurgeon, who carries out a sacral laminectomy. By monitoring intravesical pressure and simultaneously stimulating individual extradural sacral nerve roots, those roots that primarily cause detrusor contraction can be identified (Fig. 6.5). Selective section of these roots (sacral rhizotomy or sacral neurectomy)

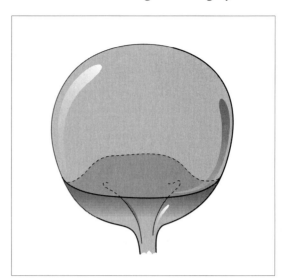

Fig. 6.6 Bladder transection, showing the line of incision used for endoscopic transection.

eliminates instability without adversely affecting the urethral sphincter (Torrens & Griffith, 1974). Anterior rootlets or 'fascicles' can be dissected from the main trunks and selectively divided (superselective rhizotomy). However, the long-term urodynamic results of complete root section seem to be more reliable than the selective operation, where it is thought that alternative neural pathways may open up. Selective intradural section of the sacral posterior roots is an alternative method of interrupting reflex activity. It has been used in cord-injured patients who are having anterior sacral root stimulators implanted to improve bladder emptying. A case could be made for using this method as a means of preventing hyperreflexia in neuropathic patients who have already lost perineal sensation; however, it is unlikely to be used in the neurologically intact. These procedures use up hours of a neuro-surgical operating list, and when the results are known to be poor and other definitive options exist their use as routine solutions cannot be justified.

Pelvic parasympathetic nerve section has been described both trans-abdominally and transvaginally (Ingelman-Sundberg, 1980), and the same plexus can be partially ablated by injection of phenol at the sacral foramina. These procedures never gained popularity and we have no experience of them. Supratrigonal transection of the bladder in a transverse plane just above the ureteric orifices divides intramural nerves and thus decentralizes the bladder fundus (Essenhigh & Yeates, 1973). The operation has also been practised endoscopically (Fig. 6.6) (Parsons *et al.*, 1984) but results of both this and the open operation have had mixed success and are no longer widely practised.

Dunn *et al.* (1974) reported the use of Helmstein bladder distension carried out under epidural anaesthesia. The balloon is inflated to diastolic blood pressure (measured with either a fluid-filled manometer or an arterial blood pressure monitor). Inflation is maintained at this pressure for four periods of 30 min interspersed with a 5-min period of deflation to allow blood to flow in the mucosa and avoid mucosal sloughing due to ischaemic necrosis. This technique arguably produces the most peripheral form of denervation, causing degeneration of nerves within the submucosa. The results from various centres have differed widely and most have found this a disappointing procedure. It may still have a place prior to major surgery but success does seem to depend on good epidural anaesthesia and an obsessional technique. Complications have included bladder rupture and sloughing of the bladder wall.

Augmentation

A more pragmatic approach for dealing with the overactive bladder has been the surgical attempt to convert a high-pressure storage system into a low-pressure one by incorporating into it a 'sump' or 'gusset', usually constructed of a segment of bowel. Early attempts to do this were conceived as a treatment for the contracted bladder of tuberculosis, but in 1969 Turner Warwick described caecocystoplasty as a means of treatment for the overactive bladder. The most basic principle of these operations is to increase functional bladder capacity. Use of caecum or sigmoid colon achieves this aim but in retaining the tubular structure of the bowel segments high-pressure bowel contractions can still occur that themselves cause episodes of urgency or incontinence. Furthermore there is also a tendency for the additional 'sump' to act as a bladder diverticulum, i.e. urine empties into the sump rather than being voided efficiently, with attendant complications of infection and stone formation.

Clam cystoplasty. Bramble (1982) described a technique where the bladder is opened widely in a coronal or sagittal plane, like a clam, and a length of bowel split along its antimesenteric border is laid as a patch into the defect that has been created (Fig. 6.7). The terminal ileum is usually used for this purpose, although in neuropathic patients there is often a high-riding and short small bowel mesentery that makes the sigmoid a much more attractive alternative.

The bladder can be divided in either the sagittal or coronal plane and it makes little difference to the results. Whichever incision is chosen, it should be extended towards the bladder neck as far as the interureteric bar, effectively slitting the bladder in two apart from the bladder neck. The sagittal dissection is easier but sewing the bowel patch into the anterior corner can be difficult. The coronal dissection is more tedious and although commencing the repair in the lateral corners is difficult, it becomes progressively

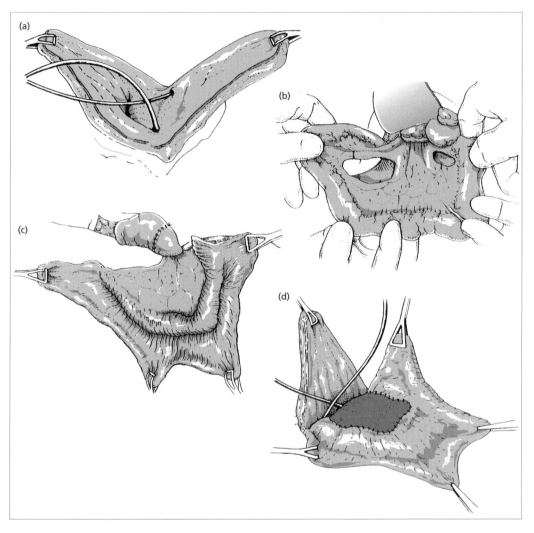

Fig. 6.7 Clam cystoplasty: (a) the bladder is bivalved in a coronal plane (note the ureteric catheters to protect the ureteric orifices); (b) a segment of ileum is isolated and (c) opened along the antimesenteric border; (d) the bowel segment has been sewn along the posterior bladder wall and is next sewn along the anterior wall to complete the cystoplasty. (From Mundy (1993), with permission.)

easier as the suturing continues. With a coronal incision the anterior bladder segment must be kept equal to the posterior segment or ischaemic shrinkage of the anterior flap occurs. Inadequate bivalving of the bladder results in shrinkage of the suture line and the patch then acts as a diverticulum.

Theoretically, the patch or gusset dissipates the effect of contraction of either half of the bladder, with little resultant increase in pressure, and the detubularized segment of bowel can no longer generate a pressure rise of

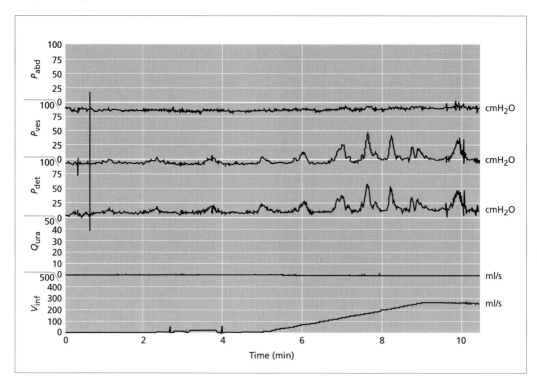

Fig. 6.8 Cystometrogram from a cystoplasty showing pressure waves generated by a 'clam' segment.

its own. Such a cystoplasty does not actually eliminate instability. It appears to act largely by increasing functional capacity, shifting the cystometrogram curve to the right and allowing unstable contractions to occur at larger volumes with a lower pressure rise. The bowel patch itself contracts and if it is too small can generate contractions measuring 20–50 cmH$_2$O (Fig. 6.8). Mebeverine or loperamide can be prescribed to reduce this motility and the pressure created, although these drugs may precipitate constipation. Better results may be obtained by doubled ileal patches, which reduce this tendency, although it can then be difficult to bring the corners low enough into the pelvis to fill the corners of the bladder defect. Patients with low functional capacities due to sensory urgency are not helped by clam cystoplasty.

For 10 years clam cystoplasty transformed the surgical treatment of detrusor instability. For the first time there was an operation with a 90–95% success rate for curing incontinence. This seemed to justify the high postoperative complication rates (early risks including cardiorespiratory and thromboembolic crises, bowel obstruction, leakage and fistula), although it is the longer-term problems that have begun to raise more serious doubts about the widespread use of this operation (Table 6.4). These are all a direct consequence of incorporating a bowel segment into the lower urinary tract. The problems

Table 6.4 Complications of clam cystoplasty.

Early complications	Late complications
Cardiorespiratory: deep venous thrombosis and pulmonary embolism	Bowel: diarrhoea
	Metabolic: acidosis, bony demineralization
Gastrointestinal: prolonged ileus, bowel obstruction, anastomotic leak	Infection: UTI, CISC, stone formation, renal failure
Urine leak/fistula	Mucus
Wound infection	Malignancy
	Spontaneous rupture of clam segment

CISC, clean intermittent self-catheterization; UTI, urinary tract infection.

occurring with this operation are the same for simple cystoplasty or complex reconstruction, as described later in the chapter.

Problems associated with bowel interposition.

1   *Bowel problems.* Bowel distur-bance due to disruption of the bile acid cycle is common (Barrington *et al.*, 1995). This usually manifests as diarrhoea and cholestyramine settles the problem.

2   *Metabolic problems.* These include vitamin B_{12} deficiency caused by loss of the ileal segment and hyperchloraemic metabolic acidosis caused by reabsorption of water and electrolytes from the interposed bowel segment. Metabolic disturbance, at least as occult metabolic acidosis, occurs in all patients and may be symptomatic requiring long-term alkali supplements (Nurse, 1991). Acidosis can always be detected with measurement of arterial blood gases, although a marked acidosis should be apparent from a venous blood sample. Acidosis leads to mobilization of calcium and decreased bone mineralization, with the theoretical risk of osteoporosis developing in older patients.

3   *Infection.* Voiding difficulty occurs in 50–95% of patients and increases the risk of urinary infection and a high risk of stone formation (Palmer, 1993). This is more likely in neuropathic patients and in patients where colon was used for the patch. One must realize that the urine in these patients is always contaminated so it is illogical to treat with antibiotics unless an infection is symptomatic. However, chronic infection may play a role in the subsequent development of malignancy by producing urinary nitrosamines, which are known carcinogens. Antibiotic therapy and CISC may be important long-term strategies to minimize the risk of malignancy.

4   *Renal function.* Systems that still produce high pressures (with leak point pressures > 40 cmH$_2$O) represent a risk to upper tract function. In addition, there is increased urinary excretion of calcium, phosphate and magnesium which, associated with mucus, infection and urinary stasis, lead to stone formation in 40% of patients. This increases the risk to renal function, although the risk is lowest in low-pressure efficiently emptying systems. Patients need to

maintain a high fluid intake, perform CISC with bladder washouts and use maintenance low-dose antibiotics to reduce these risks.

5 *Mucus* is a nuisance, often causing urethral or catheter blockage and associated pain and may be the cause of acute retention leading to bladder rupture. Effective mucolytics are hard to find. Acetylcysteine instilled into the bladder is an effective mucolytic (30 ml of 20% solution). Ranitidine and pentosan polysulphate have been used with some success. All patients take cranberry juice, although there is not much evidence to support its use as a mucolytic but it may help to reduce infection episodes. However, mucus production decreases over time in line with progressive atrophy of the villous epithelium.

6 *Malignancy.* The principal long-term worry for these patients is the theoretical risk of malignant transformation in the reconstructed bladder. Tumours are known to occur in ureterosigmoidostomies and ileal conduits; however, it has now become apparent that cancers also occur in ileal cystoplasties (Harzmann & Weckerman, 1992). These tumours vary widely with regard to their site within the reconstruction and their histological type. Buson *et al.* (1993) have shown that 50–65% of rodents with cystoplasties develop widespread metaplasia within the bladder urothelium. Urologists now face a potential barrage of cancers in 10–20 years' time and need to be vigilant in their follow-up of cystoplasty patients. Most urologists perform cystoscopy every year and urine cytology about 5 years after the operation. If the incidence of malignancy becomes higher, then we may have to begin to offer ablative preventive surgery of the bladder in order to prevent malignant transformation. Many urologists now feel that it is no longer acceptable to offer clam cystoplasty to young patients with idiopathic detrusor instability and have returned to denervation procedures or methods of autoaugmentation.

Autoaugmentation: detrusor myectomy. Much work has been done to develop an alternative to cystoplasty that increases functional capacity but without the complications of bowel interposition. In detrusor myectomy, the whole of the detrusor muscle above the bladder 'equator' is removed from the underlying mucosa while the bladder is kept partly filled to assist the dissection (Fig. 6.9). The effect is to create a broad-opening bladder diverticulum with no intrinsic contractile capacity in the diverticulum (Cartwright & Snow, 1989). It is a potentially elegant operation but often frustrating because even tiny holes in the bladder mucosa will leak and tear, making visibility and accurate dissection increasingly difficult as the operation proceeds. It can be performed extraperitoneally but if there is a lot of leakage then an omental flap should be formed to wrap over the defect. Results have been acceptable in relieving incontinence; urodynamically, the cystometrogram is shifted to the right but with little improvement in functional capacity or compliance so that there is often still frequency (Cartwright & Snow, 1996). Myectomy is a

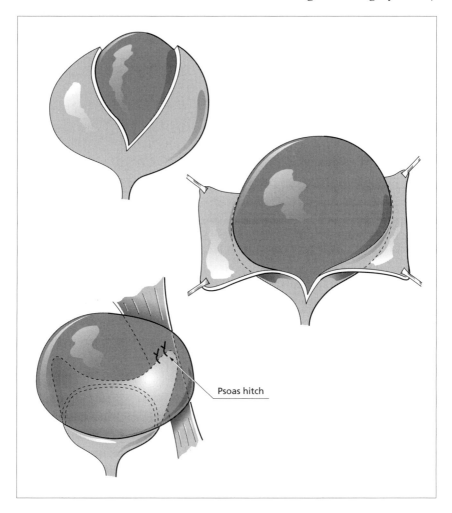

Fig. 6.9 Detrusor myectomy.

lesser operation than cystoplasty and does not produce the complications of infection, mucus production, voiding dysfunction and malignancy. It should be considered in younger patients. However, in the neuropathic patient, where the bladder is often very trabeculated, the operation is difficult because the sacculations of mucosa are easily perforated during dissection of the muscle from the bladder wall. Cystoplasty still represents the best option for this group.

Another technique, multiple detrusor myotomy, has been described by Mahone and Lafferte (1972) and Stothers *et al.* (1994) but has not been widely adopted. However, it is an attractive principle as the repeated cross-hatching of the bladder muscle down to mucosal level interrupts the ephaptic spread of excitation around the smooth muscle syncytium, preventing co-ordinated phasic bladder contraction, and the method leaves the mucosa protected by

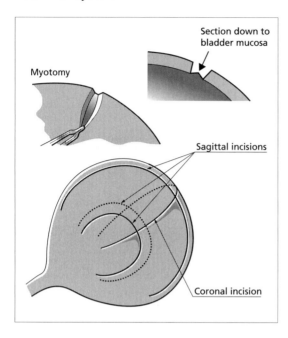

Myotomy

Section down to
bladder mucosa

Sagittal incisions

Coronal incision

Fig. 6.10 Multiple detrusor
myotomy: three sagittal
incisions and one coronal
incision leave all the detrusor
segments vascularized but
'electrically' isolated from each
other.

overlying bladder wall. We have tried a modification of this technique
(Fig. 6.10), in which no section of the bladder wall is allowed to become
devascularized, in a very limited number of patients, with early success.

Because of the intrinsic disadvantages of cystoplasty techniques there
have been attempts to invent an alternative. Gastrocystoplasty involves the
same bivalving of the bladder as clam cystoplasty. A segment of gastric
antrum is then mobilized on a pedicle of the gastroepiploic vessels and laid
into the bladder defect. The advantage of this method is that acid secretory
epithelium rather than absorptive epithelium is used so that the problems
with metabolic acidosis should be reduced. However, patients have suffered
an unacceptable incidence of haemorrhagic cystitis and bladder spasm due to
gastric acid secretions, which are not controlled with an H_2 blocker, and
hypochloraemic alkalosis has also occurred. Combined ileogastric patches
have been proposed as a way of cancelling out the undesirable metabolic
effects. The surgery involved in these procedures is technically challenging
and hence much more likely to lead to immediate postoperative failure.

Another method that has been utilized is to perform a detrusor myectomy
and then replace the excised bladder wall with a detubularized segment of ileum
with the mucosa stripped off (autoaugmentation enterocystoplasty), thus theoretically offering the advantages of compliance without the dangers of foreign
mucosa and protection of the bladder from adherence to bowel loops. However, the transitional epithelium does stick to the underlying bowel and the bowel
segment fibroses easily, so the protection is not as good as had been hoped.

Neuromodulation

Permanently implantable stimulators have been developed to provide chronic electrical stimulation directly to the S3 roots. This has been shown to reduce detrusor hyperreflexia and instability dramatically. Because of the very high cost of these prostheses their use is being strictly limited at present to clinical trials and there are only a few centres that actually perform the surgery. The precise role and ideal patient selection has yet to be determined. Preliminary trials of treatment with transcutaneous electrical nerve stimulation (see Chapter 4) seem worth while before permanent implantation, since the cost is high and the potential morbidity best avoided if the likely benefit is small. Alternatively, functional magnetic stimulation of the sacral nerve roots with a multipulse magnetic stimulator has been used for testing responses and could provide a non-invasive therapeutic alternative in its own right.

SURGERY FOR STRESS INCONTINENCE

The surgical approach to the control of GSI is bedevilled by choice. A great many procedures have been described and reported but very few rigorously compared with independent outcome assessment. Some of the procedures are outlined here in order to illustrate the underlying principles employed, although it needs to be clearly stated that surgeons may use significantly different techniques but consider themselves to be performing the same operation. The degree of dissection and tension applied to tissues and sutures can fundamentally change the results. The reported short-term and long-term outcomes of procedures are difficult to interpret. It should be remembered that when meta-analyses are employed many different surgeons are clustered together, even though each has their own success rate that may have been determined by personal surgical nuances and by subtle differences in case composition depending on referral patterns (Table 6.5). Publication bias favouring good results is doubtless a factor in the exaggeration of success and underestimation of complication rates. Conscious or subconscious polishing of data prior to publication is another unquantifiable confounding factor in trying to establish the real outcomes of various techniques. For these and other reasons we strongly encourage an external audit of all surgical outcomes. This difficult path, about which many clinicians have grave misgivings, is perhaps one way of giving our patients and ourselves the high-quality information needed to make rational decisions regarding treatment choices. Without this reliable data each clinician will continue to use whatever technique they are comfortable with.

Surgery for GSI is a balance between providing continence, by elevation or support of the bladder neck and associated structures, and the creation of

Table 6.5 Outcome of surgery for stress incontinence. From Jarvis (1994a), with permission.

Operation	No. of patients objectively assessed	Percentage continent (mean)	Percentage with urge syndrome	Percentage with voiding difficulty
Anterior colporrhaphy	490	31–96 (72)	Unrecorded	Unrecorded
Marshall–Marchetti–Krantz	384	71–100 (89)	1	3–11
Colposuspension	1773	59–100 (83)	3–18	3–32
Needle suspension	433	39–93 (70)	2–20	1–24
Bladder neck sling	365	78–100 (88)	2–27	3–15
Injection procedures	95	31–70 (63)		

postoperative morbidity, in the form of outflow obstruction and detrusor instability. Additional morbidity may result from alteration of the vaginal contour leading to dyspareunia that predisposes to further prolapse. More importantly from the continence viewpoint, the effect of tissue trauma and resultant scarring to the bladder neck and paraurethral tissues may exacerbate the intrinsic weakness that we believe is present in all patients with GSI.

In most reconstruction procedures the first attempt presents the best opportunity for a good result. This is particularly true of bladder neck surgery. It is vital to get it right first time, and recognition of this requires us to choose a procedure that has the best short-term and long-term risk–benefit profile. We believe that in each case it is essential to determine the degree of bladder neck mobility, the integrity of the lateral vaginal wall support and the significance of vaginal or periurethral scarring. These can be determined by a combination of good clinical examination and lateral bladder neck imaging. Lateral sulci support is appropriate if there is detachment but may not be needed if the bladder neck hypermobility is due to central weakness.

Patients must be made fully aware of the likely short-term and long-term results of surgery. Preoperative voiding studies may indicate possible postoperative difficulties and, if this is recognized, training in CISC before admission is advisable. No patient should have surgery before conservative methods of control have been fully evaluated and understood. All the procedures that are described have initial failure rates ranging from 5 to 50%. Added to this is the gradual deterioration of symptom control over time, which may be a function of poor surgical choice or technique and the natural gradual failure of the pelvic floor compromised at the outset. These failed patients need continued care, either further surgery or reliance on conservative measures.

All our patients are taught pelvic floor exercises before their operation. They are also made aware of what may compromise their pelvic floor function as time passes, particularly repetitive strain injury associated with chronic constipation or incorrect lifting techniques. The role of parturition in the pathophysiology of pelvic floor dysfunction has been discussed in Chapter 2. It is usually appropriate to continue with conservative measures until the family is complete but if this is not possible then future deliveries will probably require elective Caesarean section to avoid disruption of the repaired continence mechanism. (One-third of female gynaecologists would choose elective Caesarean section for themselves in order to preserve normal pelvic floor function. This high figure, which will probably rise and influence delivery patterns throughout the UK and other countries, reflects a failure to recognize the normal mechanisms that prevent damage and aid recovery. Population-based research on pelvic floor protection is urgently needed.)

Coexisting pathology in the pelvis is crucially important when advising patients on the management of their presenting complaint. There is no value in ignoring uterine prolapse or posterior vaginal wall defects, as these problems will certainly worsen after bladder neck surgery and may be dealt with more appropriately before or during the procedure. Similarly, the difficult problem of vaginal vault descent after hysterectomy should be sought and treated, for example by sacrocolpopexy at the same time. It is worth noting that subtle changes to the pelvic floor architecture can resolve problems in another area. Vaginal hysterectomy, alone or in combination with a simple anterior colporrhaphy, may be all that is required to correct minimal GSI if the uterus has been descending, dragging the bladder base downwards and pulling open the posterior bladder neck.

When hypermobilitiy of the bladder neck is not present, the role of conventional surgery should be questioned. The role of endoscopic bladder neck injection with collagen or silicone is particularly important in this clinical scenario and may not prejudice open surgery later. A clinical algorithm is presented in Fig. 6.11, which represents our own approach for choosing the surgical treatment of stress incontinence. This should be read in conjunction with Table 6.6, which presents a series of questions that must be answered in order to guide one through this algorithm. This algorithm is a simplification of a very complex decision pathway and is included in order to highlight the interplay between hypermobility, lateral vaginal wall support, previous surgery and vaginal compliance.

Supporting operations of the urethra

Anterior colporrhaphy. The standard gynaecological anterior repair involves plication of the paravaginal fascia underlying the bladder base, resulting in a

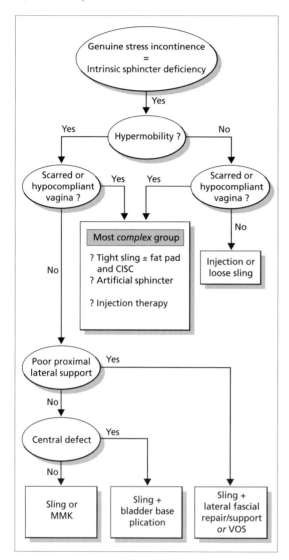

Fig. 6.11 An algorithm to demonstrate a decision pathway in the choice of surgery for women with stress incontinence. CISC, clean intermittent self-catheterization; MMK, Marshall–Marchetti–Krantz procedure; VOS, vagino-obturator shelf.

'buttressing' of the bladder neck and bladder base (Fig. 6.12). The procedure approximates two layers of intrinsically weak tissue (this is why there is hypermobility in the first place). Cosisky Marana *et al.* (1996) have reported a 79% recurrence rate with this procedure. There is still a place for anterior repair in the treatment of pure anterior wall prolapse or where stress incontinence is only a minor part of this problem. It can also be used in conjunction with another procedure, such as a sling, simply to control the cystocoele element. However, use of the anterior repair alone as treatment for stress incontinence is to be deprecated.

Table 6.6 Preoperative planning for stress incontinence surgery.

Questions to be answered before any surgery for stress incontinence	Significance of these questions
Is there genuine stress incontinence?	This always implies that there is some intrinsic sphincter weakness
Is there hypermobility of the bladder neck?	Providing new support for the bladder neck is logical
Is there scarring or rigidity of the urethra and bladder neck?	Attempting to provide further support is futile and further augmentation of closure by obstruction or injection is required
Is vaginal compliance and size normal?	If not, then colposuspension or VOS are inappropriate
Is there loss of support in the proximal lateral vaginal/paravesical fascia?	If so, failure to repair this at the same time may result in voiding failure or progressive deterioration in prolapse
Is there central prolapse of the bladder base?	If so, the comments above still apply but the surgical solution is different
Does the bladder contract normally during voiding?	If not, then the chances of voiding failure are high and the patient may need to learn CISC
Is there associated vault prolapse or anorectal disorder?	This should be investigated and possibly surgically repaired at the same time

CISC, clean intermittent self-catheterization; VOS, vagino-obturator shelf.

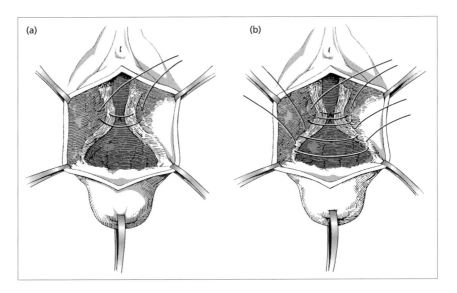

Fig. 6.12 Anterior repair/colporrhaphy: (a) a midline vaginal dissection is performed and sutures placed in the pubocervical fascia; (b) the stitches draw together the pubocervical fascia to support the bladder base. Excess vaginal skin is often excised. From Monaghan, J.M. (1986), with permission.

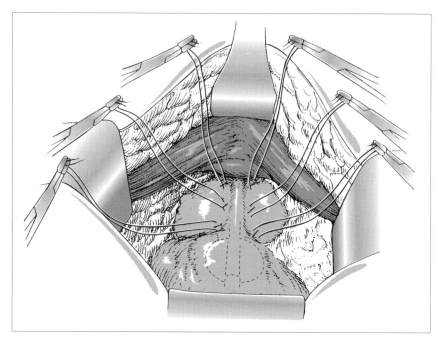

Fig. 6.13 Suture positions for the Marshall–Marchetti–Krantz operation. From Hinman jnr (1989), with permission.

Marshall–Marchetti–Krantz. This is a suprapubic operation (Marshall *et al.*, 1949) in which the bladder is mobilized from the vagina using blunt dissection and two or three sutures are placed on either side of the urethrovesical junction into the paraurethral fascia to elevate this and the proximal urethra behind the pubic symphysis (Fig. 6.13). However, inappropriate suture positioning is common. Many surgeons position the sutures too close or even into the urethral tissues or bladder neck, causing 'tenting' of the anterior urethra and adversely affecting its closure mechanism. Consequently the operation has had mixed results.

Burch colposuspension. This is another suprapubic procedure (Burch, 1961) in which the endopelvic fascia to either side of the bladder neck is elevated and secured, with a number of interrupted sutures, to the back of Cooper's ligament (Fig. 6.14). Thus a 'shelf' is formed over which the urethra passes, which prevents it from downward displacement during coughing and straining (Fig. 6.15). The techniques for performing this operation have also evolved, including variations in the number of stitches, their precise placement, whether there is any tension or bowstringing of the sutures and the amount of dissection of the endopelvic fascia allowing prolapse of the vaginal

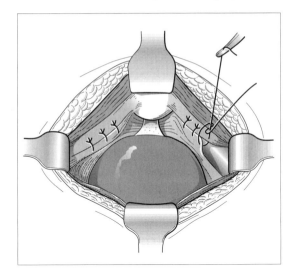

Fig. 6.14 Suture positions for Burch colposuspension. In this case the endopelvic fascia has not been breached but is being elevated by attachment to Cooper's (pectineal) ligament using three sutures on each side.

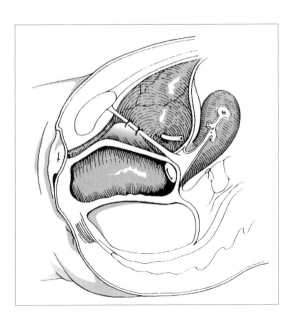

Fig. 6.15 Sagittal section to show how colposuspension elevates the anterior vaginal wall and creates a shelf for the urethra. From Monaghan, J.M. (1986), with permission.

vault towards the ligament (Fig. 6.16). Laparoscopy has now been added to the repertoire of techniques used in colposuspension, allowing less dissection and faster recovery rates, although the precise placement of stitches may be less satisfactory and the short-term results have been poor in non-controlled studies.

In the vagino-obturator shelf (VOS) the endopelvic fascia is divided to either side of the bladder neck and the underlying paraurethral fascia is

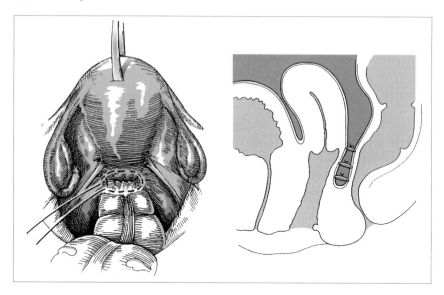

Fig. 6.19 Insertion of sequential purse-string sutures to close the pouch of Douglas and prevent enterocoele after colposuspension. From Monaghan, J.M. (1986), with permission.

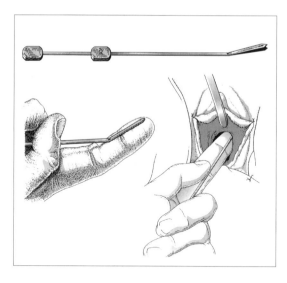

Fig. 6.20 The Stamey needle can be passed from above downwards to the vaginal incision or, applied to the index finger, from vagina to rectus sheath. Passage of sutures through the space of Retzius is facilitated.

Stamey (1973) popularized the technique by introducing a special needle that facilitated passage of the nylon thread. The sutures are threaded through a short cuff of Dacron or Silastic and are tied anteriorly over the rectus sheath so as to produce elevation of the paraurethral tissues (Figs 6.20 & 6.21). The position of the sutures and the adequacy of bladder neck support can be checked endoscopically during the operation (Fig. 6.22). Apart from improving transmission of intra-abdominal pressure, any contraction of the rectus muscles also results in further elevation of the pubovesical fascia. Theoretically,

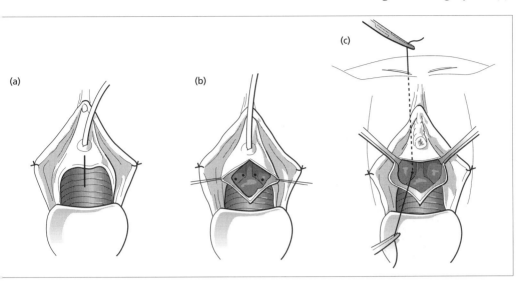

Fig. 6.21 Operative sequence showing a Stamey bladder neck suspension: (a) longitudinal vaginal incision; (b) exposure of the bladder neck and paraurethral fascia from below, indicating the points at which the Stamey needles should perforate; (c) positioning of the Dacron cuff that supports the paraurethral tissues.

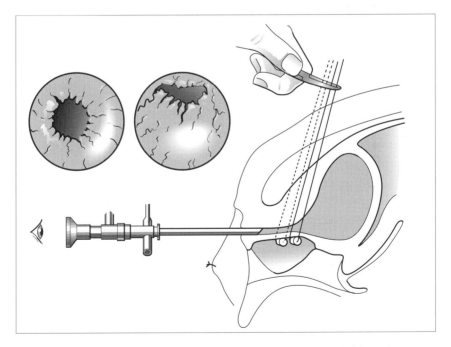

Fig. 6.22 Stamey bladder neck suspension shown in sagittal section. The bladder neck is checked endoscopically to ensure that sutures do not pass through the bladder and the effect of suture tension on bladder neck closure can be checked.

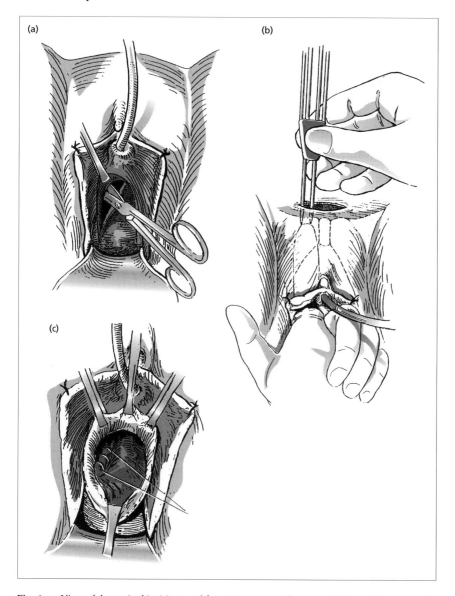

Fig. 6.23 View of the vaginal incision used for a Raz cystourethropexy: (a) lateral dissection of the paraurethral fascia; (b) a finger penetrating the retropubic space from the vaginal incision; (c) the principle of needle suspension is the same as in a Stamey procedure but the sutures are secured with helical bites to the paraurethral and vaginal tissues. From Raz (1981), with permission from Elsevier Science.

therefore, this repair is 'dynamic', allowing varying degrees of elevation, and does not interfere with the integrity of the urethrovesical junction.

Further modifications of the operation have been described. For instance the Raz cystourethropexy (Raz *et al.*, 1989) relies on the same principle of dynamic suspension with nylon threads, although the nylon is secured to

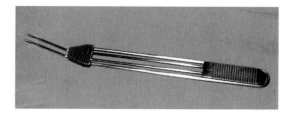

Fig. 6.24 The Peyreyra double ligature carrier facilitates placement of nylon suspensory sutures for bladder neck suspensions and slings.

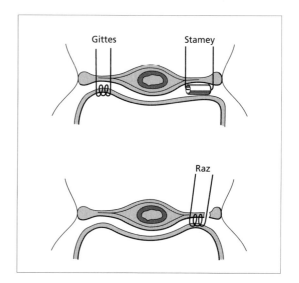

Fig. 6.25 Schematic diagram to illustrate the different suture positions of the Gittes procedure, Stamey operation and Raz cystourethropexy.

the paraurethral fascia with three helical sutures (Fig. 6.23). This makes the suture placement much more precise than the Stamey operation, an approach that appeals to some surgeons even though it cannot be supported by any objective improvement in results. The Peyreyra double ligature carrier also simplifies the procedures (Fig. 6.24). The Gittes procedure (Gittes & Loughlin, 1987) uses the principle of the Stamey operation but allows the sutures to be placed by needle passage alone and the thread simply supports the vaginal wall without any attempt to mobilize the bladder neck from the adjacent vaginal tissues (Fig. 6.25). It is a minimally invasive procedure that can be done under local anaesthesia. Although such techniques have become popular with surgeons because of their relative ease and speed, the long-term results have been poor in a number of studies (33% of patients dry at 10 years; Mills *et al.*, 1996).

'Sling' procedures. Over the last 80 years a variety of procedures have been described in which a sling is passed around the urethrovesical junction or proximal urethra in order to provide support during moments of abdominal

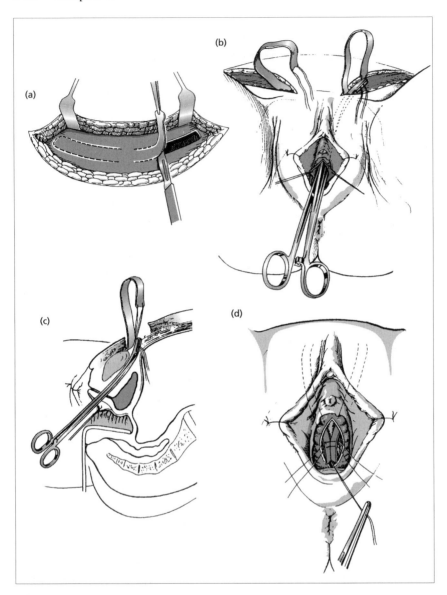

Fig. 6.26 The Aldridge sling: (a) medially based rectus sheath slings are mobilized; (b) the vaginal dissection and creation of a hernia through the endopelvic fascia proceeds as for a Raz operation using a Roberts forceps passed from below; (c) the slings are drawn through to the vaginal incision and (d) sewn together in the midline under the urethra. From Monaghan (1986), with permission.

stress. Various autogenous organic and inorganic materials have been employed for this purpose. Some surgeons reserve these techniques for the second operation, i.e. when a suspensory procedure has already failed. One of the earlier popular techniques was the Aldridge sling, in which medially based flaps of rectus sheath are mobilized and passed downwards through the space of Retzius to a central vaginal incision. The flaps are then sutured together under the urethra to provide support (Fig. 6.26).

Once again there is a problem interpreting results because of the changing philosophy of these procedures. If the sling is tight then it is obstructive and undoubtedly cures stress leakage but at the expense of voiding. This is what makes it attractive as a secondary operation. However, a sling loosely applied around the bladder neck prevents downward displacement and, in principle, interferes little with voiding. A meta-analysis of surgery for stress incontinence (Jarvis, 1994a) showed that the best long-term results were obtained with sling procedures, which had rates of voiding dysfunction similar to colposuspension (see Table 6.5). However, the range of cure rates was much narrower and more consistent for sling procedures than colposuspension. This was taken to imply that the best available operation is therefore the sling. However, since many variations of technique and objectives exist between different uncontrolled study groups such an analysis should be interpreted with great caution. However, we would suggest that, because of the placement of a sling around the urethra, there is probably less potential for interoperator variation with slings than with other procedures, except in terms of sling tension which is critical.

In our own practice the loosely applied pubovaginal sling using a free autologous rectus sheath fascia has become the standard operation for correction of stress incontinence related to hypermobility (Fig. 6.27). A pilot study of short rectus sheath 'sling on a string' has given encouraging early results and is now the subject of a rigorous randomized trial to compare it with conventional sling technique.

Raz has described a sling technique in which the existing tissues of the paravaginal fascia and paraurethral fascia are plicated on each side of the urethra and suspended from the rectus sheath using a needle technique (Rovner *et al.*, 1997). In effect this creates a suburethral sling of vaginal wall that supports the bladder neck (Fig. 6.28). Raz argues that the vaginal wall sling deals equally well with intrinsic sphincter weakness and hypermobility and that this renders obsolete the need for careful preoperative assessment of the cause of leakage. The results are good but have not been compared properly with other procedures.

Barua *et al.* (1993) described an operation devised by Wheeler in Dundee in which the medial slip of the rectus muscle is divided where it inserts into the pubic symphysis and is passed backwards into the space of Retzius to be sutured to the vaginal vault in the same position that one might apply the sutures of a Burch colposuspension (Fig. 6.29). Once again, the principle is that of a dynamic support provided by rectus muscle contraction. Small pilot studies have shown results at least as good as other suspensory procedures.

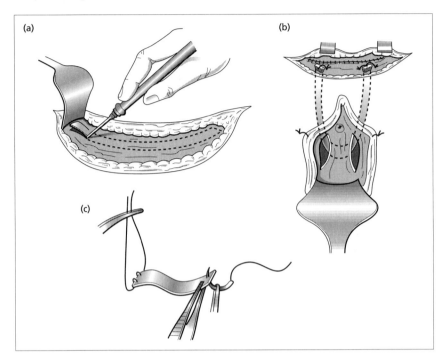

Fig. 6.27 Free rectus sheath fascia pubovaginal sling: (a) a free graft is fashioned from the rectus sheath; (b) the vaginal dissection is through two laterally based incisions connected by a tunnel under the posterior urethra. The sling is drawn through and secured either directly to the rectus sheath or (c) suspended from lengths of nylon with no tension or elevation, known as 'sling on a string'.

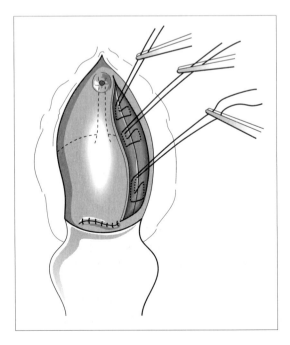

Fig. 6.28 The principle of Raz's 'six-point' vaginal wall sling procedure. This plicates and corrects a laxity in the lateral urethral, bladder neck and vesical support but downward displacement is prevented by suspension of the vaginal wall from the rectus sheath in the same way as all other needle suspensions and slings.

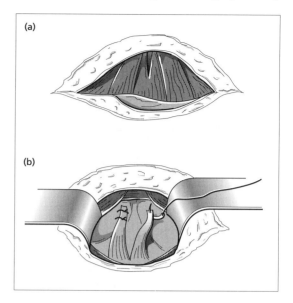

Fig. 6.29 Medial slip rectus transfer operation: (a) the medial slip of each side of the rectus abdominis is mobilized; (b) the tendinous part of the rectus slip is sutured to the anterolateral vaginal wall to prevent downward displacement.

Fixation techniques. Recently, a number of companies have seized on the concept of fixation of a needle suspension to a fixed point using nylon threads and have introduced a range of devices to pin or screw a metal fixing point into the bone of the pubic arch, either transvaginally or suprapubically (Fig. 6.30). Otherwise the principle of suspension of either Raz sutures or sling material is the same as the originally described procedure. It is essential that fixed suspension procedures are compared with supposedly 'dynamic' ones in a well-structured trial before too many bits of alloy are implanted into female pubic bones.

Procedures for sphincter weakness

Bladder neck injection techniques. Injection of Teflon paste into the submucosal tissues of the bladder neck enjoyed a vogue in the early 1980s until it was realized that migration of Teflon particles occurred. Since then the risk has been considered unacceptable.

Two materials have recently been licensed for use in controlling stress incontinence: collagen (Contigen™) and silicone (Macroplastique™). Their administration requires slightly different techniques, due to their different viscosities. With the aid of a cystoscope, both materials are injected into the tissues around the neck of the bladder, creating increased tissue bulk and subsequent coaptation of the urethral lumen (Fig. 6.31). The manufacturer of Macroplastique plans to market a simplified delivery system obviating the need for endoscopy. Both materials are designed to improve passive urethral

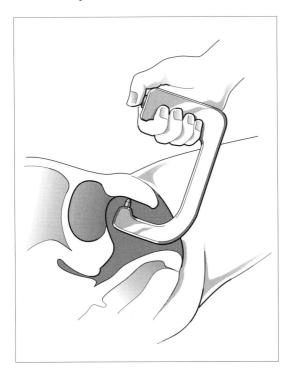

Fig. 6.30 One of the commercially available fixation systems. A metal pin is fired into the back of the pubic arch through the anterior vaginal wall and can be used as the fixed point from which any type of bladder neck support can be suspended.

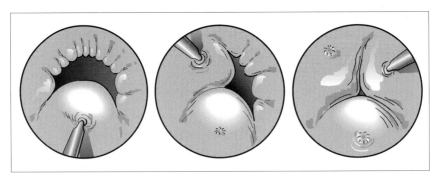

Fig. 6.31 The effect of submucosal injection in coapting the urethral walls.

closure and may lengthen the functional urethra. Surprisingly little postoperative voiding morbidity occurs despite complete apposition of the urethral mucosa. This may be due to postoperative moulding of the materials during voiding or is illustrative of the dynamic widening of the internal meatus secondary to detrusor muscle contraction during a normal void.

The techniques are rapidly gaining popularity, despite the high cost of materials, and in our practice are beginning to be used as first-line therapy for patients without hypermobility and as second-line treatment for conventional surgical failures without excessive bladder neck mobility. Others are

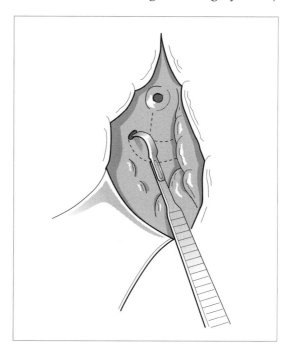

Fig. 6.32 Use of a stitch cutter to perform urethrolysis of a previously implanted sling.

promoting their use for primary treatment with hypermobility. This recognizes the role of intrinsic sphincter weakness in the pathophysiology of most cases of GSI, regardless of hypermobility. It remains to be seen from long-term follow-up how successful this strategy is and whether the materials are as inert and trouble-free as their manufacturers claim.

Reduction urethroplasty. This operation was designed for the treatment of type III incontinence where there was scarring of the urethra and bladder and there is nothing to be gained by an attempt at further repositioning. This was prior to the introduction of an effective artificial urinary sphincter (AUS) and modern injection techniques. The only possible place for this operation now would be in the repair of a particularly patulous urethra.

Role of urethrolysis. Occasionally after surgery for stress incontinence that has been too obstructive, the patient complains bitterly of voiding dysfunction or of secondary urgency and urge incontinence worse than the original problem they had with stress incontinence. In this situation release of the supporting mechanism can easily be achieved through a small vaginal incision. A tiny skin incision is made and a stitch-cutter blade mounted on a knife handle can be passed through with a sweeping motion to cut the sling or colposuspension sutures (Fig. 6.32). Remarkably, this often restores balanced

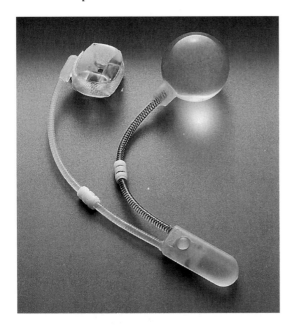

Fig. 6.33 The artificial urinary sphincter manufactered by American Medical Systems (AMS 800). With permission from AMS UK Ltd.

voiding, with improved emptying, and relieves urgency because of diminished outlet obstruction. It may cause a recurrence of the stress incontinence although, surprisingly, it often does not.

Artificial urinary sphincter. For several years there was competition to produce an implantable device for urinary incontinence that would prevent GSI but allow intermittent voiding at normal bladder pressures. Kaufman and Raz (1979) produced a device of fixed resistance that was implanted around the bulbar urethra, while Rosen (1976) produced an inflatable, non-circumferential Silastic sphincter. The results of both were poor. More recently, Brantley Scott introduced a device (manufactured by American Medical Systems Ltd) that has been consistently more reliable (Fig. 6.33). Its features include a circumferential periurethral/bladder neck cuff, which is maintained constantly inflated by a pressure-regulating balloon, and a control pump inserted in the scrotum or labia that allows complete cuff deflation for voiding (Fig. 6.34). This innovation has radically changed the management of refractory incontinence. Used initially for men with post-prostatectomy incontinence (Fig. 6.35), the device has now been widely implanted for patients with neurogenic bladder dysfunction, women after failed surgery for GSI (Fig. 6.36) and even in conjunction with major reconstructive bladder surgery (Fig. 6.37). In women with recurrent stress incontinence the ideal recipient is the patient with intrinsic sphincter weakness and detrusor failure, where any other procedure would lead to voiding failure whereas an AUS would allow natural voiding.

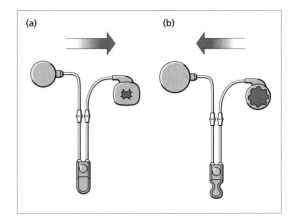

Fig. 6.34 The artificial urinary sphincter (AMS 800) showing (a) the cuff inflated in the resting state and (b) the pump having been squeezed until the cuff has deflated to allow voiding. Reproduced with kind permission of American Medical Systems UK Ltd.

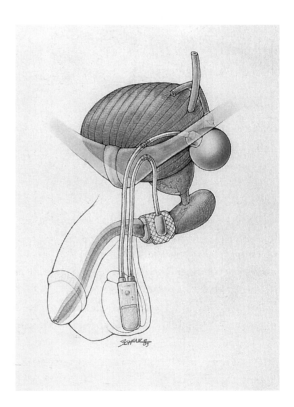

Fig. 6.35 Artificial urinary sphincter inserted around the bulbar urethra in a male (typically for post-prostatectomy incontinence). Reproduced with kind permission of American Medical Systems UK Ltd.

The chief indication for an AUS is always that there is demonstrable sphincter weakness incontinence (Table 6.7). Careful preoperative assessment with videourodynamics is mandatory. Associated detrusor overactivity must be dealt with at the same time as the implantation of the sphincter; this usually means a cystoplasty, although there is no reason why a myectomy

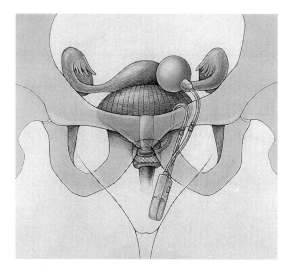

Fig. 6.36 Artificial urinary sphincter inserted around the bladder neck in a female (typically after failure of other surgery). Reproduced with kind permission of American Medical Systems UK Ltd.

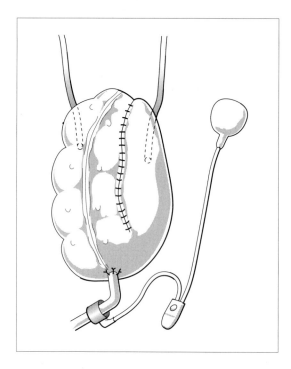

Fig. 6.37 Use of an artificial urinary sphincter in conjunction with a neobladder to control associated sphincter weakness incontinence.

should not be done concurrently with AUS placement. Any bladder outlet obstruction must be alleviated surgically prior to AUS insertion, since any future endoscopic surgery could jeopardize the integrity of the periurethral cuff or create erosion or infection resulting in subsequent removal of the device. In patients disabled with neuropathy, the placement of the pump

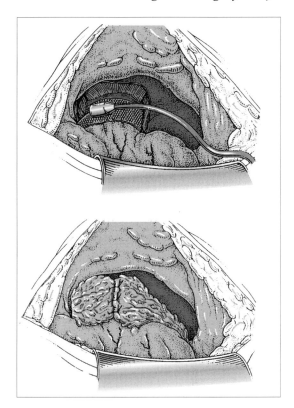

Fig. 6.38 The omentum can be mobilized to wrap inside and around the sphincter cuff to protect delicate urethral tissues (an 'omental sandwich'). From Mundy (1993).

Table 6.7 Indications for an artificial urinary sphincter.

Sphincter weakness incontinence secondary to pelvic surgery
    Transurethral prostatectomy
    Radical prostatectomy
    Orthotopic bladder reconstruction

Surgery for stress incontinence
    Failure of previous surgery, proven intrinsic sphincter weakness with normal support
    Women with poor detrusor contraction, because they may still be able to void without
        catheterization

Neuropathic bladder
    Ambulant patient
    Proven sphincter weakness

should be carefully considered with regard to dexterity and the ease of access to the scrotum or labia (Table 6.8).

However, while the surgery involved in inserting the device is not difficult, patients require very careful preoperative assessment and assiduous

Detrusor instability or hypocompliance
Bladder outflow obstruction
Urethral stricture
Poor dexterity, intelligence or motivation
Terminal malignancy

Table 6.8 Contraindications to an artificial urinary sphincter.

long-term follow-up. Long-term complications include erosion of the cuff, leakage of the device or pump failure, and atrophy of the urethra within the cuff, which results in progressive incontinence because the cuff is no longer the appropriate size for the urethra. Wrapping the cuff with omentum can reduce some of the erosive complications (Fig. 6.38). A tight fibrous sheath can form around the pressure balloon, making filling of the balloon (emptying of the cuff) increasingly difficult and leading to urinary retention. The device is expensive (about £2500) and repeat operations to correct problems are required in about 50% of patients, even in units where large numbers have been performed. The provision of such a service is a major long-term commitment and thus is outwith the armamentarium of the average urologist. Patients who have had an AUS inserted may attend a continence clinic for advice or follow-up and an appreciation of potential problems and trouble-shooting measures is therefore important (Tables 6.8 and 6.9).

The increasing use of the periurethral autologous fascial sling may reduce the need for AUS insertion. The sling can be inserted around the posterior urethra in both men and women in order to control sphincter weakness leakage. Its advantage is that avoidance of implanted material prevents erosion and the risk of mechanical failure or infection. However, the chance of voiding difficulty is higher than with an AUS. Often a patient can choose between these options.

COMBINED STRESS INCONTINENCE WITH DETRUSOR INSTABILITY

Detrusor instability is often associated with GSI. Some authors state that associated detrusor instability is a cause of failed surgery and should therefore always be treated first (Stanton *et al.*, 1978). Indeed if the high-pressure bladder is rendered compliant and given a good enough capacity the associated stress incontinence may cease to be a problem or, if mild, may even be an advantage by permitting bladder emptying (Mundy, 1993). McGuire and Savastano (1984) stated that only 13% of patients with detrusor instability plus GSI have troublesome incontinence postoperatively if the GSI is treated first. However, this study used a more liberal definition of instability than that used by the International Continence Society at the time (the definitions have since changed) and has been criticized because of this as it probably included many patients who would not have been classified by others as

Table 6.9 Troubleshooting with the artificial urinary sphincter.

Problem	Cause	Confirmation	Solution
Stress incontinence	Balloon pressure too low or cuff too big	Likely if leakage starts as soon as system is activated	Reduce cuff size or increase pressure balloon
	Atrophy of urethra	Takes months or years to develop: low leak pressure	Insert smaller cuff
	Leakage of system (most commonly the cuff): sometimes a connector loose; occasionally instrument damage to tubing	Oblique X-rays show deflated balloon and contrast in tissues. Inflation and deflation films help to clarify	Identify leaky component and replace
	Air bubbles in system	X-rays show air in tubing	Refill system
	Hypocompliant bladder	Leaks with full bladder. Leak pressure equates to closure pressure of the system. Confirm with urodynamics	May require further surgery to augment bladder
Urge incontinence	Detrusor instability	May be exacerbated by insertion of device	See treatments for detrusor instability
Pump fails to operate, resulting in inability to void	Particulate matter in system	Sudden blockage	Replace part of system
	Kinked tubing (only happens with early models)	Visible with oblique films	Explore and replace part of system
	Sheath forms around balloon	Gradual onset	Explore and reposition balloon
Acute retention despite apparently normal working system	If immediately after implantation, system not properly deactivated	Check deactivation button	
	Erosion or infection of system resulting in swelling of the urethral tissues within the cuff	Cystoscopy	See below
Excessive pumping required to deflate balloon	Failure of valve mechanism		Replace pump
Swelling or tenderness around pump, fever	Infection or erosion	Urethrography or urethroscopy demonstrates erosion	Antibiotic therapy may provide temporary relief but eventually the whole system will have to be removed

Always confirm suspicions by doing videourodynamcis and pay particular attention to the leak pressures.
Decompress the cuff before catheterization and then allow the cuff to refill before commencing bladder filling.

unstable. Abrams and Yande (1988) reported that while low-pressure instability (< 35 cmH$_2$O) often improves with corrective GSI surgery, higher-pressure instability rarely does.

Surgery for GSI is usually comparatively simpler than surgery for detrusor instability. Many surgeons, and patients, naturally favour the simpler operation first on the grounds that a proportion of patients, probably those with low-pressure instability, are improved and never require major surgery. However, in our experience a supporting operation for GSI in a patient with urodynamically proven instability often leads to severe urge incontinence, even though the stress leak is cured, and the subsequent need for augmentation after months of further suffering. This is usually extremely demoralizing for the patient. In some of these cases augmentation at the outset is undoubtedly the better option. It is simple to add a loose sling or a VOS to a cystoplasty procedure, although the addition may risk a higher likelihood of voiding difficulty and the need for CISC. It would therefore seem that there is no absolute solution and that the decision regarding surgery for any patient with combined instability and stress incontinence should include a careful explanation to the patient of the pros and cons of each approach.

SURGERY FOR VAGINAL PROLAPSE

Careful clinical examination of the patient presenting with symptoms of urinary dysfunction may reveal various degrees of prolapse of the pelvic organs into the vagina. Pelvic floor failure in one compartment is often accompanied by weakness or deficiency, if not complete failure, in another compartment. If there is significant uterine descent, with the uterus extending to the vaginal introitus or further, then surgical correction is inevitably required and can be performed as part of a urinary incontinence procedure or as a separate surgical intervention. A description of the techniques used for assessment and classification of prolapse can be found in Chapter 3. For simplicity, prolapse can be thought of as first, second or third degree or complete as shown in Fig. 6.39.

Anterior vaginal wall descent

Two types of anterior vaginal wall prolapse are recognized. The first is due to lateral fascial weakness with resultant descent of the whole bladder base, while the other is central weakness with normal lateral support and herniation of the central bladder base (Fig. 6.40). It is also important to recognize that some patients can present with a marked degree of vaginal wall descent without any evidence of detrusor instability or stress urinary incontinence. Correction of a central anatomical defect by anterior colporrhaphy can resolve the presenting problem of a vaginal lump but cause detrusor instability or

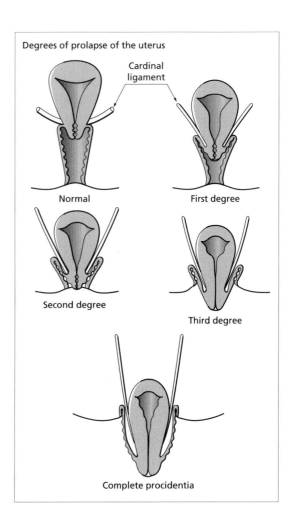

Fig. 6.39 A simple
classification of prolapse.

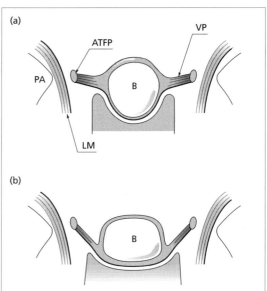

Fig. 6.40 The distinction
between (a) a central anterior
wall defect (upward pressure in
the lateral fornices does not
alter the appearance of the
prolapse) and (b) a lateral
fascial defect (upward pressure
in the lateral fornices causes the
prolapse to disappear).

stress urinary incontinence. Any dissection of the anterior vaginal wall disrupts the autonomic nerve supply to the bladder base, bladder neck and urethra. There is also disruption of the blood supply and venous return from the area that may be sufficient to modify the neurological control of the bladder and the closure pressure of the urethra. However, it is not possible to predict this side-effect of surgery and, although uncommon, patients should be aware of the possibility. Mild to moderate degrees of anterior vaginal wall descent are corrected at the time of surgery for urinary incontinence without any specific additional dissection. This is particularly true of procedures that elevate the bladder neck and bladder base, such as Burch colposuspension and VOS. A sling procedure can be accompanied by an anterior colporrhaphy and this means that any degree of central anterior vaginal wall descent can be corrected during surgery to correct incontinence.

The standard anterior colporrhaphy is not a very successful method of controlling urinary incontinence and can only be justified if there is significant anterior vaginal wall descent and the patient is made aware that further surgery may well be required to fully control her urinary incontinence. The procedure involves laying open the anterior vaginal wall using a midline incision. The vaginal wall is dissected free of the underlying pelvic fascia, which is then plicated using absorbable sutures. The number of sutures inserted depends on the size of the defect. Specific sutures placed at the level of the bladder neck raise and support the bladder neck (Kelly's sutures). Plication sutures placed between the bladder neck and external urethral meatus may cause urethral obstruction. When a large defect is present the vaginal skin will have been stretched, so that after repair of the fascial layer some vaginal skin may be redundant and need to be excised. In principle it is wise not to remove very much of this redundant vaginal skin. The anterior vaginal wall should be closed with interrupted vertical mattress sutures and over the next 4–6 weeks the vaginal skin returns to its normal conformation. Removal of too much skin may result in excessive scarring of the anterior vaginal wall and abnormal narrowing of the vaginal cross-sectional diameter. Patients with recurrent herniation of the anterior vaginal wall should be considered for a retropubic approach or a repeat vaginal approach with the interposition of a Prolene mesh between the plicated pelvic fascia and vaginal skin. Our own short-term results with mesh used in this location are encouraging, although no long-term results are yet available. Any surgery through the vagina may be accompanied by infection and for this reason great care should be employed when using non-absorbable materials.

Lateral fascial defects are recognized at operation because upward pressure in the lateral vaginal fornices causes the vaginal prolapse to disappear. Anterior colporrhaphy is illogical in these patients as it approximates two layers of intrinsically weak tissue under the bladder base, providing no effective long-term support. A more logical method is to perform a retropubic approach

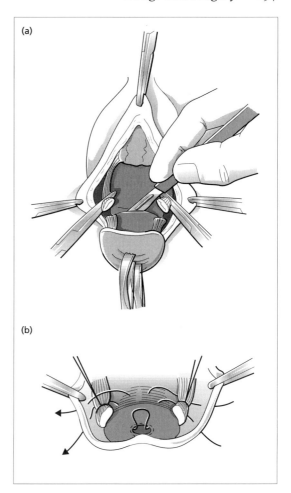

Fig. 6.41 Manchester repair:
(a) amputation of the cervix;
(b) vaginal closure and fixation
of uterosacral ligament in front
of the cervical stump.

and plicate the defect in the endopelvic fascia or to place Raz-type sutures into the middle and upper thirds of the vagina creating a six-point suspension (see Fig. 6.28). The choice between these two procedures depends on whether a suprapubic or vaginal approach to correct incontinence is being carried out.

Manchester repair (amputation of cervix plus anterior repair)

Descent of the cervix and uterus through the vagina to the vaginal introitus is usually dealt with by vaginal hysterectomy; however, under some circumstances the uterus itself may be normally positioned but accompanied by abnormal elongation of the cervix and cervical canal. This condition can be surgically managed using a combination of anterior colporrhaphy and amputation of the cervix, including shortening of uterosacral ligaments and anteversion of the uterus by suturing the ligaments in front of the cervical canal (Fig. 6.41). This procedure has the merit of preserving the uterus for future fertility in younger women but is no longer commonly employed.

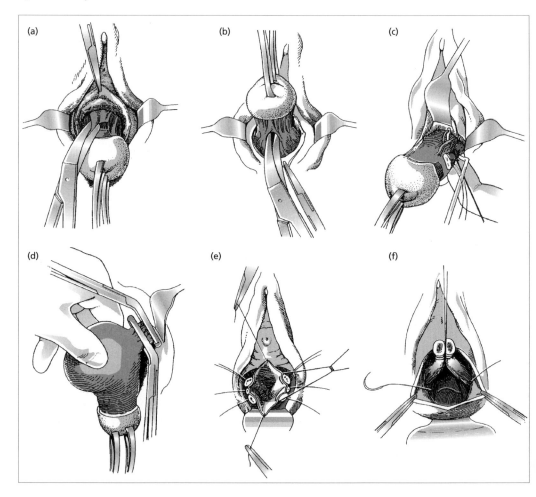

Fig. 6.42 Vaginal hysterectomy: (a) division of the 'cervicovesical' ligament anteriorly;
(b) opening the pouch of Douglas posteriorly; (c) ligation of the uterine vessels laterally as the
uterus is prolapsed further into the vagina; (d) clamping the tubo-ovarian pedicles; (e) closure of
the posterior peritoneal defect; (f) closing the enterocoele gap. From Monaghan, J.M. (1986),
with permission.

Vaginal hysterectomy

The standard vaginal hysterectomy may be accompanied by an anterior or
posterior colporrhaphy or is performed as a single procedure (Fig. 6.42). It
involves opening the vaginal skin and circumscribing the cervix at the level of
the anterior and posterior fornix. The uterovesical pouch of peritoneum is
opened. The pouch of Douglas is similarly opened and the uterus removed
by sequential clamps placed on either side of the uterus, working up from
the uterosacral and cardinal ligaments, through the lower broad ligament
uterine vessels to the upper broad ligament. The ovaries can be removed at

the same time and this should be considered in any woman over the age of 45. Additional specialized clamps and vaginal wall retractors facilitate oophorectomy. Trends in vaginal surgery are gradually changing and there is a tendency to no longer close the peritoneal cavity. However, it is important to identify an enterocoele sac and dissect this at the time of the hysterectomy. Once the enterocoele sac has been reflected, the uterosacral and cardinal ligaments should be brought together in the midline and the posterior compartment to the vaginal vault further supported by plication of the uterosacral ligaments laterally into the midline.

Posterior colporrhaphy

Defects of the posterior vaginal wall may or may not be accompanied by rectoanal dysfunction and faecal incontinence. If these are present it is essential to fully investigate these symptoms before surgery is planned (see Chapter 3). The clinical differentiation between an enterocoele and high rectocoele is sometimes difficult but an enterocoele should always be considered when repairing the proximal (upper) portion of the posterior vaginal wall. Failure to recognize the enterocoele sac results in recurrence of posterior compartment prolapse. The enterocoele sac should be closed as high as possible, with redundant peritoneum excised (Fig. 6.43). If a vaginal approach has been employed to repair the rectocoele, absorbable sutures placed into the puborectalis on either side will draw this tissue in front of the rectum, creating a definite supporting layer between the rectum and the vagina. If a transperineal approach has been employed, these sutures are more difficult to place and the rectum may be plicated longitudinally. There is insufficient evidence available to determine whether a transanal, transperineal or transvaginal approach is more appropriate for the correction of an uncomplicated rectocoele, although it is interesting to note that surgical procedures employing different principles may achieve broadly similar results.

It is important to be aware of potential vaginal scarring and narrowing when a vaginal route is employed for any surgical procedure and great care needs to be taken in sexually active women to avoid a hypocompliant vagina. In addition, tightening the posterior vaginal wall and underlying structures may cause descent of the anterior vaginal wall and bladder neck.

Posterior vaginal introitus

The vagina before childbirth is a continent structure: the anterior and posterior vaginal walls lie together with a potential space between. After childbirth the vagina may or may not remain continent and gynaecologists clearly recognize the presence of a gaping vaginal introitus (deficient perineum). The

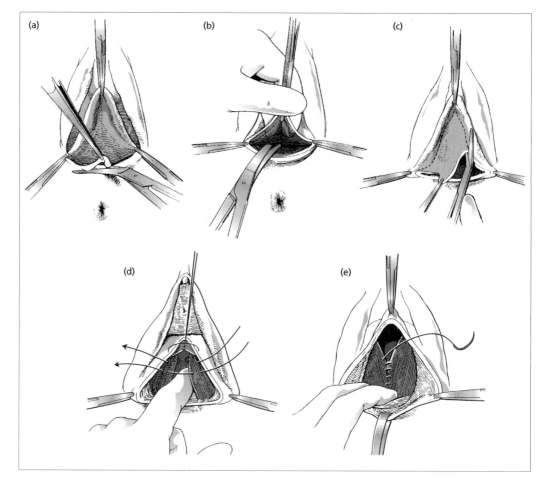

Fig. 6.43 Posterior repair: (a) excision of the perineal scar tissue; (b) exposure of the rectovaginal plane; (c) excision of vaginal skin; (d) and (e) plication of the levators/pararectal/paravaginal fascia. From Monaghan, J.M. (1986), with permission.

deficiency may or may not cause sensation of vaginal prolapse and dissatisfaction with vaginal intercourse. We postulate that the integrity of the tissue lying between the vaginal introitus and the anal canal (perineal body) acts as an important support structure for the bladder base and bladder neck.

Great care needs to be employed when repairing the perineum in order to avoid narrowing the vaginal introitus too much, thereby causing dyspareunia. Access to the perineal tissues is achieved through a transverse incision, following the curve of the vaginal introitus, between two tissue forceps that when opposed achieve appropriate reconstruction of the vaginal introitus. The procedure may be performed with or without removal of any vaginal skin after exposure of the plane between the vagina and the rectum. The

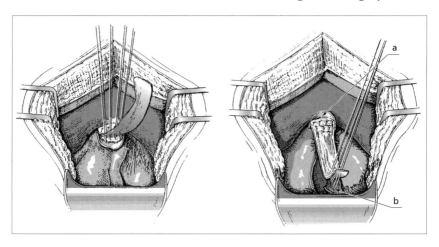

Fig. 6.44 Sacrocolpopexy: a sling of rectus fascia or prosthetic material is sewn to the vaginal vault at one end (a) and suspended from the presacral fascia at the other (b) to support the prolapsed vaginal vault. From Monaghan, J.M. (1986), with permission.

perineal body is reformed by placing lateral stitches into the levator ani and puborectalis, avoiding the rectum (Fig. 6.43d,e). The lower vaginal wall is repaired with a continuous locking suture that finishes at the introital margin. The perineal skin is best repaired using an absorbable subcuticular suture. The perineoplasty can be combined with a rectocoele repair or performed separately. If the supporting sutures are placed too laterally then a constriction ring will be formed in the vagina, usually at the level of the lower third and upper two-thirds of the vagina or 3 cm inside the vaginal introitus.

Sacrocolpopexy/sacrospinous fixation

The procedures so far described all tend to narrow and scar the vagina, which is normally a compliant organ. It is possible to repair the posterior vaginal wall defect without using a vaginal incision via either a transanal or laparoscopic approach. An alternative is to resuspend the vaginal vault on either the sacrum or sacrospinous ligament. This procedure can be performed with or without the presence of a uterus and is most appropriate for those patients who have vaginal vault prolapse after hysterectomy. Sacrocolpopexy involves the attachment of the vaginal vault to the median ligament of the sacrum, the gap being bridged with non-absorbable tape or a strip of rectus fascia harvested as described for sling procedures (Fig. 6.44). The vagina itself is not usually sufficiently long to be approximated directly to the median ligament of the sacrum. However, the vagina can be attached directly to the sacrospinous ligament and this is achieved through a transvaginal

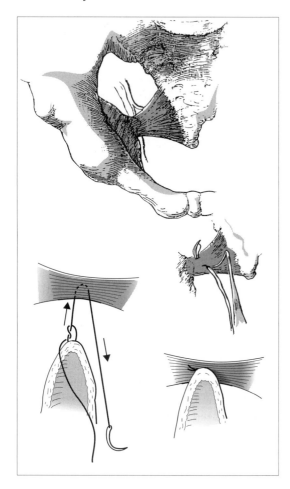

Fig. 6.45 Sacrospinous fixation: through a posterior vaginal dissection the sacrospinous ligament is exposed and a suture used to fix the highest part of the vagina to the ligament on one side only.

incision (Fig. 6.45). The rectum is reflected posteriorly and the ischial spine identified and sacrospinous ligament cleaned. Two sutures are placed through the ligament and drawn down into the vagina in such a way that when tightened approximate the vaginal vault to the sacrospinous ligament. The procedure is performed on one side only (most conveniently the right sacrospinous ligament for a right-handed surgeon). Support of the vaginal vault in this way tensions the fascia on the anterior and posterior vaginal wall and may be sufficient to deal with a small cystocoele or rectocoele. Specific consideration needs to be given to the presence of an enterocoele at the time of sacrospinous fixation.

SURGERY FOR COMPLEX INCONTINENCE PROBLEMS

Often an incontinence problem comprises more than just one type of dysfunction. In these cases careful urodynamic and pelvic floor evaluation is vital and planning of surgery needs to incorporate more than just an appreciation of the physiological or anatomical defect. Some of these problems can undoubtedly be managed by one specialist, whereas others require training in all aspects of pelvic surgery. Such broadly trained pelvic surgeons are still a rarity and a cooperative team approach is more likely to be required. Complex problems include:

- combined bladder and urethral dysfunction;
- associated bowel dysfunction and urinary incontinence;
- complex prolapse associated with incontinence;
- patients who have had multiple previous operations for incontinence;
- patients with congenital neuropathy and those with degenerative neurological disease;
- those with bladder disease such as interstitial cystitis, tuberculosis or post-radiation cystitis or contracted hypocompliant bladders associated with neuropathy;
- patients in whom preservation of renal function is of primary importance, e.g. transplant recipients.

In some of these it is possible to correct the functional abnormality by addressing each of the elements of the problem in turn. For example, 'reconstruction' may involve an abdominal rectopexy and sacrocolpopexy for rectorectal intussusception and vault prolapse, a sling to deal with intrinsic sphincter weakness and a cystoplasty or myectomy to deal with detrusor instability. All of these can be performed at the same time but necessitate careful preoperative evaluation, counselling and planning of the surgery.

The options for urinary tract reconstruction are, essentially, always the same but are influenced greatly by the circumstances of the case. The choice lies between orthotopic reconstruction (bladder reconstruction with preservation of the normal bladder outlet) or urinary diversion, which can be either incontinent or continent. The choice depends more on the underlying disease, general fitness, intelligence and motivation than it does on the precise urodynamic abnormality being corrected.

Orthotopic bladder reconstruction

The aims of orthotopic reconstruction are to (i) provide a good-capacity low-pressure reservoir for urine storage; (ii) protect the upper urinary tracts if possible by preventing reflux; (iii) provide urinary continence during filling but normal voiding through the urethra and complete emptying of the neobladder; (iv) offer the highest level of independence for the patient; and (v) achieve these objectives with the lowest morbidity, complication and reoperation rates. The latter two objectives are crucial to the choice of surgery. The obese wheelchair-bound patient who works in an office where

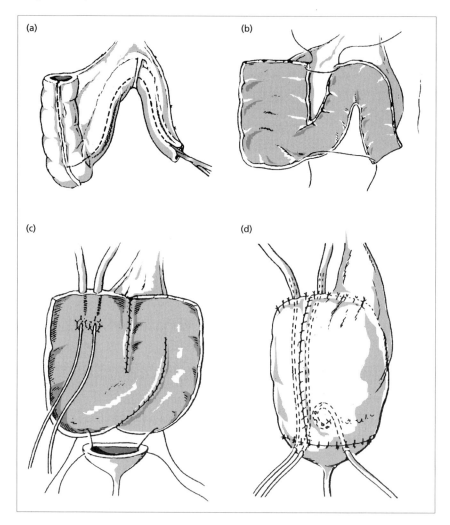

Fig. 6.46 (a) The Mainz pouch: an orthotopic bladder reconstruction using the right colon and terminal ileum fashioned as an S-shaped pouch (b). The ureters are reimplanted through submucosal tunnels in the posterior wall of the caecum (c). The pouch may lie most comfortably in the normal anatomical position, as shown (d), or the caecum may reach the urethra more easily if turned upside down.

there is no disabled toilet will not be grateful for the provision of a 'normal' bladder if he or she is unable to empty the bladder at appropriate times. Similarly, the patient with rapidly degenerative neurological disease would not be well served by such a solution.

The ingenuity of surgeons in designing new and varied methods of sewing a bag and a couple of valves from a tube of bowel is quite remarkable. Common types of orthotopic reconstruction are illustrated in Figs 6.46 and 6.47. Even more remarkable is that many surgeons appear always to perform

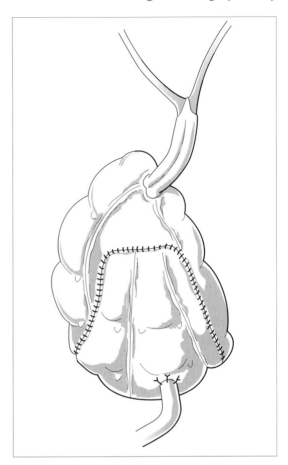

Fig. 6.47 The Studer
neobladder: the whole right
colon is detubularized and used
to create the pouch. The ureters
are implanted into an
isoperistaltic ileal segment and
reflux is prevented both by
peristalsis and the ileocaecal
valve.

the same operation in the same way. In our experience the ease with which
one particular loop of bowel can be reconfigured and laid into the pelvis
varies from patient to patient and it is vital to have a number of surgical tricks
up one's sleeve. This does not make for a 'clean' operative series but does
mean that solutions are tailored more to the individual's particular problems. However, certain basic principles can be applied and these have been
summarized by Woodhouse as the *Mitrofanoff principle* (Table 6.10).

The reservoir. If the bladder is simply unstable, cystoplasty augmentation or
even myectomy may be sufficient to create a low-pressure reservoir. However, patients with severe neuropathy with thickened bladders or patients
with diseased bladders (radiotherapy, interstitial cystitis) should undergo at
least subtotal supratrigonal cystectomy and substitution cystoplasty or, if the
whole bladder is affected by disease, total cystectomy and bladder substitution. Substitution can be achieved by using a 'pouch' of intestine; this can be

The reservoir
Must be large capacity
High compliance/low pressure
Non-refluxing ureters ideally
Options
   Bladder
   Augmented bladder (ileum or colon)
   Neobladder pouch (ileal or colonic pouch, tubular or detubularized)

The outlet
Orthotopic
   Normal urethra
   Labial skin tube
Catheterizable stoma
   Appendix
   Ureter
   Tapered ileum
   Skin tube
   Fallopian tube

The continence mechanism
Urethral sphincter (if it is normal)
Artificial sphincter
Implanted conduit
   Submucosally tunnelled, e.g. appendix
   Flap valve/nipple, e.g. Koch pouch, Indiana pouch
   Hydraulic system, e.g. Benchekroun

Table 6.10 The Mitrofanoff principle. The following three considerations must be dealt with in any bladder reconstruction. Any combination of solutions is possible but the principles must be fulfilled.

constructed in countless ways using, for example, ileum, ileum plus caecum, or colon. There has been much debate about whether the pouch should be detubularized in order to create U-, N- or W-shaped configurations. The theoretical advantage is that increasing numbers of folds more nearly approximate a sphere, thus resulting in the best capacity for a given surface area (Fig. 6.48). In addition, the effect of contractions due to circular muscle of the bowel wall is diminished and better compliance results. Unfortunately, in practice the theoretical physical advantages outlined above are not always achieved.

Tubular segments of right colon have been used extensively for bladder substitution by Mundy (1993) and shown to provide better pouch emptying, although higher rates of night-time incontinence are caused by higher resting pressures. Most surgeons now feel that a detubularized pouch with high compliance requiring self-catheterization for emptying is a preferable outcome.

Supratrigonal substitution allows the ureters to be left untouched, while total substitution requires reimplantation of both ureters into the pouch wall. Paradoxically, however, the rates of reflux after supratrigonal cystoplasty are

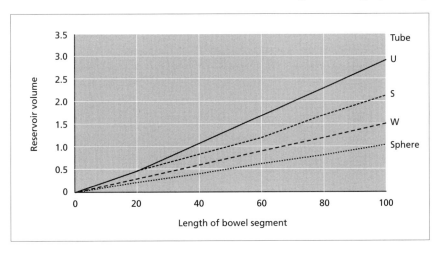

Fig. 6.48 The principle that, with increasing numbers of folds in the reconfiguration of bowel segments to form a pouch, the volumes achieved for a given length of bowel more nearly approximate the geometry of a sphere.

higher, presumably because of distortion of the intravesical segment of the ureter during suturing of the cystoplasty, while with total substitution the ureters are consciously reimplanted.

The outlet. Continence of the bladder outlet can be managed using any of the procedures already described for increasing urethral resistance. The choice depends very much on the preoperative evaluation. An AUS can be inserted at the same time as a cystoplasty, or alternatively a bladder neck suspension or sling can be performed. In this situation the AUS has the advantage that natural voiding through the urethra may be achieved, where-as supportive or sling procedures are much more likely to result in self-catheterization post-operatively. However, this advantage is achieved at the cost of a higher risk of mechanical failure, infection and erosion, etc. (see pp. 188–193). Later placement of an AUS cuff via a suprapubic approach is likely to be exceptionally difficult when a cystoplasty has been performed. Thus if there is any suspicion preoperatively that the sphincter needs to be augmented then the cuff component alone should be placed at the time of cystoplasty and left sealed so that it is available for future use. In its empty state the cuff actually increases outlet resistance slightly in much the same way as a very loose sling procedure and is often effective in controlling stress leakage without the other components ever being required.

Incontinent urinary diversion

Theoretically, one of the simplest methods of bladder diversion is urethral closure and suprapubic vesicostomy (Fig. 6.50). This technique has been

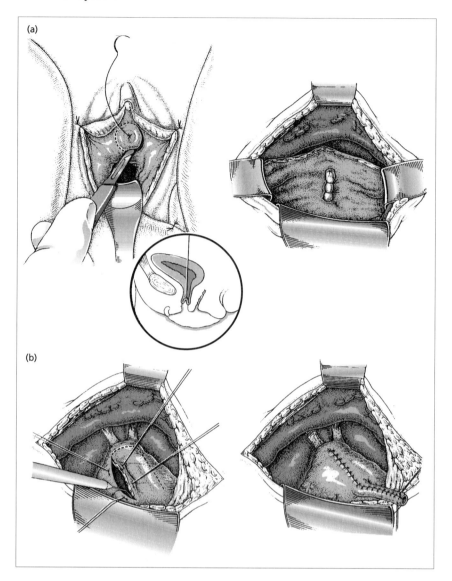

Fig. 6.49 Bladder neck closure and suprapubic vesicostomy: (a) the urethra is circumcised and drawn upwards into the bladder; (b) an anterior bladder wall flap is used to create a tube that will reach the skin. From Mundy (1993).

particularly recommended for women with multiple sclerosis. Provided that the urethral tissues are fairly healthy and the patient is not too obese then the operation is quicker and easier than any other form of diversion. However, the urethra is often badly eroded and this precludes adequate closure. Also most patients with multiple sclerosis have a hyperreflexic bladder and this simply results in incontinence through the vesicostomy instead of the urethra. The usefulness of the method is therefore limited.

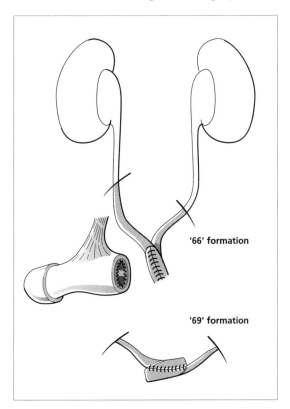

Fig. 6.50 Conventional ileal conduit with ureters joined in '66' or '69' formation ready for anastomosis to the ileal segment. The distal end has been everted and will form a stoma in the right iliac fossa.

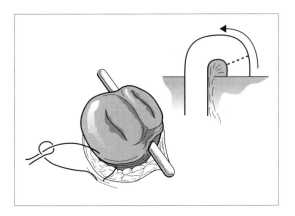

Fig. 6.51 The technique of loop ileostomy (Turnbull) is useful if there is a thick mesentery. A loop is formed and the distal antimesenteric border is incised and folded back to expose the proximal lumen. The end-result is little different to a conventional stoma.

Bricker (1952) first described the creation of the ileal conduit to create an incontinent abdominal stoma for urinary diversion. The technique has evolved little since that time. Variations include alternative methods of anastomosing the ureters to the ileal segment (Fig. 6.50), the loop ileostomy (Fig. 6.51) and the use of jejunal or colonic segments. The operation is technically simple compared with other reconstructive options and offers reliability and a low likelihood of reoperation. However, there are significant complications, including parastomal hernia, stomal prolapse and fistula, infection and stone formation, and apparent upper tract deterioration over several years, which may be related to the fact that the bowel segment used is tubular, develops high segmental pressures during peristalsis and is usually refluxing (Singh *et al.* 1997). Ileal conduits should be short and are best laid through the mesentery of the small bowel, which facilitates a tension-free stoma and the shortest length possible.

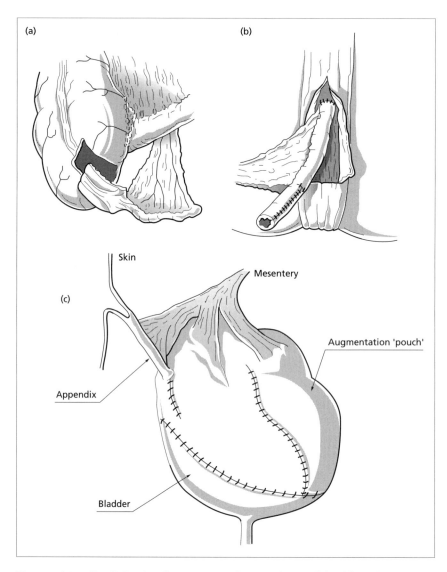

Fig. 6.52 Appendiceal Mitrofanoff operation: (a) the appendix is mobilized from the caecum on its mesentery and (b) implanted into the bowel patch/pouch; (c) it provides a catheterizable conduit to an augmented pouch.

Continent urinary diversion

As described under the Mitrofanoff principle above, continent urinary diversion follows the same rules but simply places the outlet on the abdominal wall rather than using the urethra. If the bladder itself is to be sacrificed then the stoma can be placed virtually anywhere on the abdominal wall in order to facilitate catheterization. A huge number of different techniques have now been described for creating a continent urinary reservoir and the literature is swamped with a plethora of information about each one, although very little has been based on properly randomized studies. Thus it is difficult to decide which type of operation to choose as each has its enthusiastic proponents and vigorous opponents.

Virtually any intra-abdominal tube can be used to create a stoma that can be catheterized. The commonest used are the appendix, tapered small bowel and ureter (in association with a transuretero-ureterostomy). The appendix, provided it can be catheterized, is the most reliable of these and can almost always be made to lie in a position that both implants generously into the neobladder and yet reaches the skin. Tapered tubes work well but are more likely to lead to difficulties with catheterization that may need further surgery (often major) to rectify.

The continence mechanism can be created in one of two ways. A flap valve mechanism can be fashioned, where the catheterized tube is implanted in such a way that any bladder filling results in compression of the tube within the bladder wall tunnel (e.g. appendiceal Mitrofanoff, Figs 6.52 & 6.53). Alternatively, the mechanism may be hydraulic, where the filling pressure of the bladder itself compresses the catheterized stoma (e.g. Koch pouch).

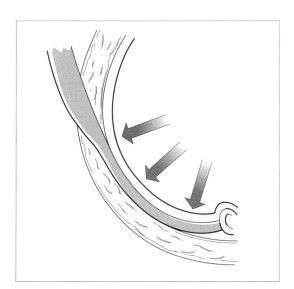

Fig. 6.53 The appendix is implanted through a submucosal tunnel, creating a flap valve for continence.

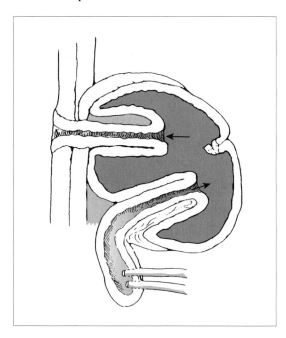

Fig. 6.54 The Koch pouch uses approximately 40 cm of ileum to create a pouch with two intussuscepted nipple valves, one for antireflux and the other for continence of the catheterizable stoma.

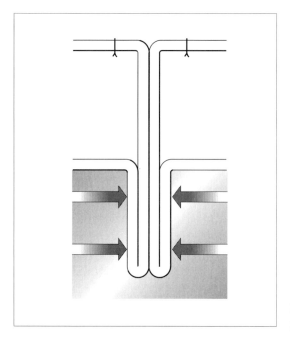

Fig. 6.55 The hydraulic principle of the nipple valve.

Failure of the continence mechanism is one of the commonest early complications of these operations. Because of their proven track record, the most widely used methods are the appendiceal Mitrofanoff procedure, the Koch pouch (Figs 6.54 & 6.55) and the Indiana pouch (Fig. 6.56).

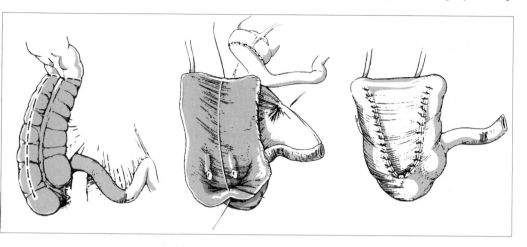

Fig. 6.56 Formation of the Indiana pouch depends on a right colonic pouch with implanted ureters. The terminal ileum and ileocaecal valve are used for the continent catheterizable stoma. For Hinman jnr (1989), with permission.

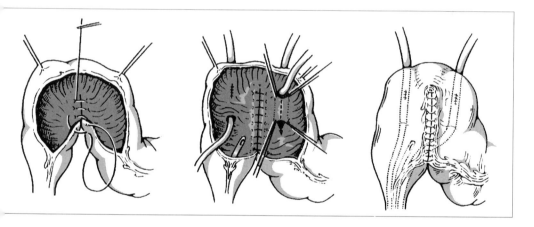

Fig. 6.57 Rectosigmoid neobladder: a low-pressure pouch is created from detubularization of the rectosigmoid and the ureters are tunnelled to prevent reflux.

Rectal bladder. The earliest form of urinary diversion was ureterosigmoidostomy, which relied for continence on control of the anal sphincter. However, the operation has fallen from favour because of problems with pyelonephritis, hyperchloraemic acidosis, incontinence and a high incidence of adenocarcinoma at the anastomotic line. New techniques of ureteric implantation, antibiotics, better suture materials and development of pouches with low-pressure urodynamics have led to a resurgence of interest, particularly in parts of the world where stoma bags are either unavailable or culturally unacceptable. The sigmoid rectal pouch uses a side-to-side linking of the sigmoid posteriorly, a nipple or submucosal tunnel implantation of the ureters and anterior formation of a rectosigmoid pouch (Fig. 6.57). While this obviously

Table 6.11 Summary of outcomes for urinary diversion.

	Ileal conduit	Neobladder	Continent diversion
Mortality (%)	1–14	1–6	2
Early complications (%)	28–49	7–17	16–50
Late complications (%)	20–52	15–24	16–38
Reoperation (%)	10	9–15	13–69
Incontinence (%)	58	Day: 3; Night: 80	18

requires a good sphincter beforehand, authors have reported high continence rates. Repeated surveillance with colonoscopy and barium examination is essential for these patients.

Choice of reconstruction

The debate about which reconstruction is best also revolves around reported complication rates. These are highly dependent on surgical technique so it is unwise to extrapolate the experience of others to one's own practice. Many individual series have been presented and usually reflect the bias of the authors. A number of 'comparisons' of technique can be found in the literature but none are randomized trials so that the differences reflect as much about patient selection as they do about the particular techniques employed. Table 6.11 shows the continence, complication and reoperation rates collated from a Medline search of series with more than 200 orthotopic reconstructions or ileal conduits and more than 50 continent diversions. There seems little doubt that the complications of continent diversion, while numerically little different to those of ileal conduit or orthotopic reconstruction, are usually more complex and difficult to resolve. The Koch pouch seems to be fraught with more problems than the appendiceal diversion or the Indiana (tapered ileum) pouch. Orthotopic reconstruction, provided the patient is sufficiently independent to use his or her own urethra for voiding, provides the best functional outcome, with lower complication rates than continent diversion but higher rates than ileal conduit.

Many issues need to be resolved: ideal pouch geometry, continence mechanism, prevention of reflux, and stoma characteristics with minimal complications. In the planning of any reconstruction the surgeon has to consider several important points, some of which are preoperative and others perioperative.
- What is the basic functional defect that needs to be corrected?
- What are the patient's prime objectives: to protect renal function, to be dry using the simplest method or to achieve maximum functional and social independence whatever the cost?

- What is the patient's physical and emotional fitness for surgery and recovery or the possibility of future surgery?
- What needs to be removed?
- What is available for reconstruction?

All these variables provide a multitude of solutions and cleverly devised operations for any one individual. It is vital for any surgeon who takes on such problems to have a full appreciation of the various techniques that can be employed, an ability to perform them and the flexibility to change his or her mind at the time of surgery and adapt to unpredictable circumstances. The patient's wishes and the prime objectives of surgery are paramount at all times and outweigh the natural desire of an enthusiastic surgeon for one particular operation or another. The patient with degenerative multiple sclerosis is not well served by a continent diversion, however beautifully created, if within the year she needs further surgery for catheterization problems and within 2 years can no longer self-catheterize or remains incontinent of faeces because nobody thought to address the bowel problem as well as the bladder problem.

Those whose surgical experience or facilities means that they can only offer a limited range of the surgical options available should not undertake this sort of work. To do so will inevitably result in compromises being made for a patient where a better surgical solution existed. The decisions should ideally be made in full discussion with the patient and/or their carer or closest relatives. A nurse counsellor always brings a degree of objectivity to decision-making, which can otherwise be greatly influenced by a persuasive surgeon.

POORLY EMPTYING BLADDERS

The bladder may empty ineffectively because of bladder outlet obstruction, which may be mechanical or functional in origin, or inadequate detrusor contraction; both situations can coexist. Incontinence in such patients is usually improved by improving their bladder emptying. It follows that where there is mechanical obstruction, for instance due to prostatic hypertrophy, relief of obstruction is required. Where there is functional obstruction caused by detrusor sphincter dyssynergia the obstruction can be relieved by endoscopic sphincterotomy, although this increases incontinence rather than decreasing it. The indication for sphincterotomy is to protect renal function and continence is usually a casualty of this decision.

If detrusor contractions are poorly sustained or inadequate there are two manoeuvres that may help. In patients with suprasacral cord injuries who have poorly sustained hyperreflexic contractions, implantation of a sacral anterior root stimulator has provided an effective means of bladder emptying.

Electrodes are placed around selected sacral nerve roots (S2–S4) in the dural canal. These are connected to a remote radio receiver implanted into the chest wall. The patient is taught to hold a radio transmitter over the implanted receiver. Rapid, repetitive, square-wave signals induce an electrical stimulus in the electrodes sufficient to stimulate the nerve roots and result in bladder contraction. Bladder emptying occurs during the relaxation phase when bladder pressure temporarily exceeds intraurethral pressure. Careful adjustment of stimulation parameters is vital to the success of this technique. However, root stimulation is painful and so the procedure is really only of value to patients with complete cord lesions, no sensation and good dexterity.

In patients with multiple sclerosis who have detrusor sphincter dyssynergia and loss of volitional control of voiding, a suprapubic pressure-sensitive vibrator has been developed at the National Hospital for Nervous Diseases. Mechanical stimulation at the appropriate frequency facilitates a bladder contraction with relative sphincter weakness, thus improving emptying. The pressure-sensitive pad can be activated by patients with quite limited manual dexterity. Our preliminary experience with this device has been encouraging.

For all patients in whom emptying is inadequate one option is to learn CISC, which has revolutionized the management of poorly emptying bladders. Not only does the technique relieve overflow incontinence but it may also restore renal function and alleviate persistent urine infection by the elimination of residual urine or upper tract dilatation. While good manual dexterity, intelligence and relatively normal anatomy are an advantage in learning, the converse is not necessarily so. We have taught patients with learning difficulties and others in their nineties, some blind or severely disabled with rheumatoid arthritis or multiple sclerosis, to perform the technique successfully and thus avoid permanent catheterization. Teaching the technique requires skill and patience but also determination to succeed. Severe adduction deformity of the hips and urethral stricture or false passage are about the only absolute contraindications.

Surgery for anorectal incontinence

This section is concerned with the principles of anal sphincter reconstruction and the current techniques at the disposal of the surgeon for the achievement of this goal. Some standard and proven operations are described in detail as it is the responsibility of surgeons who wish to establish an incontinence practice to understand the indications, principles and techniques for anal sphincter augmentation. The term 'anorectal incontinence' (ARI), as opposed to 'faecal incontinence', has been used deliberately because the constant leakage of mucus and severe urgency may be just as incapacitating to the patient as the passive leakage of solid stool. In ARI, one of the major problems in selecting patients for surgery and comparing the results of different series has been the lack of a uniform continence scoring system. The Cleveland Clinic Incontinence Scoring System has done much to correct these indiscrepancies and is recommended (see Chapter 3).

It should be remembered that ARI may be only one manifestation of pelvic floor failure. The coloproctologist has to appreciate that ARI may coexist with other disorders of anorectal function, such as obstructive defaecation and rectal prolapse (see Chapter 2), as well as urogenital dysfunction. Hence surgery for ARI has to be tailored to other anorectal problems because the surgical correction of one set of symptoms may often exacerbate others.

It is against this background that the specific procedures for ARI need to be considered. The aims of surgery are to reconstruct an intact muscle ring in those patients in whom this has been disrupted by anal surgery or obstetric trauma. A further aim in patients with neurogenic incontinence but an intact sphincter has been to re-establish the anorectal angle. A final group of operations involves using transposed muscle, synthetic materials or artificial sphincters to replace lost or irreparably damaged muscle. It may also be prudent to correct causes of obstructive defaecation, such as symptomatic rectocoele, at the same time.

GENERAL POINTS

Some general points apply to several of the operations described in this section. Preoperative measures include full mechanical bowel preparation and prophylactic antibiotics, such as metronidazole and a cephalosporin. Although some surgeons prefer the prone jacknife position, it is our practice to position the patient in the lithotomy position. In any event, the coccyx should be easily palpable as it provides a major landmark. External sphincter injury due to previous anal surgery can be situated anywhere on the circumference of the anus and technique has to be modified accordingly. The operative field should be widely infiltrated with 1 in 200 000 adrenaline solution to reduce bleeding and assist in identification of planes (Fig. 6.58).

Postoperatively, the surgeon may decide to employ temporary faecal diversion using a sigmoid loop colostomy, fashioned by an open, trephine or laparoscopic technique depending on the patient's physique and surgical preference. The patient requires adequate pain relief and a urinary catheter; if not faecally diverted, an elemental diet may be instituted for 7 days followed by stool softeners. Complications are suprisingly uncommon, although bleeding may occasionally occur and some degree of wound infection is not uncommon (Fig. 6.59). Complete dehiscence is fortunately rare.

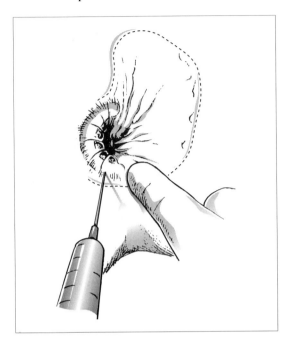

Fig. 6.58 Prior to any anorectal reconstruction it is important to infiltrate the operative area with 1 in 200 000 adrenaline solution. From Mann & Glass (1997), with permission.

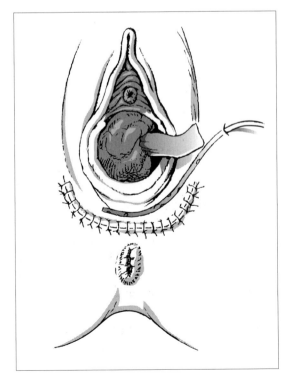

Fig. 6.59 Wound collection is prevented after anterior levatorplasty by insertion of a suction drain and a vaginal pack. From Mann & Glass (1997), with permission.

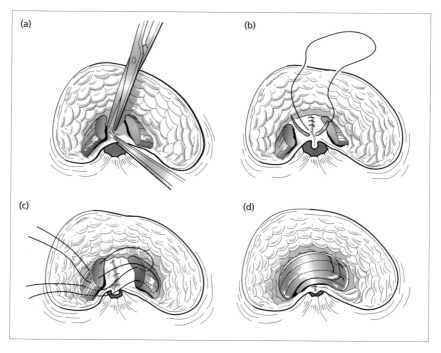

Fig. 6.60 Anal sphincter repair/sphincteroplasty: (a) the separated ends of the external sphincter have been exposed through an anterior perianal incision and are being freed up by sharp dissection; (b) the internal sphincter is imbricated; (c,d) the external sphincter is overlapped with interrupted sutures. Fibrous tissue is left on the cut ends to assist in holding the sutures.

ANAL SPHINCTER REPAIR (SPHINCTEROPLASTY)

The indications for this procedure include disruption of the external anal sphincter due to obstetric or other trauma. The operation may be performed at any time after the injury once it has been recognized. Careful evaluation of the site of injury preoperatively using anal endosonography is mandatory and has superseded electromyographic mapping.

Through an anterior perianal incision the ischiorectal fossae are entered on both sides, avoiding damage to the neurovascular bundle (Fig. 6.60). The intersphincteric plane is entered in order to separate the internal and external components of the sphincter. This has the advantage of allowing access to the supralevator space for performing a concurrent levatorplasty. The internal sphincter is imbricated with absorbable monofilament sutures and the external sphincter repaired using an overlapping technique. If the repair has been performed correctly it is impossible to close the skin in the direction of the original incision and it may be necessary to leave the centre of the wound open to heal by secondary intention.

Most patients who undergo sphincter repair experience an improvement in continence, providing that the site of repair does not become infected and that there is minimal evidence of neuropathy in obstetric-related cases. The wide range of success reported is due in part to the relative proportions of patients with obstetric-related injury in each series. Other factors that adversely affect outcome include age, previous failed repair and length of time between injury and repair. In general, an excellent result can be anticipated in two-thirds of patients.

POSTANAL REPAIR

This operation was originally designed by Sir Alan Parks to recreate the anorectal angle by approximating and plicating the posterior 'slings' of the levators around the back of the rectum. Current evidence suggests that the procedure has no influence on this and probably works by increasing the functional length of the anal canal or possibly by improving anal canal sensation. The main indication for this operation includes neurogenic incontinence with an intact muscle ring.

The key to this operation lies in identifying the intersphincteric plane, which is most easily accomplished laterally on either side. The internal sphincter in these patients is often thin and atrophic and can be difficult to identify. Waldeyer's fascia is opened transversely by sharp dissection (Fig. 6.62) and the rectum lifted off the levator plate and lowered as far forwards as possible, as far as the ischial spines. A layered repair of the levator 'defect' is made with interrupted Prolene sutures, beginning as far anteriorly as possible and working posteriorly and finishing with a plication of the puborectalis and the external sphincter. It is usually not possible to approximate the most anterior parts of the levators. Wound infection and disruption remain the most serious complications and may be accompanied by failure of the repair. Haematoma, bruising and skin necrosis may also occur.

In the early postoperative period, continued incontinence is common due to pain and the use of laxatives. In those patients who achieve a satisfactory outcome, continence is apparent by 6–8 weeks after surgery. A successful outcome after postanal repair has been variously attributed to greater anal canal length, improved anal sensation, higher anal pressures, changes in tissue compliance after surgery and reconstitution of the anorectal angle. Many of these claims are now refuted and it is now believed that only the length of the high-pressure zone in the anal canal is improved by postanal repair. The effect of postanal repair on continence has been reported by several authors (Table 6.12). Early, enthusiastic results have not stood the test of time and it is suggested that failure is the result of continuing and progressive neurological damage to the pelvic floor muscles.

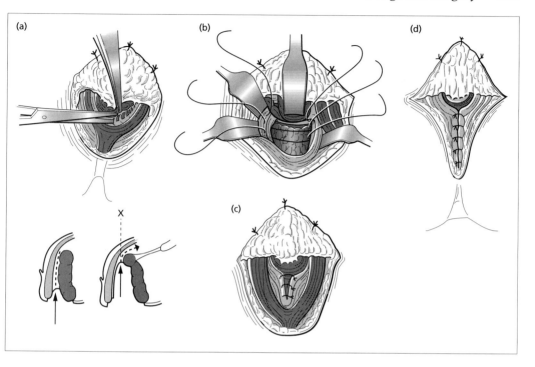

Fig. 6.61 Postanal repair. (a) A posterior horseshoe incision has been made and the skin flaps sewn over the anus. The intersphincteric plane (X) has been entered to expose Waldeyer's fascia, which is opened by sharp dissection for access to the supralevator space. (b) The levators are being drawn together with interrupted sutures starting high and anteriorly. (c) Usually the most anterior suture cannot be tightened and is left bow-stringed. (d) The more superficial layers of the levators are closed separately.

Table 6.12 Results of anal sphincter repair and postanal repair.

	Percentage of patients continent to solid and liquid stool	Percentage of patients continent only to solid stool	Percentage of patients no better
Anal sphincter repair (series with more than 30 patients)	25–85 (mean 59)	15–55 (mean 30)	5–20 (mean 11)
Total no. of patients	234	122	33
Postanal repair (series with 40 or more patients)	34–74 (mean 51)	12–57 (mean 23)	8–30 (mean 14)
Total no. of patients	256	127	83

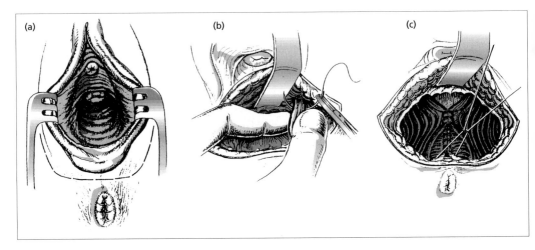

Fig. 6.62 Anterior levatorplasty: (a) the anterior perianal incision is used for access to the intersphincteric plane as described for anterior sphincter repair; (b) the highest and most anterior stich is inserted into the puborectalis on the left side; (c) the puborectalis has been drawn together and the external sphincter is being plicated. From Mann & Glass (1997), with permission.

ANTERIOR LEVATORPLASTY AND EXTERNAL SPHINCTER PLICATION

In patients with neurogenic incontinence the disappointing results of post-anal repair and the fact that this operation has no effect on the anorectal angle, whose role in maintaining continence remains open to question, have led some surgeons to adopt an anterior procedure. An added advantage of this approach is that rectocoele and obstetric injuries to the external sphincter can be dealt with at the same time.

Through an anterior perianal incision the vaginal wall is dissected off the external sphincter as far as the anorectal junction (Fig. 6.62). It is easy to identify this point because the dissection becomes more difficult and the planes less well defined than further caudally. There is a real danger of entering the anterior wall of the rectum here, particularly in patients with rectocoele where the rectal wall is often very thin and supporting fascial layers attenuated. The ischiorectal fossae are entered and the external sphincter separated from the anterior arches of the puborectalis. The supralevator compartment is entered via the intersphincteric plane. This is embryologically and anatomically correct and provides far greater access than the limited access provided by dissecting outside of the sphincters. In difficult circumstances, vertical division of the posterior vaginal wall allows easy access into the supralevator compartment and avoids unpleasant dissection in the region of the anorectal junction from below. Plication of the levator mechanism and external sphincter is accomplished under direct vision. Prior to skin closure one or two sutures approximating the anterior arches of the puborectalis complete the reconstructive procedure.

The immediate complications of this operation parallel those of sphincter repair. Unrecognized injury to the rectum may present with severe sepsis in the immediate postoperative period or the later development of a fistula. Adequate pain relief and avoidance of straining are of paramount importance in the immediate postoperative period. Although the long-term effects on continence are unknown, early reports of this operation indicate that they are at least as good as postanal repair (see Table 6.12). Clearly, longer-term series will answer this question.

TOTAL PELVIC FLOOR REPAIR

As a means of circumventing the problems of isolated repair of either the posterior or anterior levator mechanism, Keighley has described a procedure that essentially consists of a postanal repair and an anterior levatorplasty. The procedure was originally performed in two stages in a group of 14 patients who had poor results after postanal repair. More recently, a synchronous approach has been adopted and medium-term results indicate that outcomes are superior to those of postanal repair alone.

MUSCLE TRANSPOSITION

The object of these procedures is to augment the physically disrupted or neuropathic external sphincter and puborectalis with somatic muscle from the leg or gluteal region. Gracilis has been the most widely used muscle graft, although other authors have reported the use of gluteus maximus, sartorius and adductor longus. Puborectalis may also be employed though experience with this is limited. Recent developments with gracilis transposition include the use of bilateral grafts and the neostimulated graciloplasty, in which the muscle is converted from a fast-twitch to a slow-twitch muscle by continuous electrical stimulation, thereby allowing it to resist fatigue and maintain continuous contraction. The main indications for muscle transposition procedures include patients with incontinence due to failed previous repairs, extensive loss (> 50%) of external sphincter due to trauma or infection and congenital lesions of the anorectum in children.

Gracilis transposition

The results of graciloplasty (Fig. 6.63) are variable and difficult to interpret because of the small numbers of patients in any individual series and the lack of objective preoperative data concerning pelvic floor function. Nevertheless,

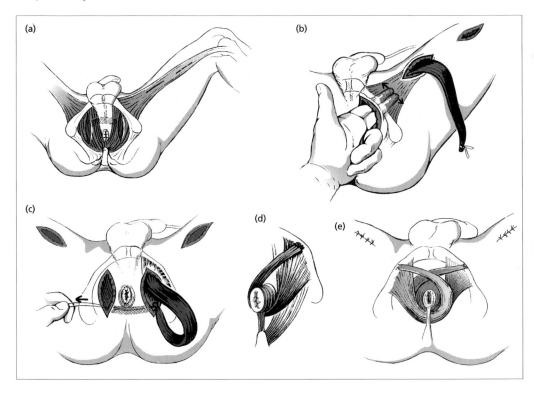

Fig. 6.63 Gracioplasty: (a) the gracilis is mobilized by making separate longitudinal incisions on the medial aspect of the thigh and a large incision to expose the ischiorectal fossa on both sides; (b) a tunnel is fashioned by blunt finger dissection through which the gracilis will be drawn; (c) the muscle is drawn posteriorly through the tunnel from one ischiorectal fossa to the other and (d) fixed to the ischial tuberosity (if length permits) or the pubic ramus; (e) a bilateral gracilis wrap. From Mann & Glass (1997), with permission.

the best functional outcome has been achieved in patients with congenital lesions or traumatic sphincter loss. In contrast, results in patients with neurogenic incontinence have been less satisfactory. Early results of bilateral gracioplasty have been encouraging despite small patient numbers. The mechanism by which gracioplasty works is unclear; however, it has been suggested that the transposed tendon and muscle serves as a living Thiersch wire.

Gluteus maximus transposition

There has been a recent resurgence of interest in the use of transposed gluteus maximus. Indications are similar to those of gracioplasty. Using this technique, it is possible to place a thick muscular ring around the anus, in contrast to gracioplasty where much of the wrap consists of the distal tendinous portion of the muscle. Preliminary results using this technique have been encouraging in small numbers of patients and both resting and squeeze pressures may attain normal levels, indicating tonic and voluntary activity of the transposed gluteus maximus. An intriguing development has been the introduction of dynamic gluteoplasty, based on similar principles to stimulated graciloplasty. Functional outcome in a handful of patients has been excellent.

SALVAGE OPERATIONS

Despite accurate preoperative assessment and the best efforts of the surgeon, there remains a group of patients who are either unsuitable for definitive sphincter reconstruction or in whom repeated attempts at some form of repair fail. These patients can be treated using the procedures outlined below.

Dacron-impregnated Silastic sling

The principles of this operation are similar to those of the Thiersch wire technique, which was formerly used for the treatment of rectal prolapse in patients deemed unsuitable for more major procedures. Many of the problems associated with the use of wire, nylon or other unyielding material have been overcome by the choice of Silastic, which has elasticity in the circumferential vector. This has reduced the tendency for the material to fail and has also decreased postoperative faecal impaction by allowing the anal canal to dilate during the passage of a faecal bolus. Theoretically, continence is maintained by the tonic elastic component of the implant.

Wound infection can be minimized by ensuring complete bowel preparation prior to surgery and the use of prophylactic antibiotics. Incisions are made about 2 cm from each side of the anal canal so that they can be easily deepened into both ischiorectal fossae. A tunnel is then developed below the levator plate but as high as possible and outside the external sphincter. A ribbon of Dacron, 2 cm wide, is then passed around the sphincter complex and tightened until the anal canal can admit the tip of the surgeon's index finger. The two ends of the Dacron ribbon are then secured with a linear stapler.

Artificial sphincter

Although artificial sphincters have been used by urologists for many years as a means of improving urinary incontinence, they have been less popular with proctologists in attempts to correct ARI. This is largely because of the known risks of technical failure and because the device was designed to close a narrow tube at relatively low pressures (the urethra) and not a wide, thin-walled viscus that can generate high pressures (the anorectum). Recently, the AMS 800 prosthesis has been redesigned for implantation around the anal canal and there is now renewed interest amongst coloproctologists for evaluating this method of treating end-stage anal sphincter failure. Sepsis is still the main complication of the procedure and it is suggested that all patients should have temporary faecal diversion. Sporadic case reports concerning the use of this device have been followed by more firm reporting of longer-term results. Two recent studies report a success rate of 70% at follow-up of up to 60 months. These results seem encouraging and it is likely that the use of this device will be explored with great vigour in the future.

Faecal diversion

Despite repeated surgical attempts to reconstruct the anal sphincter complex there are some patients who remain incontinent. More often than not these patients have undergone many operations and are only too pleased to accept a stoma as a form of palliation; there is a further group of patients who have very severe symptoms initially, are medically unfit, or are on the basis of clinical judgement and physiologically unsuitable for attempts at sphincter surgery. It is important to point out that the construction of a stoma should not be viewed by either the patient or surgeon as a failure but as a sensible solution to the problem of intractable ARI. The support of a stomatherapy service within the hospital and community is most important in ensuring the success of this method of treatment.

Most authorities, including ourselves, suggest that a left iliac fossa end colostomy is created, assuming that there is no upstream motility disorder when a loop ileostomy may be more appropriate. Either stoma may be raised through a small trephine, laparoscopically or by laparotomy, depending on the patient's physique and the surgeon's preference. An uncommon but well-documented problem seen in a minority of patients is diversion proctitis. This condition can mimic inflammatory bowel disease and histologically the features may be difficult to distinguish from Crohn's disease. Clinically, this condition produces troublesome discharge of mucus and occasional bleeding. Instillation of short-chain fatty acids into the bowel lumen has been suggested as a method of treatment, although this is seldom convenient in the long term. Witchhazel suppositories may also offer symptomatic relief. More definitive treatment includes proctectomy and we and others have found this necessary on occasion.

SURGERY FOR INCONTINENCE COMPLICATED BY
OBSTRUCTIVE DEFAECATION

Surgery for incontinence associated with obstructive defaecation due to rectocoele, rectorectal intussusception and rectal inertia requires special consideration. The techniques at the surgeon's disposal remain the same but the added problem of preoperative difficulty in faecal evacuation is not corrected by sphincter reconstruction. Indeed, the need for continued straining due to the inability to evacuate rectal contents is not only distressing for patients but also a potent cause of failure of the repair. Assessment of rectal sensation and videoproctography are important preoperatively. Several surgical strategies have been designed to cope with these functional problems.

Correction of the anatomical abnormality with or without sphincter reconstruction

Up to 70% of patients with neurogenic incontinence or ARI associated with obstetric disruption have evidence of rectocoele. If these lesions are symptomatic, then they may be corrected at the same time as anterior levatorplasty or sphincter repair. However, despite anatomical correction of the defect rectal emptying only improves in about 50% of patients and the need for suppositories or other measures to facilitate evacuation may persist. Another commonly encountered situation is ARI in association with rectorectal intussusception. This ill-understood condition may produce the symptoms of obstructive defaecation as well as blood and mucus discharge from the anus. It is likely that ARI occurs as the result of diastasis of the levators and stretching and denervation of the sphincters. Under these circumstances, it is prudent to perform abdominal rectopexy in order to avoid further sphincter compromise.

Antegrade colonic enema procedures with or without sphincter reconstruction

In principle, antegrade colonic enema procedures involve the creation of a conduit that can be used for irrigating the colon or rectum and hence mechanically evacuating faeces. The appendix (Malone procedure) was the first organ to be used as a conduit; modern alternatives include caecal flaps, transverse colon, sigmoid colon with nipple valves to prevent reflux and even button caecostomy. This intriguing idea has been successfully employed for the treatment of overflow incontinence in children with intractable constipation or ARI due to spina bifida and congenital anorectal malformations. Colonic irrigation can be accomplished in a short period of time and is effective in keeping patients clean between irrigations. It is logical that these procedures should be applied to adults in some situations, including patients with evacuation problems and ARI due to failed previous repairs where further sphincter surgery is not appropriate, and also those patients who have successful sphincter surgery but are plagued by the inability to defaecate.

Table 6.13 Operations for
rectal prolapse.

Perineal operations
Encircling devices
   Thiersch wire
   Silastic-impregnated mesh
   Silicone collar (Angelchick)
   Muscle (gracilis)
Mucosal reduction procedures
   Delorme's operation
   Gant–Miwa plication
Resection
   Rectosigmoidectomy
   Pouch perineal resection
Perineal rectopexy with or without postanal repair

Abdominal operations
Sigmoid excision
   Lahaut's operation
   Posterior extraperitonealization
Rectopexy
   Anterior sling (Ripstein)
   Posterior fixation with Ivalon sponge
   Posterior fixation with mesh
   Posterior sutured rectopexy
Resection
   Anterior resection
   Coloanal pouch
Resection and rectopexy
   Sigmoidectomy and sutured rectopexy
   High anterior resection and sutured rectopexy
   Segmental colectomy and sutured rectopexy
   Total colectomy, ileorectal anastomosis and sutured
     rectopexy

SURGERY FOR RECTAL PROLAPSE

The primary aim of surgery is to control prolapse. Although there is current
evidence to suggest that other functional problems such as incontinence
and slow-transit constipation should be corrected at the same time, this
issue remains controversial. Many operations for rectal prolapse have been
designed (Table 6.13). While this may demonstrate surgical ingenuity, it is
more likely that the wide spectrum of operations that has evolved for the
treatment of rectal prolapse attests to the inadequacies of any one procedure
for solving the problem.

    Surgery for rectal prolapse is a perineal or abdominal procedure. There
is much individual surgeon variation in terms of preference but the type
of operation chosen should be carefully tailored to each patient. For example,
a Délorme's procedure may be entirely appropriate for an elderly infirm

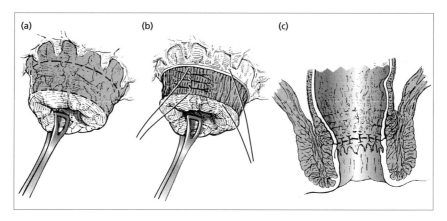

Fig. 6.64 Delorme's operation: (a) a sleeve of mucosa is resected from the prolapsed portion of the rectum; (b) sutures are placed to plicate the muscular layer and bring the mucosal edges into apposition; (c) appearance after the sutures are tied. From Dietzen (1989).

patient where the main aim is to make the patient more comfortable and make life easier for the carers. By contrast, a younger patient with prolapse associated with slow colonic transit may be better served by sutured recto-pexy and segmental colectomy. Notwithstanding these comments, the peranal plication described by Delorme and transabdominal sutured rectopexy with or without resection of the sigmoid and upper rectum are the most popular methods of treatment in the UK. Perineal rectosigmoidectomy with levator repair is more commonly performed in the USA than in the UK. However, there has been a recent resurgence of interest in this technique. Operations that involve the placement of prosthetic material behind the rectum (Ivalon sponge or Marlex mesh) or anterior slings (Ripstein's procedure) via the transabdominal route are falling out of favour because of their poor func-tional results.

Delorme's procedure

This is an excellent operation for the elderly, medically unfit patient in whom laparotomy is felt to be unwise. It also has a place in the surgical treatment of male children and adolescents with rectal prolapse where deep pelvic dissec-tion carries the risk of injury to hypogastric nerves and nervi erigentes and subsequent sexual and bladder dysfunction. The operation can be performed in either the lithotomy or prone jacknife positions and involves stripping the mucosa from the redundant rectum that forms the prolapse and plicating the denuded muscle to form a 'doughnut' (Fig. 6.64). The recurrence rate after Delorme's operation varies from 15 to 30% and this seems to increase with longer-term follow-up. Nevertheless, this procedure remains useful in

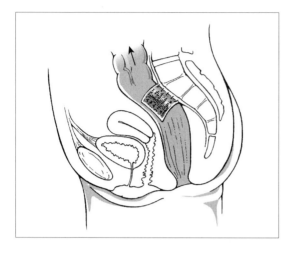

Fig. 6.65 Mesh rectopexy: a mesh has been used to fix the mobilized rectum to the presacral fascia. From Wassef & Rothenberger (1986), with permission.

patients with limited longevity; moreover, the operation may be repeated with minimum morbidity. It is our belief that Delorme's operation is the procedure of choice for patients deemed unfit for abdominal rectopexy.

Perineal proctosigmoidectomy

This alternative technique offers the advantage of anterior or posterior levator repair if this is deemed necessary, as well as resection of the prolapsed rectum. Despite the fact that a peranal coloanal anastomosis is performed in this operation, anastomotic failure rates are reported to be low and morbidity minimal. The reasons for this remain unclear. Results in terms of prolapse control seem to be excellent and recurrence rates low.

Abdominal approaches to rectal prolapse

These operations involve the use of prosthetic meshes or suture of the lateral ligaments to the ala of the sacrum with or without resection of the sigmoid colon (Figs 6.65 & 6.66; see Table 6.13).

Functional results of prolapse surgery

Objective data concerning the effects of prolapse surgery on continence are difficult to acquire. Many surgeons perform prolapse surgery without preoperative investigation, there is no standardized definition of incontinence and few clinicians differentiate between constipation, i.e. infrequent call to stool, and obstructive defaecation, i.e. difficulty in evacuation of stool with normal frequency of evacuation. It is our belief that patients with rectal

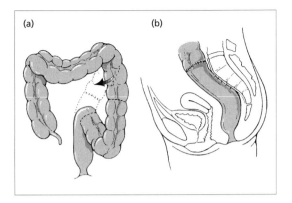

Fig. 6.66 Presacral rectopexy with sigmoid resection: (a) the redundant sigmoid loop is resected; (b) the mobilized rectum is fixed to the presacral fascia. From Wassef & Rothenberger (1986), with permission.

Table 6.14 Results of rectal prolapse surgery in improving anorectal incontinence using cumulated data from 19 separately published series.

Operation	No. of patients	Percentage with preoperative incontinence	Percentage improved by surgery
Abdominal procedures			
Sutured rectopexy	111	39–64	68–93
Resection rectopexy	156	40–67	38–94
Anterior sling	232	43–62	57–78
Posterior sling	190	58–80	75–78
Perineal operations			
Resection alone	138	23–60	25–55
Resection plus levator repair	52	100	78–91
Delorme's operation	45	50–67	44–83
Rectopexy and levator repair	24	63	100
Resection, rectopexy and repair	25	100	100

prolapse should undergo proctography, anal endosonography and anorectal physiology prior to surgery. It is only by adopting this policy that the correct operation can be selected for each patient. Currently, there is no ideal operation for patients with rectal prolapse.

The effects of correction of rectal prolapse on incontinence are variable and to some extent governed by the type of procedure undertaken (Table 6.14). Moreover, there is no general agreement as to whether procedures aimed at correcting continence should be performed at the same time as rectopexy. After fixation rectopexy without resection about two-thirds of patients who are incontinent preoperatively can be expected to improve. Results after excisional rectopexy are less impressive, raising the question as to whether resection of the sigmoid and upper rectum leads to more frequent and more liquid stool. On the basis of existing data it seems that perineal resection with concurrent levator repair offers the best chance of improving continence.

INTERNAL ANAL SPHINCTER FAILURE

The surgical management of internal anal sphincter (IAS) dysfunction as a cause of incontinence has received less attention than somatic muscle failure. The IAS may be disrupted as part of obstetric trauma and resting pressures are low in neurogenic incontinence. Nevertheless, under these circumstances, surgery is directed towards correction of the somatic component of the sphincter mechanism.

However, in certain situations the IAS may be divided while the integrity of the external sphincter is maintained. For example, intersphincteric anal fistulae and anal fissures are treated by deliberately sacrificing the IAS. Furthermore, the IAS may be inadvertently injured during the course of haemorrhoidectomy. Not only is resting pressure within the anal canal lost after these procedures but a physical gutter (keyhole deformity) is created as the result of retraction of the divided ends of the IAS. Moreover, contraction of a divided sphincter mechanism results in an increase in aperture rather than the constriction produced by contraction of the intact sphincter. The result of IAS division is ARI consisting of uncontrollable leakage of mucus and flatus that produces considerable disability.

Surgical management presents major problems. The ends of the divided IAS retract widely and direct repair is difficult without producing anal stenosis. Moreover, in those cases where repair has been achieved, the functional outcome has been poor in our experience. This has led to a different approach to the surgical treatment of IAS deficiency. It is well known that the internal and external anal sphincters contribute 85 and 15% of resting anal pressure respectively; however, when there is zero tension within the anal canal, it is theoretically open. These findings contributed to the anal cushion theory, which postulates that the haemorrhoidal complexes and soft tissues of the anal canal seal the canal when closed. These observations prompted the development of anoplasty to treat ARI caused by discrete injury to the IAS. In principle, the operation involves excision of the skin and scar tissue directly over the defect, which should have been accurately localized by anal endosonography. This excision is continued cephalad until intact IAS is encountered. An island flap of skin and subcutaneous tissue is then raised and advanced into the anal canal to fill the defect. The effect of this operation is to fill the gutter deformity in addition to allowing the anal canal to remain closed at rest. Postoperatively, wound infection can occur and cause dislodgement of the flap. Under these circumstances, the patient should be returned to the operating theatre and have the flap resutured, with the formation of a temporary colostomy. Early and medium-term follow-up indicates that the majority of patients experience an improvement in continence after this procedure. Although these results need to be confirmed by other workers, it is our belief that anoplasty should be part of the armamentarium of surgeons who treat ARI.

7: Research and Audit

Ian W. Mills, Alison F. Brading & Tim Stephenson

We have only a relatively superficial understanding of the mechanisms involved in the behaviour and control of the lower urinary and gastrointestinal tracts in normal humans, and an even poorer understanding of what exactly goes wrong when incontinence occurs. This lack of knowledge clearly hampers development of rational treatments of the clinical disorders and prevents the design and implementation of strategies to minimize the risks of developing them.

Both clinical and basic science research is still needed. Although a great deal of research has been carried out in this field, sadly much of it is relatively trivial and poorly substantiated. The need for research has clearly been appreciated by clinicians and many practising urologists do undertake research, although inevitably this is limited by the time constraints imposed by the clinical practice, the descriptive nature of the research (since the majority of potential experimental interventions are unlikely to be ethical) and the heterogeneity of the population studied. Furthermore, basic scientific research on the mechanisms of micturition and defaecation is relatively unfashionable and is hampered by difficulties in obtaining funding and the obvious ethical limitations associated with experimental work on humans.

In this chapter we consider what it is that basic scientists and clinicians can contribute to incontinence research, as well as the best ways for clinicians and scientists to collaborate in order to advance understanding and the potential value of clinical and basic scientific research for pharmaceutical companies.

Basic scientific research

The tasks of the basic scientist are to increase understanding of the normal mechanisms involved in the maintenance of continence and of the normal processes of micturition and defaecation, as well as to investigate the changes that occur in the various types of incontinence and to devise ways of studying the aetiology of the conditions. Understanding the normal processes is often an essential precursor in establishing the necessary foundation for determining what goes wrong in the incontinent patient and for subsequently devising novel treatments that can be tested using the same experimental methodologies. In the following sections we spell out in more detail the information that we need and then go on to consider the types of material that can be used for the studies, the experimental approaches available and how these methods have helped us to penetrate some of the mysteries of incontinence.

What do we want to know from basic science?

What is responsible for normal urinary and faecal continence?

This requires knowledge of the detailed anatomy of the outflow tracts, the functional roles of the constituent parts and the factors controlling the contractile activity of the muscular elements in the resting state. The latter includes determination of any spontaneous myogenic activity (including tone), the involvement of any continuous neuronal input (including the transmitters released from the various nerve endings, the receptors they activate and the functional response of the postsynaptic cells) and the balance between excitatory and inhibitory inputs.

What neuronal pathways are involved in micturition and defaecation and what triggers the reflexes?

This requires tracing of afferent and efferent neuronal pathways, using both anatomical methods and stimulation and recording techniques, and the monitoring of defaecation and micturition behaviour. It also requires appreciation of the relative roles of the somatic, sympathetic and parasympathetic nervous systems and of the neurotransmitters involved.

What are the important cellular mechanisms?

We need a more detailed understanding of the cellular mechanisms involved, for instance in the generation of mechanical activity in the various muscles during the filling and voiding cycle, and of the receptor–effector coupling mechanisms involved in modulating contractile activity (ion channels, G-protein-linked receptors, factors controlling intracellular calcium concentration, modulation of the contractile machinery sensitivity to calcium, etc.).

What changes occur with various types of incontinence?

These include behavioural changes, macroscopic and microscopic structural changes (hypertrophy, degenerative changes, denervation, etc.), changes in cellular structure at the electron microscopic level, changes in the contractile activity of the muscular elements, changes in sensitivity to neural stimulation and applied agonists, and changes in intracellular mechanisms (mitochondrial function, calcium storage, etc.).

What is the aetiology of various types of incontinence?

We can try to generate or find animal models of the various types of pathology and look at the factors underlying their development.

Material available for study

The vast majority of basic research that has been undertaken to investigate the physiology, pharmacology and pathology of the lower urinary and gastrointestinal tracts has been carried out on small mammals. This is inevitable in basic science laboratories, where experiments are carried out on a daily basis, requiring a ready supply of homogeneous material. A few basic science laboratories work in close collaboration with clinicians and can obtain human material from biopsies taken during clinical procedures. However, the amount of material is limited, the population that it comes from is heterogeneous, the donors varying in age and medical history, and little of this type of material is from people with normal urinary or gastrointestinal tracts. Moreover, non-therapeutic experimental studies in humans are likely to be unethical, unless risks are minimal and informed consent obtained. Similarly, it would not be acceptable to subject humans to screening of novel drugs for efficacy. For these and many other reasons animals are used, and various animal models of pathological conditions thought to mimic those seen in humans have been developed. Basic scientists working in isolation from clinicians are rarely qualified to carry out work on human volunteers and will thus use animals for *in vivo* work. In principle, experiments can be carried out on the following preparations.

SMALL BIOPSIES

These are usually human tissue samples obtained from consenting patients under either local or general anaesthesia. Biopsies can be removed by simple incision, as in the case of internal anal sphincter biopsy obtained at lateral sphincterotomy for anal fissure. Alternatively, they can be obtained using biopsy forceps, particularly from the bladder at cystoscopy or the rectum at colonoscopy; in the former, detrusor muscle may be obtained safely, but in the latter only mucosa can be biopsied in view of the risk of perforation of the rectum. Such specimens can be used to isolate cells for patch clamp studies or tissue culture. They are also often suitable for preparation of muscle strips for tension recording with sensitive transducers and can be used for histological studies, immunohistochemical identification of intrinsic nerves, autoradiographic localization of receptors and molecular biological techniques.

LARGER SAMPLES

These are taken from freshly killed animals or from patients during operative procedures. They or cadaveric dissections can be used for the preparation of muscle strips for more detailed investigation of the contractile and electrophysiological behaviour of the tissues and for study of cellular mechanisms, such as the production of second messengers (cyclic nucleotides, inositol phosphates) or the phosphorylation of target proteins, etc.

ISOLATED ORGANS

These are often necessary for working out the detailed anatomy of the structures present and their arrangement. Whole bladders isolated from small animals can be studied *in vitro* in order to investigate their behaviour during filling and their ability to empty in response to activation of the detrusor.

WHOLE ANIMALS

Experiments on whole animals allow studies of the reflexes and the behaviour of the organs *in vivo* and can also permit investigation of the aetiology of different types of incontinence, via the development of animal models, and study of the effects of pharmacological and surgical interventions. The use of live animals for scientific research in the UK is controlled by the Animals (Scientific Procedures) Act 1986, in accordance with which such experiments are carefully monitored by the Home Office. All experiments on live animals must be performed under a specific project licence, at a place designated by the Secretary of State, and all individuals involved must hold a personal licence; both types of licence must be granted by the Home Office.

The animals used for basic research vary depending on many factors, in particular the type of technique to be used. Small mammals provide a relatively cheap source of material for the production of single cells or for *in vitro* muscle strip experiments and have bladders that may also be thin enough to remain viable *in vitro* as whole organs. In a large basic science department, it is often possible to arrange for organs removed from a single animal to provide experimental tissue for a number of different researchers with interests in different physiological systems, thus reducing the number of animals sacrificed for experimental purposes. Larger animals are more suitable for studies requiring more tissue or for *in vivo* studies of conscious animals with implanted lines or telemetry systems for recording of pressures in the lower urinary and gastrointestinal tracts. The macroscopic and microscopic structure, ultrastructure and physiological properties of the lower urinary and gastrointestinal tracts following *in vivo* exposure to conditions potentially involved in the aetiology of incontinence may then be compared with those from normal control animals.

An important consideration is the relevance of the results obtained from animals to the human condition. The presumed common ancestry of mammals and the common problems faced with regard to the storage and release of waste products make it likely that very similar overall solutions have been found during evolution. However, there are some obvious differences between most animals and humans. The upright stance of humans means that the outflow tracts have to prevent leakage due to gravity and thus they may be required to generate larger outflow resistances. Another difference is that many animals use waste products for territorial marking and may have specific neuronal mechanisms designed for rapid expulsion of small amounts of urine or faeces. A recent article in the *British Journal of Urology*, which considered the excretory behaviour of the wombat, exemplifies this point (Johnson, 1998). This contrasts with the complete evacuation that normally occurs in humans. In spite of these differences, experimental evidence shows that there are many similarities in the mechanisms involved in storage and release of waste products in all mammals studied and that common changes occur when the systems are disrupted pathologically, by accident or experimentally. It is thus legitimate to extrapolate to a certain extent from one species to another. However, one should be aware that the number of cellular mechanisms available to achieve the same overall patterns of behaviour may be considerable. Furthermore, during evolution the chances are that mutations have changed the amino acid sequences of the proteins so that even if the main function has been preserved it is likely that the detailed structures differ between species. Thus the precise details of these mechanisms, such as receptor subtypes or channel subunit composition, disclosed in one species may be of little value in predicting the situation in humans.

Techniques

ANATOMY

There is still a surprising amount of ignorance of the anatomy of the outflow tracts. Even if the properties and control of the muscular components can be elucidated, their overall role in the whole animal cannot be established without knowledge of the distribution and orientation of the various muscle layers. Perhaps the most powerful methodology available for these studies is the use of serial sectioning and computer-aided three-dimensional reconstruction. For this to be successful, freshly obtained specimens are essential. To preserve detailed structure, the specimens should be fixed. If experimental animals are used, two fixation methods are available: perfusion fixation (using the cardiovascular system to deliver the fixative to the tissues in anaesthetized or brain-dead animals) or immersion fixation (using a suitable fixative such as formal saline). For small animals, the whole organ can be processed and embedded in paraffin for sectioning. With larger organs, the specimens have to be cut into smaller sections for embedding and a system of artificial reference points employed in order to allow correct positioning of the sections during reconstruction. The blocks can then be sectioned, mounted and appropriately stained. For small organs, it may be possible to view whole sections under the microscope at sufficient magnification; using a digitizing camera, the images can then be 'grabbed' and stored by a computer for later analysis. For larger sections, it may be necessary to photograph the sections at a lower power and project them on to a digitizing pad. This allows the relevant areas of muscle to be outlined (using the microscope for confirmation) and again stored on the computer. There are several software packages available for image analysis and three-dimensional reconstruction. The techniques are time-consuming, laborious and require considerable skill to achieve good results, but they can provide valuable information. Plate 8 (opposite p. 148) and Fig. 7.1 show some of the information that can be obtained by these techniques.

HISTOCHEMISTRY AND IMMUNOHISTOCHEMISTRY

These are methods for the identification of particular enzymes or antigenic sites in a section. For example, histochemical localization is useful for identifying acetylcholinesterase (the enzyme that breaks down acetylcholine at endplates in striated muscle and at postsynaptic terminals in parasympathetic nerves) and different classes of striated muscle fibre using ATPase or phosphorylase. Often these techniques require use of rapidly frozen specimens sectioned using a cryostat to avoid the use of a fixative, which might destroy enzyme activity. In some cases sufficient activity may be retained in fixed material to allow more precise localization of the sites than is usually possible with frozen sections. Histochemical methods use an enzyme substrate that can be cleaved, either directly to a coloured product or indirectly to one that can react specifically with another reagent to give a coloured product. If the product is insoluble, good localization can be achieved (soluble products run the risk of diffusion away from the site of formation).

Immunohistochemistry uses localization of a bound antibody to identify specific sites. Indirect methods are most commonly used (direct identification can be achieved if the antibody can be cross-linked to an enzyme for

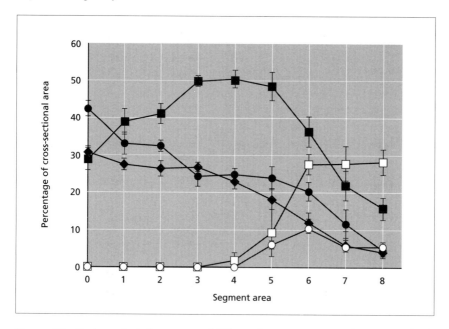

Fig. 7.1 Distribution and relative amounts of different tissue components in the vesicourethral junction and along the length of the female pig urethra ($n = 6$). The urethra was divided into nine segments; segment 0 corresponds to the vesicourethral junction and segment 8 corresponds to the distal urethra. The cross-sectional area of tissue components is expressed as a percentage of the total cross-sectional area of the histological section ± SEM. The different tissue elements quantified include circular (■) and longitudinal (●) smooth muscle, circular (□) and longitudinal (○) striated muscle and lamina propria (◆).

histochemical localization). Indirect methods incorporate an amplification step that allows good labelling with low concentrations of antibody (thus reducing non-specific staining). A common method is the ABC (avidin–biotin–peroxidase complex) method (Fig. 7.2). An example of the use of immunohistochemical localization of antigenic sites is the recognition of different nerves, where antibodies can be raised against the transmitters themselves or specific precursors or enzymes involved in their synthesis. Other useful sites that may be identified are specific receptors or channels or structural proteins expressed in particular cells (e.g. antibodies against neurofilaments for identification of any nerve or against smooth muscle actin for identification of smooth muscle).

Secondary antibodies coupled to fluorescent molecules can also be used (Fig. 7.3). Many fluorescent markers are available that each emit light of a particular wavelength. A section can thus be labelled with several antibodies, each coupled to a different marker. Using the appropriate filters to screen out particular wavelengths, it is then possible to determine the position of each marker separately, allowing co-localization of antibodies to be established. An example of this is shown in Plate 9 (opposite p. 148), which shows co-localization of nitric oxide synthase and haemoxygenase in a small ganglion

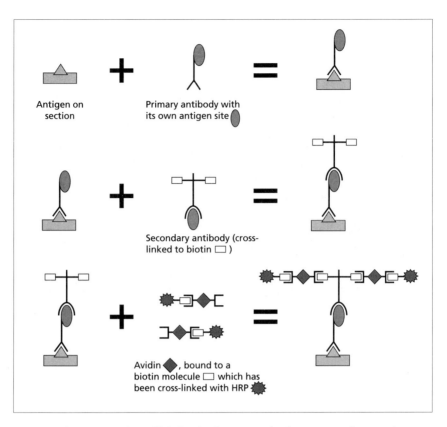

Fig. 7.2 Indirect immunological labelling by the ABC (avidin–biotin–peroxidase complex) method. The primary antibody is raised in one species and, after applying it to the section, the bound antibodies are further labelled with secondary antibodies (cross-linked to biotin). Avidin, a protein that binds avidly to several biotin molecules, is mixed with biotin that has been cross-linked with horseradish peroxidase (HRP) and the slides are treated with this mixture. This results in several molecules of HRP becoming attached to each of the secondary antibodies, thus enabling the production of a dense reaction product.

Fig. 7.3 The immunofluorescence method. Secondary antibodies are coupled to fluorescent molecules, such as fluorescein isothiocyanate (green) or rhodamine (red). Labelled sections may then be studied with the fluorescence microscope.

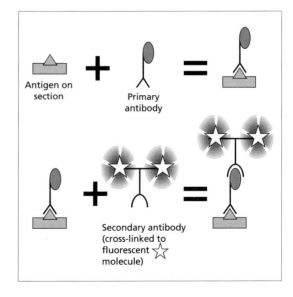

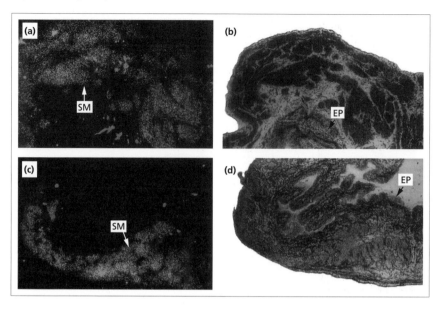

Fig. 7.4 Example of the application of autoradiography. These photomicrographs demonstrate the distribution of muscarinic receptors in bladder sections from female rats that were untreated (a,b) and neonatally treated with capsaicin (c,d); (a) and (c) are dark-field photomicrographs of bladder sections incubated with QNB, and (b) and (d) are light-field photomicrographs of the bladder sections stained with cresyl fast violet. Autoradiographic grains are seen over the smooth muscle (SM) but not the epithelium (EP). Magnification × 16. From Gunasena *et al.*, 1995 with permission.

in the wall of a human female urethra. Fluorescent labels are also ideal for imaging nerves within preparations using confocal microscopy.

Ligands labelled with a radioactive isotope can be used to identify the positions of target receptors or enzymes by autoradiography (Fig. 7.4). In this technique the section with the radioactive label applied is placed in contact with a film of photographic emulsion in the dark. Ionizing radiation released as the isotope decays exposes the emulsion (reacting with it to generate metallic silver). For precise localization of the ligand low levels of tritiated ligand are used, since the electrons emitted by decay of tritium have little energy and only interact locally with the emulsion. However, the relatively long half-life of tritium means that the sections have to remain in contact with the emulsion for days or weeks. The density of the silver grains can be measured using a densitometer and their localization established by histological staining and microscopic examination of the underlying structures.

ELECTRON MICROSCOPY

This is used for ultrastructural studies of cells in the organs responsible for the maintenance of continence. It allows examination of the intracellular organelles of the different cells and of the intercellular junctions between cells and thus identification of characteristic patterns associated with storage or voiding dysfunctions. Tissues must be cut and fixed soon after removal from the body, in order to cross-link and thus immobilize the proteins, before being processed for electron microscopy. Scanning electron microscopy may be employed to view the surfaces of unsectioned specimens, thus giving a three-dimensional appearance; this permits resolution to about 10 nm. Transmission electron microscopy, in which an electron beam is directed through an ultra-thin section of a specimen, is preferred for ultrastructural studies since it gives finer intracellular and pericellular detail, allowing a resolution of approximately 0.1 nm. Using this technique, the ultrastructural appearance of the detrusor in detrusor instability has recently been described, with evidence of a characteristic pattern of intercellular connections and demonstration of protrusion junctions and ultra-close abutment of cells resembling a quasi-syncytium (Fig. 7.5).

CONTRACTILE ACTIVITY: MUSCLE STRIPS

A great deal of information can be obtained by recording contractile activity from strips of smooth muscle. Strips can be cut from any of the smooth muscles available, although care should be taken to cut the strips following the orientation of the muscle bundles. A dissecting microscope allows this to be determined easily for smaller bladders, but with samples from larger animals or from the sphincters it is not easy to see the orientation. However, if the sample is pinned down at one end and fine forceps are used to grasp the muscle, gentle pulling usually reveals the orientation of the fibres running from the forceps. Experience shows that activity may be surprisingly variable, even in strips taken from the same preparation, and it is sensible to record from several strips at the same time if possible. In our laboratory we use continuous and simultaneous superfusion of six strips mounted separately in small chambers for recording contractile activity. The apparatus is shown in Fig. 7.6 and a diagram of an individual chamber is shown in Fig. 7.7. With this approach precisely timed applications of agonists can be achieved simply and reproducibly and the consequent tension generated in the strip recorded. Platinum ring electrodes embedded into the walls of the chambers allow electrical stimulation of the preparations.

We routinely use samples of about 7 × 1 × 1 mm, weighing 2–5 mg. Strips even of this small size contain large numbers of cells (about 1.5 million if the cells are considered as cylinders with a length of 300 μm and a diameter of 4 μm) and are likely to have many postganglionic nerve fibres running in them. Selective activation of the nerves can be achieved by using short-duration

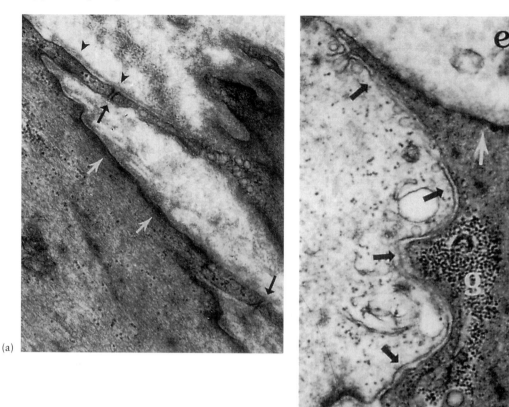

(a)

Fig. 7.5 Distinctive features of detrusor overactivity demonstrated using transmission electron microscopy. (a) Protrusion junction (flat tip-to-tip contact between two cell processes) indicated by black arrows. Magnification × 49 850. (b) Ultra-close abutment between the bump of one cell surface and the matching shallow depression on the surface of another, indicated by black arrows. g, glycogen particles in sarcoplasm; e, elastic fibre; white arrows, dense bands; arrowheads, basal laminae. Magnification × 38 400. From Elbadawi *et al.*, 1993, with permission.

current pulses. In our hands, stimuli need to be as short as 0.05 ms to be selective for intrinsic nerves in the bladder. It is essential to check that select-ive activation of the nerves is being achieved and this can be done by using tetrodotoxin (5×10^{-7} M is usually sufficient), a poison derived from the puffer fish that blocks voltage-sensitive Na^+ channels and prevents action potential generation in nerves while leaving smooth muscles unaffected. Thus any responses to electrical stimulation in the presence of tetrodotoxin are probably due to direct stimulation of smooth muscle cells rather than being evoked by transmitter released from the nerves. In this way it is pos-sible to construct frequency–response graphs to nerve stimulation of smooth

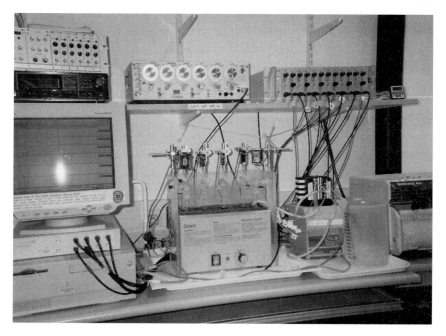

Fig. 7.6 Organ bath set-up for recording contractile activity in smooth muscle strips. Six organ baths are suspended above a heated water bath (centre of picture), through which tubing passes from the peristaltic pump (right) to the organ baths. Tension recording can be performed via either a pen chart recorder (far right) or MacLab software on the Apple Macintosh computer (far left).

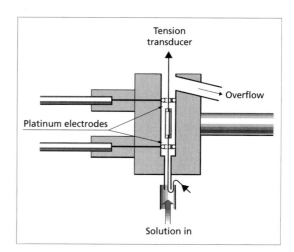

Fig. 7.7 An individual organ bath.

muscle taken from the lower urinary and gastrointestinal tracts of patients or animals with various types of incontinence. This can aid in the assessment of whether denervation is a pathophysiological feature. Similarly, concentration–response graphs to agonists can be constructed. Such studies

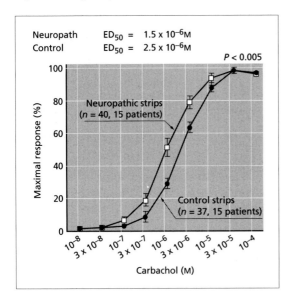

Fig. 7.8 Comparison of the dose–response curves obtained with carbachol for muscle strips taken from neuropathic and control bladders. There is a leftward shift in the dose–response curve from neuropathic strips, indicating a degree of supersensitivity.

led to the identification of denervation supersensitivity in the neuropathic unstable detrusor (Fig. 7.8).

Judicious use of specific receptor-blocking drugs or specific nerve toxins (such as guanethidine, which blocks release of transmitters from sympathetic nerves) can help to establish the types of nerve innervating the strip and the transmitters used by the nerves. Information about receptor subtypes can be obtained by studying the effects of specific agonists or the potency of specific antagonists in blocking the receptors; the mechanisms involved in mediating their effects can be studied by applying various channel-blocking drugs or drugs that interfere with the production of second messengers (Kenaki, 1997).

CONTRACTILE ACTIVITY: ISOLATED ORGANS

The bladders from small mammals can be removed from the animal and set up *in vitro* to study the behaviour of the whole bladder (Fig. 7.9). This technique was pioneered by Levin and Wein (1982) using rabbit bladders and is now being extended to other animals (rat and guinea-pig). The bladder needs to be small enough to ensure that it can obtain the necessary oxygen and metabolic substrates from the bathing fluid. The bladder can be filled transurethrally and intravesical pressures recorded under constant volume conditions or the bladder can be allowed to empty. The response of the bladder can be recorded on activation of its smooth muscle by addition of agonists to the bath or by transmural stimulation. Electrical stimulation can be achieved by passing current between an intravesical electrode and large 'paddle' electrodes in the bathing solution. Figure 7.10 shows records from

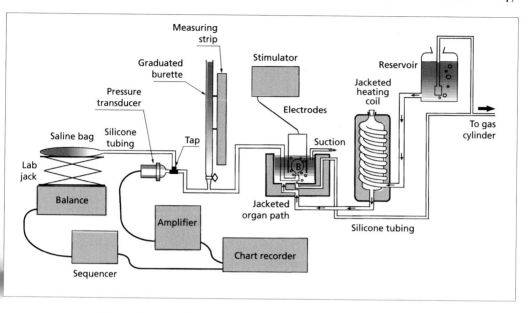

Fig. 7.9 Apparatus for recording from isolated guinea-pig bladder. The bladder (B) is cannulated transurethrally and mounted in a jacketed organ bath heated to 37°C. The bladder can be filled to a desired volume from the graduated burette and is then connected via a three-way tap to either a pressure transducer or a large partially filled saline bag. When connected to the pressure transducer, isovolumic changes in pressure can be recorded; when connected to the saline bag, the isotonic fluid movement into or out of the bag can be recorded by continuous monitoring of the change in weight of the bag. The height of the bag, and thus the pressure to which the bladder is exposed, can be varied. The bladder smooth muscle can be activated by either addition of agonists to the bathing solution or electrical stimulation of the intrinsic nerves.

Fig. 7.10 Examples of isotonic and isovolumic recordings from isolated guinea-pig bladder stimulated with carbachol (CCh), electrical field stimulation (EFS) and to αβ-methylene ATP (αβ-MeATP).

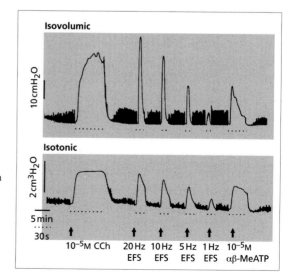

an isolated guinea-pig bladder. This methodology can give important information about the effectiveness of the smooth muscle contractions in emptying the bladder, information not available from muscle strips. It is also possible to record from afferent nerves in some species, if the nerve trunks are removed with the bladder. In this case an isolating partition is needed through which the nerves can be threaded in order to allow activity to be recorded from them.

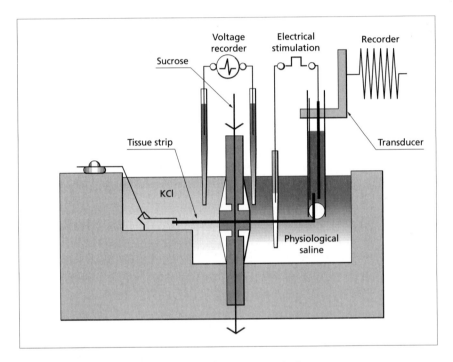

Fig. 7.11 Sucrose gap recording apparatus: this version is a single sucrose gap apparatus as used by Carol Maggi and his colleagues. The tissue strip is threaded through a 'sucrose gap' separating two compartments. The gap is a thin tube through which ion-free iso-osmotic sucrose solution is slowly perfused, which prevents extracellular current flow between the chambers. Current can only flow from cell to cell through the tissue in the gap. The left-hand chamber is filled with iso-osmotic KCl solution in order to depolarize the tissue and stop spontaneous activity in this part. The right-hand chamber is filled with physiological saline solution. The voltage difference between the two chambers recorded across the sucrose gap monitors the electrical activity of the tissue in the physiological saline solution, while its mechanical activity is recorded with a transducer. Stimulating electrodes in the right-hand chamber allow activation of the tissue either directly or via activation of the intrinsic nerves. If the tissue is threaded through two sucrose gaps, with a small node between them perfused with physiological saline solution, then current can be injected into cells in this node across one gap and the potential change elicited in the nodal cells recorded across the other gap. This is then a double sucrose gap.

RECORDING ELECTRICAL ACTIVITY

Ideally, electrical activity should be recorded from strips of smooth muscle. This can be achieved using the single or double sucrose gap technique (Fig. 7.11), which allows simultaneous recording of electrical activity and tension and the response of the tissue to applied depolarizing or hyperpolarizing currents. Alternatively, sharp microelectrodes can be used for intracellular recording. Unfortunately both techniques are difficult when applied to smooth muscles and normally only yield useful information in the hands of experts. Such studies can establish the basic electrical properties of the cell membranes, demonstrate the effects of stimulating the intrinsic nerves and help to elucidate the mechanisms of action of various transmitters. Examples of the results of such studies on urinary tract smooth muscles are shown in Figs 7.12 and 7.13.

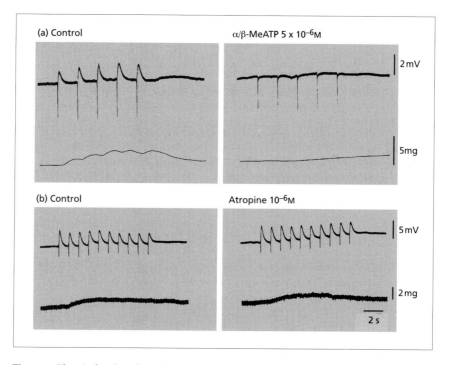

Fig. 7.12 Electrical and mechanical activity recorded from a strip of guinea-pig detrusor using the double sucrose gap method. Each pair of traces shows electrical activity (upper trace) and mechanical activity (lower trace) of the smooth muscle cells in the node. Short depolarizing current pulses activate intrinsic nerves and elicit excitatory junction potentials and contraction. (a) The excitatory junction potentials are abolished by pretreatment with the P_{2x} purinoceptor desensitizing agent α,β-methylene ATP ($\alpha\beta$-MeATP). (b) The excitatory junction potentials are unaffected by the muscarinic receptor antagonist atropine. Tracing kindly supplied by K. Fujii.

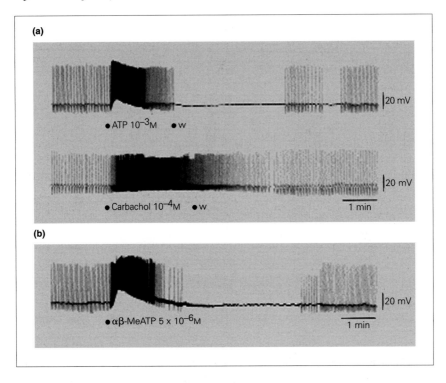

(a)

ATP 10^{-3}M   w

20 mV

Carbachol 10^{-4}M   w

20 mV   1 min

(b)

αβ-MeATP 5×10^{-6}M

20 mV   1 min

Fig. 7.13 Microelectrode recordings of the effects of agonists on the electrical activity of guinea-pig detrusor. Note that the P_{2x} agonists ATP and α,β-methylene ATP (αβ-MeATP) both depolarize the tissue and increase the frequency of action potentials, while the muscarinic agonist carbachol causes little depolarization but also increases action potential frequency. In (a) the drugs were applied for 2 min and washed off (w), whereas in (b) αβ-MeATP was applied continuously from the dot and recovery of the normal action potential frequency occurred showing the complete desensitization of the receptors. From Fujii, 1988 with permission.

Single cells isolated from the various smooth muscles can be studied using patch electrodes. These are glass micropipettes, usually with a larger tip diameter than microelectrodes, that have polished tips to ensure a good seal with the cell membrane. The pipette tip is placed on the surface of a cell and slight suction exerted through the electrode, which pulls the glass and membrane together to form a high-resistance seal (in the giga-ohm range). Several recording methods are then available (Fig. 7.14). To record from the whole cell (Fig. 7.14a), rapid suction can be applied that breaks the membrane patch within the electrode and allows continuity between the intracellular environment and the fluid filling the electrode, thus providing a low-resistance pathway. With this technique spontaneous electrical activity of the cell can be measured and the effects of drugs on the membrane potential or membrane resistance can be investigated (Fig. 7.15a).

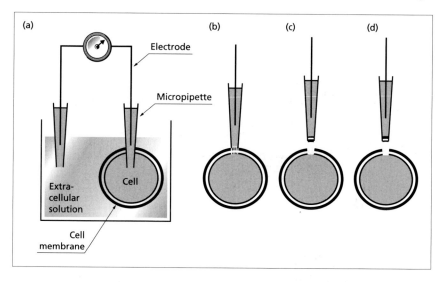

Fig. 7.14 Patch clamp techniques: (a) whole-cell recording; (b) permeable patch technique; (c) 'outside-out' isolated patch technique; (d) 'inside-out' isolated patch technique.

The disadvantage of these whole-cell recordings is that the cell can lose soluble molecules that may normally regulate the activity of membrane channels. To reduce this, the permeable patch technique can be used (Fig. 7.14b). In this case, the patch of membrane within the pipette is not broken but small holes are made in it by applying ionophores (such as valinomycin or gramicidin) to the membrane in the pipette solution. This can increase the permeability to ions, thus preserving the important low-resistance pathway into the cell but preventing diffusion from the cell of larger molecules. Figure 7.15b shows an example of currents recorded in response to a potassium channel-opening drug (levcromakalim) using whole-cell and permeable patch techniques.

The properties of individual ion channels can also be studied using patch clamp techniques. In this case the channels must be in the patch of membrane within the pipette. Recordings can be made from cell-attached patches, in which case the inner leaflet of the membrane is in its normal environment, or the patch can be detached from the cell, allowing manipulation of the solution bathing either side. It is possible to generate isolated patches either in the 'outside-out' or 'inside-out' configuration (Fig. 7.14c,d). The high-resistance seal between the membrane and the pipette means that currents flowing in response to applied voltages flow almost exclusively through the patch of membrane, and high amplification can be used to visualize small blips of current flowing through individual channels as they open and close (Fig. 7.15c).

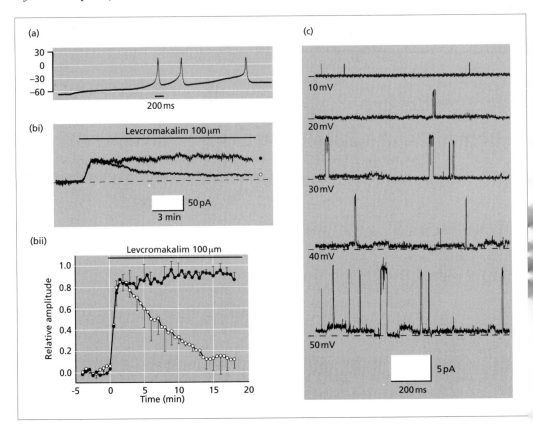

Fig. 7.15 (a) Spontaneous action potentials recorded from a single human detrusor myocyte using the current clamp mode of the whole-cell patch clamp technique. (From Montgomery & Fry, 1992 with permission.) (b) (i) Outward currents recorded from single myocytes from a pig urethra in response to application of the potassium channel-activating drug levcromakalim. (ii) Comparison of the results from a conventional whole-cell recording (open circles) and one using a nystatin perforated patch technique (filled circles). The former method allows free diffusion between the cell interior and the patch electrode, while the latter only allows diffusion of small ions and molecules through the nystatin-derived pores. Loss of some necessary intracellular constituent probably accounts for the current run-down in the whole-cell mode. (c) The opening of large- and small-conductance Ca^{2+}-activated potassium channels in an inside-out membrane patch from a pig urethral myocyte, with 140 mM KCl on both sides of the membrane. The size of the current pulses increases linearly with the voltage across the patch. The large-conductance channel has a relatively brief open time, while the small-conductance channel has a longer mean open time. Figure kindly supplied by N. Teramoto.

PHARMACOMECHANICAL COUPLING

Investigations into the mechanisms involved in mediating the effects of receptor activation can encompass many techniques. The various second messengers can be studied by rapid freezing of tissue samples at timed intervals after activation of particular receptors, followed by homogenization of the frozen tissue and extraction and measurement of the second messengers (e.g. inositol trisphosphate or cyclic nucleotides) by appropriate methods. The functional roles of various elements in the pathways between receptor activation and mechanical effect can be established by administration of substances that block or enhance the various steps in the potential pathways. For instance, the involvement of G-proteins can be studied using non-hydrolysable analogues of GTP (such as GTPγS) to permanently activate G-proteins, or administration of GDPβS to inactivate G-proteins by high-affinity binding to the GDP site. The involvement of cyclic nucleotides can be implicated by inhibiting the various phosphodiesterases that break down these molecules. Specific kinase inhibitors or activators are available, as are relatively specific phosphatase inhibitors.

MONITORING INTRACELLULAR CONCENTRATIONS IN REAL TIME

The intracellular concentrations of individual ions (Ca^{2+} being particularly important) and pH can be measured using fluorescent or luminescent probes. A common approach is to use a lipid-soluble form of a specific fluorescent or luminescent binding molecule that can be cleaved by intracellular enzymes to leave a charged lipid-insoluble molecule trapped inside the cell. The intracellular molecule can then bind specifically with the ion of interest, resulting in concentration-related changes in the emission or absorption of the probe. A molecule with the right properties can be used to signal the concentration of the ion in real time, either by quantifying light emission or the changing absorption or emission of monochromatic light shone on the specimen. These techniques can be carried out in single cells, allowing the opportunity to record both electrical activity and, for instance, intracellular free calcium concentration, although this is rather sophisticated. Experiments can be carried out most easily on tissue cultured cells, although it is possible to record signals from strips of smooth muscle, in which case tension might also be recorded. Recent studies have applied such techniques to tissue cultured cells in order to investigate the effects of agonists on intracellular calcium concentrations, examining differences between cells cultured from biopsies of normal bladders and those from unstable bladders.

IN VIVO ANIMAL STUDIES

A number of species have been used, each having their individual merits. Small mammals such as rats, guinea-pigs and rabbits have the advantage of being easy and cheap to keep in relatively large numbers and easy to handle. Each basic science research group has its favoured small mammal and this usually reflects the animal used in the majority of its laboratory-based research. Similarly, pharmaceutical companies usually favour small mammals, especially the rat, for *in vivo* studies of the effects of compounds that have shown promise in laboratory screening using a number of the techniques described above. While some useful information can be obtained from these animals, their differences from humans must be considered in the interpretation of results. For example, the rat bladder has a number of significant features that distinguish it from the human bladder: it has a primarily purinergic excitatory innervation, in which ATP is the neurotransmitter, in contrast to the exclusively cholinergic excitatory innervation of the normal human bladder; it has no ganglia in its wall, whereas many of the pre-ganglionic efferent nerves to the human bladder synapse with ganglia in the bladder wall; and a gradual rise in baseline detrusor pressure, with phasic increases in pressure superimposed on this, are features of the normal rat filling cystometrogram, while such findings would indicate a diagnosis of hyperreflexia or instability if seen on a human cystometrogram. So despite the greater expertise required, more difficult husbandry (animal care and housing) and higher costs, larger mammals (e.g. pig and dog) can provide information more obviously relevant to the human condition. This is especially true in the context of incontinence research, where the anatomical considerations associated with size of the animal mean that pressures in the lower urinary and gastrointestinal tracts are more similar to those in humans. Live animals are used for three aspects of incontinence research: understanding features of normal micturition and defaecation, creation of animal models of different types of incontinence, and investigation of the diverse effects of potential drugs for the treatment of incontinent patients.

Much has been learned about the innervation of the lower urinary and gastrointestinal tracts and the reflexes involved in normal micturition and defaecation by the application of retrograde neuronal tracing techniques, which involve a tracer that is taken up by nerve endings and transported to the cell bodies of the respective nerves by axonal transport. The tracer can be injected into a site of interest in an anaesthetized animal, which is sacrificed after 24 hours or so. Tissue is then processed for cryostat sections in order to localize the injection site and for whole-mount preparations in order to localize transported tracer. For example, this technique has been used in the guinea-pig to demonstrate that tracer is taken up from the internal anal sphincter and transported to neurones in the rectal myenteric plexus, which also stain positively for nitric oxide synthase-containing neurones. This provided strong evidence for the presence of an intrinsic nitrergic rectoanal neuronal pathway, which is probably involved in the rectoanal inhibitory reflex.

Once the distribution of the afferent and efferent innervation of the bladder, urethra, rectum and anus has been described for a particular species, it is feasible to record activity in relevant nerves during the normal filling

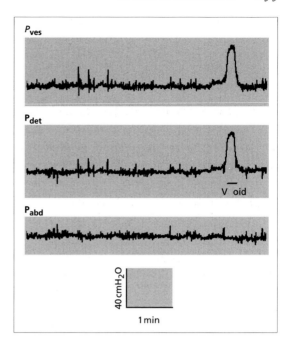

Fig. 7.16 Cystometrogram obtained from a normal, ambulatory, unstressed female pig using implanted pressure-sensitive telemetry equipment. P_{ves}, vesical pressure, from implanted catheter with its tip in the bladder; P_{abd}, abdominal pressure, from implanted catheter with its tip in the peritoneal cavity; P_{det}, detrusor pressure, obtained by subtracting P_{abd} from P_{ves} using MacLab and Chart 3.4.2 software.

and voiding phases of micturition and defaecation. It is also possible to determine the effects of stimulation of individual nerves in the anaesthetized animal and the effect of sectioning of particular nerves on normal micturition and defaecation behaviour. This is relevant because of the apparent importance of denervation injury in both stress and urge urinary incontinence and in faecal incontinence. Such studies usually involve dynamic filling and voiding of the bladder or anorectum similar to those methods used in humans but adapted to the specific problems posed by large or small mammals. The majority of studies employing these techniques are necessarily performed under anaesthesia or sedation, which can affect the results obtained. A conscious recording model in the pig has been designed for the performance of cystometric studies, using chronically implanted abdominal and vesical cannulae tunnelled to emerge in the lumbar dorsal midline of the animal, thus allowing easy access for attachment to fluid-filled lines for pressure recording and bladder filling. The pig is then restrained in a cage during the period of study. Better still is a recently developed system that uses an implanted radiotelemetric device attached to pressure transducers, which can provide constant monitoring of vesical and abdominal pressures. Thus cystometric data from unstressed unprovoked animals may be collected in a way similar to the ambulatory cystometrograms obtained from humans (Fig. 7.16).

The creation of an animal model of a particular disease is informative since it can provide insight into the aetiology of that disease. In the context of incontinence research, much advancement in our understanding of detrusor

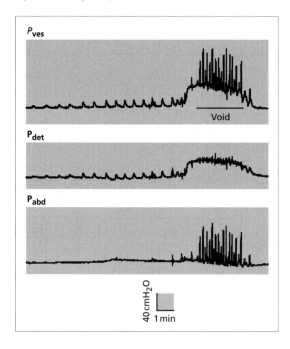

Fig. 7.17 Cystometrogram from a conscious large white female pig 4 months after surgery to implant a silver ring around the proximal urethra. This recording was made using chronically implanted abdominal and vesical fluid-filled silicone cannulae, which had been tunnelled from the peritoneal cavity to emerge in the lumbar dorsal midline. The bladder was filled with sterile saline at 37°C via a separate cannula at a rate of 50 ml/min. P_{ves}, vesical pressure; P_{abd}, abdominal pressure; P_{det}, detrusor pressure, derived by subtracting P_{abd} from P_{ves}. Detrusor pressure is significantly increased and prolonged in obstructed animals and there are phasic rises in detrusor pressure during the filling phase in this animal, indicative of detrusor instability.

instability as a cause of urge incontinence has come from studies using a model of instability secondary to outflow obstruction. This is created by implanting a ring around the proximal urethra of immature animals, which develop outflow obstruction as they grow (Fig. 7.17). Changes during the development of the instability, such as reduced vesical blood flow during micturition, can be assessed and the pathophysiological properties of the unstable bladder subsequently investigated in the laboratory following sacrifice of the animal. It has also been found that detrusor instability can be induced in pigs by performing a bladder transection, thus interrupting the innervation of the bladder, and by repeated bladder distensions, which probably also damage the nerves in the bladder wall. It would be possible to establish a model of artificial rectal filling, via the mucus fistula portion of a split sigmoid loop colostomy, using a material that mimics faeces.

Drug development and studies of the effects of currently marketed drugs are the final applications of *in vivo* animal studies. As described below, pharmaceutical companies test a number of potentially marketable compounds on animals during the development of drugs for urinary incontinence, measuring the effect of administration of test compounds on filling and voiding cystometrograms, bladder capacity and flow rate of normal animals and on other indicators of incontinence, such as volume threshold for onset of unstable contractions in a model of detrusor instability. The effects of the compounds on other important vital functions, such as heart rate and blood pressure, are also assessed in order to test their safety as well as their potential efficacy. All such studies essentially require comparison with a control, such as the drug delivery vehicle (e.g. saline), and with a standard, such as a drug that has a known effect on the parameters being recorded. As well as being involved in such studies through collaboration agreements, basic scientists perform *in vivo* studies of currently available drugs, particularly autonomic agonists and antagonists, in order to continue to contribute to our understanding of neural pathways and neurotransmitters involved in normal and incontinent lower urinary and gastrointestinal tracts.

Clinical research and audit

In an ideal world it would not be necessary to subject patients to any form of unproved technique or experimental scenario. However, because of the inevitable limitations of studies performed on non-human species, it is essential that any intervention that appears to work in an animal is subsequently scrutinized using well-designed clinical research before it is declared effective and safe for human application. Similarly, it is not practical to perform some types of research on animals, particularly those that address questions of disease epidemiology or subjective patient assessment (e.g. quality of life).

It is vital to apply the principles of non-maleficence ('do no harm') as much as possible in the design of studies that require patient involvement and cooperation and to always secure approval from local ethical committees before embarking on a particular study or trial, other than those based on retrospective data analysis. The most important feature of an ethical trial and one that should always be included is obtaining informed consent from patients/individuals, who decide whether they wish to be included after considering relevant information for a reasonable period of time (at least 24 hours). Patients should understand that treatment is in no way conditional upon giving consent to their participation in the trial, and should they at any time decide that they wish to withdraw, their treatment will not be compromised. Obviously, coercion must be avoided and patient confidentiality maintained.

In this section we consider the information that clinical studies can be used to obtain and the various techniques of study available to the interested clinician as well as to the pharmaceutical company involved in drug development.

What can clinical research tell us?

What are the incidence, prevalence and risk factors for urinary and faecal incontinence?

A lot of epidemiological data of this type have been obtained over the past few decades even though there are still some enigmas, such as the risk factors for idiopathic detrusor instability and the associations between urinary and faecal incontinence. Furthermore, in a dynamic population, the incidence and prevalence of the different types of incontinence vary and it is necessary to follow these changes in order to allow us to predict what modifications in clinical provision will be required in the future.

How should the incontinent patient be assessed and investigated in order to define the cause of their incontinence and guide treatment?

We recognize different patterns of bladder and anorectal dysfunction and the accurate identification of these inform decisions about treatment. Improvements in methodology are constantly being developed but these must always be rigorously evaluated by assessing their reliability, reproducibility, sensitivity and specificity (and predicitive value) as well as comparing them with existing gold standards. An example is the introduction of computerized pattern recognition into urodynamics and anorectal monitoring.

How should the incontinent patient be treated?

Most clinical research is directed at finding solutions to this question. Such research includes phase I to phase IV drug studies and retrospective and prospective studies of surgical, medical, behavioural and physical therapeutic interventions.

What outcome measures should be used?

Many earlier studies concentrated on obtaining objective data, such as number of pads used per day, in order to assess the effectiveness of treatment. However, in the area of incontinence, patient satisfaction is the most important outcome and therefore it is necessary to produce good quality-of-life questionnaires that are properly validated.

Is the service provided by each individual, each department and each hospital as efficient and effective as it should and could be?

To answer this question, it is necessary to be involved in ongoing audit in order to help provide reassurance to healthcare personnel, their patients and managers that the best quality of service is being achieved with regard to the resources available.

Techniques

EPIDEMIOLOGICAL STUDIES

These seek to identify the prevalence and incidence of urinary and faecal incontinence, and of the conditions associated with them, in a population. Prevalence is defined as the total number of cases in a population at a given time, while incidence is the number of new cases in a population per unit time (usually per year). Each is usually expressed as cases per 100 000 or as a percentage of the population affected. It is important to elaborate on the definitions used, the target population and the study design, since these affect the figures obtained. For example, in 1976 the International Continence Society defined urinary incontinence as 'a condition in which involuntary loss of urine is a social or hygienic problem and is objectively demonstrable'. If this definition is employed, the incidence rate of incontinence is less than if the definition used is the one given by Diokno *et al.* (1986), i.e. 'any uncontrolled urine loss in the prior 12 months without regard to severity'.

Prevalence studies require assessment of a population at a given time. In practice, it is not feasible to assess the whole population unless it is relatively small (e.g. studying the prevalence of faecal incontinence in women in nursing homes in the catchment area of a particular hospital). This problem is overcome by sampling the population, for which one usually requires the assistance of an epidemiologist, who can advise on sample size and method in order to prevent selection bias and ensure that the power of the study is sufficient to allow sound data interpretation. Incidence studies require prospective evaluation of a sample of the chosen population (with the above caveats also applying) over a prolonged period, during which they are assessed, usually yearly, for presence or absence of the disease. Thus, in any one year the number of *new* cases in the study population can be identified.

Studies of risk factors for a particular disease can be performed using either retrospective or prospective study design. Retrospective studies take the form of case–control observational studies, in which a patient sample is chosen on the basis of the presence (cases) or absence (controls) of the disease. Information is then collected about risk factors. An example is the work showing a correlation between obstetric injury and subsequent development of faecal incontinence due to external sphincter disruption, the presence of external sphincter defects visible on anal endosonography being more common in the incontinent group (Deen *et al.* 1993). Some risk factors may be less obvious but might be revealed by case–control population studies. For instance, a study of the risk factors involved in the development of stress incontinence might include weight, whether pelvic floor exercises had been performed during the first trimester of pregnancy, details of diet and bowel habit, and smoking habit. Multivariate statistical analysis can then provide relative risks with reference to each factor. Relative risk is a description of the disease risk in the group exposed to a risk factor compared with the disease risk in the unexposed group.

Retrospective studies are less epidemiologically sound than prospective studies since they rely on historical data, which may have been collected haphazardly, if at all, and may be subject to reporting biases. Thus, when a potential risk factor has been identified, a prospective cohort study should ideally be performed. This involves choosing samples based on the presence or absence of risk factors and then following the subjects over time for development of the disease.

RETROSPECTIVE TREATMENT ASSESSMENTS

Unfortunately, the majority of papers published on incontinence fall into this category, which is fraught with methodological inadequacies. Such studies are carried out in a similar way to the case–control method described above and usually involve junior members of staff trawling through patient notes in an attempt to derive some meaningful data that can be analysed in a quasi-scientific manner and provide a relatively easy publication. These techniques often rely on deficient patient assessments and non-standardized diagnostic criteria, incomplete patient records often lacking follow-up information, poorly defined inclusion and exclusion criteria, patient selection bias and variable treatment regimens. In view of these flaws, we will not consider such studies further and urge readers to avoid them if possible, except in the context of audit addressed below.

PROSPECTIVE CLINICAL TRIALS

In a recent meta-analysis of publications on the surgical treatment of stress incontinence, 263 papers were reviewed (Jarvis, 1994a). Of these only seven were randomized prospective trials and only 23.5% of patients had been objectively assessed postoperatively. In a similar cohort study (Black *et al.*, 1997), although most women appeared to be improved by surgery and were usually declared as cured by the surgeon, critical analysis showed that only 28% were completely continent at a year. Both groups stressed the need for properly constructed clinical trials to compare the treatments used for stress incontinence. In an editorial the same year the value of high-quality clinical databases was emphasized (Black, 1997) as has been achieved in other specialties such as intensive care. It is thus imperative that future research concentrates on well-designed clinical trials, although it is beyond the scope

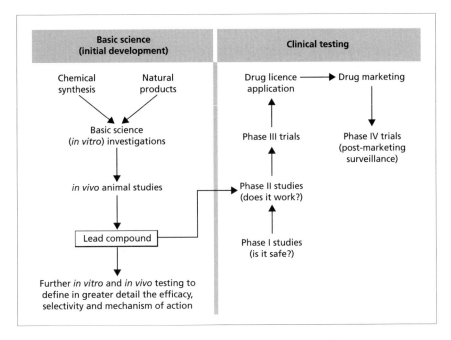

Fig. 7.18 The investigatory steps involved in the development of a novel drug by a pharmaceutical company.

of this chapter to focus much on trial design. The involvement not only of statisticians but also health outcome specialists/economists is now an important ingredient of clinical trials if they are to answer clinical questions reliably and use scarce research and development resources in a responsible manner.

In the development of a drug for treating a particular condition, there are basically four types of clinical trial (Fig. 7.18). Phase I and II trials remain the remit of pharmaceutical companies, although phase II trials may be carried out by incontinence specialists via collaboration agreements. However, the principles of phase III and IV trials are applicable to most types of clinical trial, whether of a drug, surgical intervention, behavioural treatment, etc., so they are given more attention in the ensuing paragraphs.

Phase I trials are designed to assess the safety of a novel compound that has appeared safe and potentially efficacious in preclinical trials involving a number of the basic science techniques described above. Healthy volunteers are recruited and given the compound for a period of time, during which pharmacokinetic data are collected and safety is assessed using many different clinical measurements, such as heart rate, blood pressure, ECG, haematological and serum biochemical studies. These provide information on the optimal route of drug administration, dose range and safety profile, and indicate whether the compound should progress to phase II trials. These address the question of whether the drug works and involve its administration to

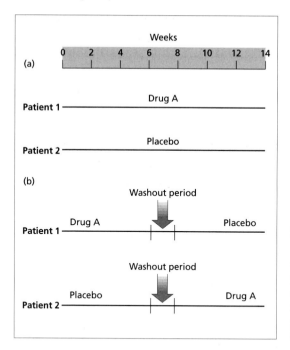

Fig. 7.19 Two common clinical trial designs. (a) Parallel study: patient 1 is randomized to receive drug A for the study period, while patient 2 is randomized to receive the placebo. (b) Crossover study: patient 1 is randomized to receive drug A first, followed by the placebo after a 2-week washout period; patient 2 is randomized to receive the placebo first, followed by drug A after the washout period.

consenting patients with the target disease. Such trials are essentially a form of pilot study, which pharmaceutical companies employ to decide whether the time and financial investment required for further drug development are warranted. They also provide essential information to help decide on the ethics of further trials.

Phase III and IV trials often have very similar designs but are distinguished by the fact that the former are part of the drug development programme carried out before it receives a licence, while the latter are carried out after a drug has been marketed in order to provide additional information about a drug's efficacy and safety profile. It is remarkably common for drugs developed for one indication to reach phase III studies and be found to have more beneficial effects in a completely different area; they are then re-evaluated in phase II studies. Both phase III and IV trials depend upon the comparison of the drug with placebo and/or with another drug currently in use for the treatment of the condition. Thus the clinical trials of the new antimuscarinic agent for treating detrusor instability and urge incontinence, tolterodine, involved comparison with either placebo or oxybutynin. Patients should be randomized to one of the treatment groups and this can be done using, for example, random number tables. The two most common designs are parallel (non-crossover) or crossover and both have advantages and multiple possible variations (Fig. 7.19). The parallel design has the advantage of being more tolerant of inevitable missed visits and of missing data.

The crossover design has the advantage of generally requiring fewer patients to detect differences in response between two treatments compared with a parallel design, but does have innate flaws, especially the requirement for identical baselines at the crossover and often patient withdrawal in the 'washout' period. There is a current vogue for having a placebo 'run-in', which is not popular with patients, and different-sized patient populations in the wings of the trial (if the statistician permits).

Overall there is a laudable increase in statistical training and knowledge amongst clinicians that should improve drug trial design and quality. However, it has to be said that many trials, especially multicentre trials initiated by drug companies, are seriously flawed. This is partly because those in the commercial environment may not understand the clinical problem sufficiently and partly because of the innate difficulties of running multicentre and often multicultural endeavours.

As previously mentioned, the principles of phase III and IV trials can be applied to most aspects of research involving a form of treatment, investigation or even patient questionnaire. For example, investigation of the efficacy of sacral transcutaneous electrical nerve stimulation in the treatment of urgency and urge incontinence can be made by comparing it with a form of placebo (electrodes placed so that they stimulate the cervical area) or with another form of treatment, such as percutaneous S3 nerve root stimulation.

Audit

There is often confusion as to what is audit and what is research. Essentially, research is the study of what constitutes good care and what should be done (i.e. the standard of care), while audit is the study of whether standards are being met. Clinical audit is defined by the Department of Health as 'the systematic, critical analysis of the quality of medical care, including the procedures used for diagnosis and treatment, the use of resources, and the resulting outcome and quality of life for the patient'. This can take many forms and is not intended to be as scientifically rigorous as clinical trials, so long as it is able to highlight opportunities for improvement and to provide a mechanism for bringing them about via the audit cycle (Fig. 7.20). It should be used to support investigation into those areas of clinical care that are considered as high risk or high cost, which are, preferably, common, or where there is perceived or proven lack of effectiveness. Despite the low risk of incontinence, it certainly fulfils the latter three criteria. Most hospitals in the UK have audit departments, who should be able to provide support in the areas of audit activities, preparation of audit programmes, planning of audit studies and performance of literature searches, screening of case records against clinically determined standards and preparation of audit reports.

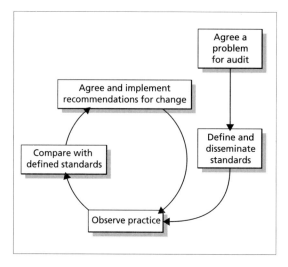

Fig. 7.20 The audit cycle.

Current status of clinical research into incontinence

The greatest difficulty standing in the way of scientific progress at the moment is financial. Drug companies, who have been our main source of funding over the years, have become less generous (despite great profitability) partly because everyone involved in (usually multicentre) phase III or IV drug trials demands remuneration and partly because patients are reluctant to take part in placebo-controlled trials where they know they may receive non-active treatment. Similarly, the major funding bodies, such as Wellcome and the Medical Research Council, have had to tighten the purse-strings and thus limit the award of research grants, even to projects that they acknowledge merit funding.

Clinical research: where is it going?

Perhaps the most important development in clinical incontinence research recently has been the realization of the importance of well-defined validated outcome measures, including patient satisfaction and quality-of-life orientated scoring systems. Despite the quasi-scientific value of urodynamic evidence of treatment efficacy, improvements in the quality of life of patients are our real objective and must therefore be the focus of incontinence research in the future.

The Urodynamic Society has produced two excellent résumés on classification of incontinence and evaluation of treatment outcomes (Blaivas *et al.*, 1997a,b). However, the authors point out that these techniques are still in their infancy, even though it is 10 years since the International Continence

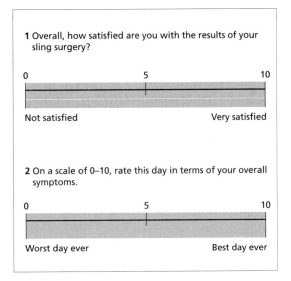

Fig. 7.21 Example of a visual analogue scale. The scale is 10 cm long; patients are asked to place a mark on the scale at a position to indicate the severity of a particular symptom or the extent to which they agree or disagree with a particular statement. The far right of the line indicates absence of the symptom, while the far left indicates extreme severity of the symptom. The position of the mark from the left of the scale is then measured and symptom severity can be expressed numerically (in millimetres).

Society produced an update on standardization of lower urinary tract function (Abrams *et al.*, 1988). Quality of life has been thoroughly reviewed by Sells and McDonagh in Chapter 1 of this book. Questionnaires tend to use categorical response items, although the visual analogue scale is possibly more 'patient friendly' (Fig. 7.21); however, the two are often interdependent. The problem with these techniques of determining patient satisfaction is that however patient friendly the design, it remains patient dependent. Answers thus depend to an extent on patient mood, patient expectation and to some extent their intelligence and understanding. Hence in this quite complex assessment a patient may give an answer to a direct question that is different to their answer on a questionnaire and this may be further at variance with objective findings. This is why scoring systems must have been through a rigorous process of validation before they are used in the context of clinical trials.

Nevertheless, it is of great importance, since in the field of incontinence (except in the neuropathic individual with a 'hostile' bladder and renal impairment) patient satisfaction is the most important outcome and this particularly applies to surgical procedures. Thus, for example, a continence rate of 89.5% at 3 years after surgical intervention for stress incontinence is meaningless unless other factors affecting patient satisfaction are taken into account, such as the effect on the urge syndrome if present and the effect or otherwise on sexual intercourse. Inevitably the number of satisfied patients will always be lower than the objective assessment findings would suggest. For example, in a recent series of rectus fascial slings, 91% of patients were cured of their stress leakage but only 78% were satisfied with the result

(Fulford *et al.*, 1997). Questionnaire data indicated that this was almost entirely related to persistence of the urge syndrome: of those in whom the urge syndrome had resolved 100% were satisfied, whereas over half of those with persistent urgency were not.

However, there are two important areas where progress has been extremely limited and sometimes confusing and where the scientist is most likely to assist in production of both scientific and practical solutions, namely the urge syndrome and the treatment of urge incontinence.

URGE SYNDROME

The urge syndrome remains an extremely common problem, both on its own and in patients with stress incontinence. In the latter group it may occur in as many as 70% of patients, although it is rare to demonstrate objective instability or poor compliance (Fulford *et al.*, 1997). It has been shown that up to 84% of such patients may show instability in ambulatory testing (Heslington & Hilton, 1996), although this has not been our experience and it does not appear greatly to affect the results of surgery. The urge syndrome is undoubtedly a multifactorial problem and somewhat unpredictable in its response to surgery when associated with stress incontinence. However, in our hands the achievement of bladder neck closure at rest seems to be the most important aspect of any surgery aimed at eradicating the urge element. Nevertheless, persistence of the urge component (or *de novo* symptoms) remains the most likely cause of patient dissatisfaction following intervention, particularly by the surgeon. The combination of conventional and ambulatory urodynamics with more sophisticated basic science techniques is the most likely way of predicting outcome in this rather confused condition. For the clinician and the scientist, it would be interesting to see whether the *in vitro* behaviour of detrusor muscle strips and their response to available drugs might also be of value in this prediction. This has previously been difficult because of the problem of achieving complete washout of the drug from the superfusion apparatus, thus potentially affecting further experiments.

TREATMENT OF URGE INCONTINENCE

This has had a high profile in the urological press recently because of the launch of a new antimuscarinic drug, tolterodine. It is salutary that such marketing hype was justified because no useful new drugs have come on the market in the past 15 years, despite this being such a common problem. This paucity of therapy is underlined by the publication of well-designed, virtually identical trials on oxybutynin 11 years apart (Moisey *et al.*, 1980;

Thuroff *et al.*, 1991). Despite the much heralded arrival of a more bladder-specific antimuscarinic drug there is still a large gap in our pharmacological armamentarium, which current basic research, in collaboration with the pharmaceutical companies, must be aimed at. Exactly how this should be approached is not easily determined.

In an otherwise excellent paper on the epidemiology and pathophysiology of urge incontinence (Payne, 1998), no mention is made of the effect of changing hormonal environment, and there is no reason why research in this area should remain in the domain of the gynaecologist. Currently, there is also a leaning towards the importance of pelvic floor weakness in the aetiology of urge incontinence. Since, from the point of view of the patient, there is a world of difference between urgency and urge incontinence, the integrity of the pelvic floor is very important. Whether it is part of the causation remains unproved. It should be added that one of the great values of effective drugs in patients with urge incontinence and limited mobility is that such drugs may give the patient time to reach a suitable voiding environment. It should also be emphasized that drugs in this field at best control symptoms but never cure the disease. Thus treatments covered elsewhere in this book, such as neuromodulation and biofeedback (greatly underused), that are aimed at both controlling symptoms and curing the patient are obviously desirable.

Summary

With a few notable exceptions, the relationship between the basic scientist and the clinician has, until recently, been one of mutual mistrust or at least lack of mutual understanding. The key to progress in understanding and treating incontinence must be for scientists to begin to comprehend the nature of the clinical and pathological problems and for clinicians to perceive the potential for basic science to answer burning questions.

One important area where collaboration between basic scientist and clinician is imperative is the provision of human tissue and the application of the basic science techniques described above to this. Most anorectal repair procedures offer such an opportunity for muscle sampling. In recent years, with the more widespread use of augmentation cystoplasty, and more recently of detrusor myectomy, it has been possible to exchange adequate amounts of bladder tissue between the urologist and the basic science laboratory and indeed amongst a number of different laboratories. If stored at 4°C in a physiological saline solution such as Krebs' or Hartmann's solution (Fig. 7.22), this human tissue can be studied for at least 24 hours after harvesting. Thus there is ample time to arrange delivery of the specimen to the laboratory, whether this be in-house or miles away. The goodwill of the laboratory

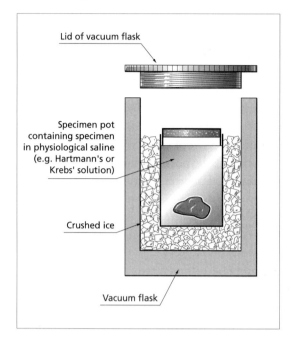

Lid of vacuum flask

Specimen pot
containing specimen
in physiological saline
(e.g. Hartmann's or
Krebs' solution)

Crushed ice

Vacuum flask

Fig. 7.22 A method of storing tissue specimens for transportation to the basic science laboratory. The tissue is placed in a specimen pot containing a physiological saline solution as soon as it is removed from the body. This pot is then placed in a vacuum flask containing crushed ice, which ensures that the specimen is kept at a temperature just above freezing point. Thus it is exposed to warm ischaemia, which can significantly affect the *in vitro* responses, for as little time as possible. It is important to prevent ice entering, or forming in, the saline solution since this can also damage the specimen.

is essential and there is clearly a feeling in many laboratories that relationships with clinical colleagues are mutually beneficial.

In most North American units, the basic science laboratory is in-house and this has the merit of permitting day-to-day contact; however, in the UK the problem of finance precludes this type of contact, except in the field of oncology. Furthermore, it is our belief that symbiosis with a major laboratory is especially beneficial and current methods of communication make geographical separation irrelevant. This does not preclude clinicians from being directly involved in basic science research. The Oxford muscle strip system (see Fig. 7.6) is very 'user friendly' and setting up properly dissected muscle strips can be quickly learned by the clinician as well as the scientist. The Oxford Continence Group is a model of how this cooperation can work well within one city yet the more distant relationship between Cardiff and Oxford illustrates how fruitful such collaboration can be, yielding much benefit to local research fellows in terms of both skills learned and understanding of the mechanisms of disturbed bladder function, particularly the neuropathic bladder. With the principle of 'shared tissue' this cooperation has also been beneficial to the scientists in Oxford. Geographical separation of busy clinical units from high quality laboratory work is no bar to productive collaboration in this field.

There is also a need for the involvement of pharmaceutical companies in this symbiotic relationship, since they can benefit from clinical and scientific acumen that is often more critical and up to date than that available within the individual companies. Moreover, the perspectives of each group are somewhat different, so that collaboration can potentially stimulate novel ideas that may lead to the establishment of new lines of research and thus the greater possibility of breakthroughs being made.

Thus mutual respect and understanding between all those involved in incontinence research are required, since this is where real advance is likely to be made in our understanding of the pathophysiological processes associated with various types of incontinence, the potential targets for future drug development and the pharmacological actions of novel compounds.

8: The Economics of Incontinence

Kirsten A. Major & Noreen R. Shields

In order to explore the economic issues surrounding urinary incontinence, it is first necessary to explore the tools that economics can offer researchers in this area before going on to summarize the prevalence and economic burden of urinary incontinence. It is then possible to explore the impact on quality of life imposed by the condition and the treatments available. Finally, it is possible to explore issues of efficiency drawing on two recent studies in Glasgow, allowing us to form some conclusions on the economics of incontinence.

What is economic evaluation?

Decision-making regarding resources in the healthcare sector is becoming increasingly complex. The source of this complexity is the number of competing demands for limited resources. Even if the resources allocated to the NHS were substantially increased, scarcity would still persist due to the finite availability of funds. One way of assessing the 'value' of competing programmes is to employ techniques of economic evaluation. A full economic evaluation in the healthcare sector is one that considers both the costs *and* consequences of a particular programme. This information is then compared across two or more programmes to assist decision-makers in selecting the 'best' option.

Economic efficiency

From an economist's perspective, 'best' is defined in terms of efficiency. There are two types of efficiency: technical and allocative. Technical efficiency is where a given outcome is maximized or cost minimized between two or more programmes. For example, in considering two screening programmes for urinary incontinence in women aged 20–45 years that both had the same health outcomes, then a technical efficiency rule would recommend that the one with the least cost was selected. Similarly, if both programmes had the same costs then the one with the greatest health gain, however that may be defined, would be selected. This type of efficiency is often referred to as cost-effectiveness and is inherently comparative. An underlying assumption within technical efficiency is that the health outcome is worth achieving;

in the above example the assumption is that women should be screened for urinary incontinence.

Conversely, allocative efficiency does not make such an assumption and explores if an outcome is worth pursuing at all. This involves often complex methods of valuing health benefits. Returning to the above example, while screening programme A may be technically efficient compared with programme B, an analysis may show that it is not allocatively efficient and neither should in fact be pursued. Assessing allocative efficiency involves techniques using quality-adjusted life year (QALY) league tables or cost–benefit analyses.

Types of economic evaluation

In attempting to measure and achieve technical and allocative efficiency, economists use a number of types of economic evaluation (Drummond *et al.*, 1990). These are discussed in detail in the following sections.

Cost-minimization analysis

To conduct a valid cost-minimization analysis (CMA), the health outcomes must be identical. If this is the case, and can be demonstrated to be so, then the costs are calculated for each programme and the one with the least cost recommended. If active consideration is not given to demonstrating that effectiveness is the same, then the study is reduced to a costing analysis and decision-makers run the risk of selecting a programme that may be cheaper but which has much lower effectiveness.

Cost-effectiveness analysis

Cost-effectiveness analysis (CEA) considers the benefits of programmes in relation to their cost, using natural units as measures of effectiveness. Common natural units used include life years saved, strokes averted, etc. If an intermediate outcome is used as the natural unit then careful consideration must be given to its relationship with final outcome, for example if reductions in blood pressure in millimetres of mercury is selected then there must be clear evidence that it relates to a final health outcome such as strokes averted. Clearly CEA, as with CMA, can only be used to compare programmes that have a common effect of interest and measure to technical efficiency.

Cost–utility analysis

Cost–utility analysis (CUA) uses utility as the measure of value for health benefit. However, measures of utility or satisfaction are difficult to obtain as no single 'satisfaction index' exists. The utility used in CUA is the value placed on a particular health status, measured by respondents' preferences for different sets of health outcomes. In practice, CUA has focused on the quality of health outcomes created or avoided by a particular programme or treatment. CUA provides a common denominator for comparing costs and consequences for very different programmes. This common denominator is almost universally the QALY. A QALY is obtained by taking the length of time affected by the health outcome and adjusting it by the value placed on that health outcome. For example, 1 year in full health would be equivalent to 1 QALY, while any health state worse than full health would be valued at some level less than 1 QALY. Consequently, CUA encompasses not only quantity of life but also health-related quality of life. When two or more programmes are compared, CUA provides measures of technical efficiency. However, if the results of CUA are entered into a comprehensive table of results (a QALY league table), then it is possible to achieve allocative efficiency if those programmes with the lowest 'cost per QALY' are pursued.

Cost–benefit analysis

Cost–benefit analysis (CBA) provides a common denominator for the comparison of costs and consequences of alternative programmes. In CBA this denominator is provided by money. The benefits, or otherwise, of a programme are expressed in terms of money, which allows direct comparison with the costs. This does not mean that costs incurred are set against those saved: these are both part of the costing side of the evaluation. CBA places a monetary valuation on the health intervention, e.g. specialist continence nurses, pelvic floor exercise training sessions, etc. CBA only recommends a programme when the benefits that accrue to those who gain are greater than the benefits forfeited by any losers.

The problem with CBA in these situations is that in most countries heathcare is at least partially subsidized by governments and so individuals do not trade it like a normal commodity where the value placed on interventions can be observed from behaviour. This is particularly true in the UK, where consumers often face no cost at the point of consumption. As a result, CBA requires individuals to estimate their maximum willingness to pay for a healthcare intervention so that monetary valuations can be obtained. An additional benefit of this approach is that it encompasses the whole range of benefits from health intervention by asking individuals to value the whole programme; other types of evaluation tend to focus exclusively on health outcome and ignore these additional benefits, such as information. CBA recommends that a programme should be pursued where the relationship between costs and benefits is most favourable and can produce allocative efficiency where these comparisons are made across a number of programmes.

Clearly, there are a number of economic techniques that could be applied to research and decision-making when considering services for individuals with incontinence. In the absence of a substantial economics literature on the subject, it is now possible to explore the economic burden imposed by incontinence by first assessing the size of the problem.

Prevalence

A MORI poll found that in the 1883 men and 2124 women interviewed in their homes throughout the UK the rate of urinary incontinence was 6.6 and 14.0% respectively. In three age groups, 30–49 years, 50–59 years and 60 years and over, the rates for men were 2.0, 5.4 and 13.3%, whereas for women they were 10.9, 15.4 and 16.8% (Brocklehurst, 1993). In the latest report by the Agency for Healthcare Policy and Research (AHCPR) (Fantl *et al.* 1996), the quoted figure is 15–35% of all subjects over 60 years of age. This clearly shows that urinary incontinence is more prevalent amongst women in all age groups and that its incidence increases with age. It has also been shown that incontinence is associated with childbirth (Jolleys, 1988). In a study of nursing homes, Peet *et al.* (1995) found that 44% of a sample of 5758 were incontinent of urine and/or faeces. Clearly, urinary incontinence is an extremely common condition, particularly amongst women. Despite the size of the problem, health services have tended to be erratic and poorly specified (Norton, 1996).

Costs

The overall cost of incontinence is difficult to estimate in one all-encompassing statement as much of the cost is borne by patients themselves on the purchase of pads and appliances. The AHCPR report estimated a cost in the USA of $16 billion per year, which is in excess of the costs of renal dialysis and coronary artery bypass surgery combined. The costs can be considered in terms of 'direct' costs, including treatments, staffing, supplies, hospitalization, etc., and 'indirect' costs to society, which encompass loss of productivity and welfare support for sufferers.

Work carried out in Glasgow that investigated the cost of pads found significant resource use. The cost of bed-pads provided by primary care services was almost £52 000 (1994 prices) per year, while products supplied by community services had a full-year value of almost £900 000 (1994 prices). Given that the Greater Glasgow Health Board area has a population of

Controlled/normal days or nights	**Table 8.1** Outcome measures
Quality of life/symptom scores	of economic evaluation of
QALY	incontinence. (From Kobelt,
Willingness to pay	1997.)
Number of leaks/volumes leaked	

QALY, quality-adjusted life year.

916 600 (1994 mid-year estimate), this would imply that the potential costs of pad supplies alone may be in the region of £57.3 million across the UK (based on 1994 UK population). Clearly, a number of assumptions enter into such an extrapolation regarding consistency of clinical practice, prescribing rates and prevalence of incontinence. What can be concluded without doubt is that the costs associated with symptom management for incontinence are likely to be substantial.

Interventions and treatments

A number of treatments for incontinence have been shown to be highly effective, but very few have been assessed by robust research methodology. Reproducible and easily determined outcome measures are as important for proper economic evaluation as they are for clinical research and audit (Table 8.1). None the less there is a wealth of clinical literature indicating good results from conservative therapies in the majority of patients and the requirement for surgical intervention applies only to the few. Pelvic floor exercises have shown improvements in up to 70% of cases and continence in 40% of those with stress incontinence. In urge incontinence, behavioural treatments such as bladder training have produced continence rates of up to 90%. Drug treatments are also effective in urge incontinence, with improvements in 70% of cases. Specialist urinary incontinence nurses have also been shown to improve levels of continence as well as improving understanding (Badger *et al.*, 1983; O'Brien *et al.*, 1991). In the context of an increasingly technology-intensive health service, these interventions are minimally intensive with apparently high rates of effectiveness and therefore merit more detailed economic evaluation.

Hence, from an economics perspective incontinence is highly prevalent, incurs substantial long-term costs in symptom management and has a number of seemingly effective and minimally intensive interventions as well as more complex and costly procedures. There would appear to be potential to improve economic efficiency, although it is vital that improvement is assessed using rigorous clinical and economic outcome measures.

Studies of efficiency

Conservative therapies

A multidisciplinary team was established in Glasgow to review local services. A crucial aspect of the review process was a study of a nurse-led continence service being conducted within primary care in the south-west of the city (McGhee *et al.*, 1997). This pilot study examined the impact of a nurse-led continence promotion service that operated as a domiciliary service within the community (62 patients) as well as within a large local nursing home (57 patients). The nursing home provided two levels of care: the residential wing, where 27 of 63 patients (43%) were incontinent; and the hospital wing, where 30 of 32 patients (98%) were incontinent. The nature of interventions provided by the specialist nurse varied widely depending on the level of patient involvement and cooperation that was possible.

In the community group, a 69% improvement in the severity of incontinence was noted, while a 30% improvement was achieved in the residential group and a 13% improvement in the residents of the hospital wing as measured by the Lagro-Janssen *et al.* (1991) classification. The resource use in the nursing home setting was in excess of £6000. The savings in the residential wing are likely to be more representative of nursing and residential homes generally and amounted to £4152, a saving of £66 per resident per year. Savings were achieved through improved levels of incontinence and more efficient garment management programmes. When extrapolated to the whole of the Greater Glasgow Health Board area, potential savings were estimated to be in the region of £157 500 per year. Changes in resource use in the community were more problematic as a number of patients referred to the new service were indeed 'new' patients and thus had not previously incurred costs to the NHS; as a consequence an increase in costs was observed in the community. The authors felt this was probably not as a consequence of the type of service but because patients were new to the NHS.

The primary care pilot has been expanded further to test if the results are replicable across a number of areas in the city. Since 1995, a continence support team has been funded by the Greater Glasgow Health Board to cover community and nursing home services for half of the city and to undertake rigorous evaluation of the economic implications of this implementation. This evaluation is still underway and is assessing clinical, psychosocial and economic outcomes. Early data from the hospitalized sector at 12 months showed that savings to the NHS of £7.16 per patient had resulted from changes in product use. Greater efficacy was confounded by a number of factors, including the high incidence of dementia (52%) and high mortality (51%) in the hospitalized group and a reluctance of other staff to implement

Table 8.2 Cumulative costs of long-term stoma care and predicted costs of dynamic gracioplasty.

	Costs pet year (£)	Total cost over 10 years (£)	Total cost over 5 years (£)
Stoma			
First operation		4 500	4 500
Appliance costs	1 500	15 000	7 500
Stomatherapy visits five times per year	60	600	300
Total		20 100	12 300
Annual cost		2 010	2 460
Dynamic gracioplasty			
Initial implant equipment		5 900	5 900
Operation cost and hopital stay (12 days)		7 500	7 500
Replacement of stimulator (6–8 years)		4 000	
Total		17 400	13 400
Annual cost		1 740	2 680

the advice that had been given on product use by the continence advisor. Interim results for the 633 patients who attended community clinics found that the changes advised should result in savings for the NHS of £14.13 per patient per year. Data are as yet unavailable on the 12-month follow-up for this group.

Clearly, the interim results from this wider study suggest substantial cost savings and it is hoped that later data will demonstrate improvements in continence level and quality of life. If we assume that specialist continence nurses would not make quality of life or severity of incontinence any worse, then from a technical efficiency perspective this is a more cost-effective mode of service delivery.

Specialist therapies

Similar economic evaluations are essential when considering high-technology interventions for incontinence. An example is shown in Table 8.2 and Fig. 8.1. This constitutes an evaluation of the predicted costs of dynamic gracioplasty for faecal incontinence based on the assumption that the neostimulator would need to be replaced after about 6 years. This has been compared to the cumulative costs of long-term stoma care. The graph illustrates that for more expensive high-technology interventions there is a break-even point beyond which costs effectively reduce. This is obviously an over-simplification

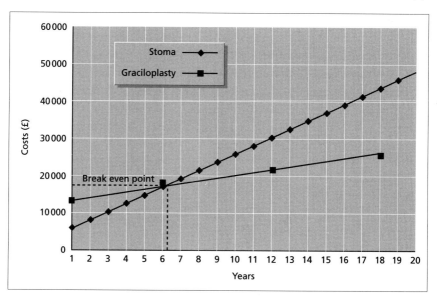

Fig. 8.1 Comparison of costs of long-term stoma care and gracilopasty, showing a break even point in costs at around 6¹/₂ years.

and makes assumptions about life expectancy for a particular patient cohort and that complication rates are predictable and similar in different hands. None the less, evaluation of specialist therapies in health economic terms must utilize this form of assessment backed up by the best available data on outcomes.

Summary

This brief examination of the economic issues surrounding urinary and faecal incontinence has shown that substantial demands are currently placed on scarce NHS resources to manage the symptoms of incontinence, despite highly effective and minimally intensive interventions being available. Furthermore, studies of economic efficiency are limited and thus researchers in this field should ensure that economic evaluation is an inherent part of any project. Decision-makers in the NHS should be provided with the fullest information on the relative costs and benefits of tackling urinary incontinence, which currently consumes significant resources.

Economic studies are often criticized for identifying 'savings' in resource use that cannot actually be realized, e.g. shortening the length of stay in hospital by 1 day does not actually release resources unless, for example, a ward is actually closed. However, in this case the resources released by improved management are genuinely available for other activities as products are no longer purchased from the private sector.

Nevertheless, against this encouraging backdrop are the perceptions of individuals who suffer from incontinence. Several studies have found that an inappropriate leakage of urine is perceived by many women as common and therefore not serious; thus it is often not reported to practitioners. Failure to seek help for continence problems, due to lack of awareness, low expectation of services available or embarrassment, is a problem. As a result, there is clearly a need for information to be relayed to the public on the availability of services. Attempts should also be made to convey the high prevalence of the problem as well as the wide range of simple and effective treatments that can substantially improve quality of life. Methods for promoting continence awareness and prevention strategies also need to be adopted. Given the high association between childbirth and continence problems, promoting continence would be particularly appropriate where young women and mothers meet. A further element of the study in Glasgow was promotion work carried out in family planning clinics, which found that between 28 and 33% of women experienced continence problems. The main problem encountered was mild stress incontinence (69%), which could be treated effectively with minimal intervention.

In conclusion, therefore, the economic burden imposed by incontinence is substantial, in addition to its highly negative impact on quality of life. Decision-makers in the NHS should closely examine their services against this backdrop and seek to improve the efficiency of care available. In parallel, attempts should also be made to increase public awareness of the problem, the interventions available as well as its prevention.

9: How to Develop an Integrated Approach to Continence Care

Mark J. Speakman

Traditionally, primary care physicians have referred patients with incontinence to urologists, gynaecologists or coloproctologists, depending on their local availability. Long waiting lists to be seen in consultant clinics have meant that there is a need for more immediate access to advice closer to a patient's home. In this potentially complex area of medicine, relatively simple investigational and management measures can be effective in a majority of patients. The artificial separation of primary and secondary care is clearly inappropriate and leads to a delay in treatment and unnecessary diagnostic pathways being followed for some patients. This division has resulted, in some areas, in a simple community-based service with little involvement of secondary care. In other areas there is a complex continence service within the hospital but little integration in the community. Shared care, with co-operation between general practice and hospital departments, is the most appropriate model. There are already several strong precedents for this in antenatal care, diabetes, cardiac care, mental health and management of lower urinary tract symptoms (Isaacs, 1992). With appropriate training the important role of the specialist nurse should continue to evolve. Whether in the form of a continence advisor, a nurse specialist, a hospital-based nurse or a practice nurse, the nurse has a pivotal role in the provision of continence care. Shared care should utilize the strengths of both primary and secondary care and not make one more important than the other.

Current situation

At present there is sometimes a lack of cooperation between primary and secondary care. Whether the primary continence team is managed by the community or hospital directorate, the two sectors must liaise to understand each other's priorities and then develop a combined philosophy for overall care in the community. With regard to management control, there are advantages to both sides. If managed by the community, the continence team may feel they have more autonomy and easier direct access to the patients, although they need good links and strong support from the GP services. If managed by the hospital directorate structure, the continence team have stronger links with hospital departments, such as urology and gynaecology, and more

279

Table 9.1 Standards of continence care.

Patient seen within a reasonable time (perhaps 6 weeks, depending on local circumstances)

Patient seen close to home (GP surgery or community hospital preferable to district general hospital)

Services provided by an appropriately trained nurse able to provide the correct level of care

Access to more detailed advice and investigations

Access to referral centres where appropriate

---

rapid access to detailed investigations, such as urodynamics, and easier contact for discussing detailed treatment plans such as surgery. However, the staff can feel less valued and may feel torn between hospital and community priorities.

Vision for continence care

This should be to provide an integrated team delivering seamless care, from the patient's home, through primary care and local community services to secondary hospital care. The service should be modelled around the current facilities, building on the known strengths in any area and developing further provision based on local opportunities. Training should include both district and practice nurses and physiotherapists. This should provide an integrated service and not just a limited number of well-trained individual continence advisors. It is important to avoid duplication in the services. The target should be to achieve an early diagnosis; clinics should also provide rapid diagnosis, rather than always aiming for 'one-stop' facilities. If this is to succeed there is a need for minimum national standards of continence care, which should be set by evidence-based medicine. These standards should include factors such as those listed in Table 9.1.

Management control of the continence team

Whichever group has overall control, there is a need for a unified management structure that covers both community and hospital services. Proper provision of adequate numbers of staff with appropriate training and proper equipment is essential. Most mobile teams need flow machines, bladder scanners and easy access to urodynamics. The staffing hinges on the nursing profile of the service. Most units work best with two or more nurses working together, one mainly located in the hospital and the second based more in the community. This model should work for units with a catchment population of about 300 000. Beyond this, it is likely that three or more staff would be necessary. A suggested programme is presented in Table 9.2. The provision of community hospital and GP surgery-based clinics providing dynamic links between primary and secondary care is the crux of an efficient service.

Table 9.2 Possible work programme for a two-nurse incontinence unit, based in the community and hospital

	Specialist nurse 1 (community based)	Specialist nurse 2 (hospital based)
Monday a.m.	Community hospital I clinic	Hospital assessment and specialist clinic
Monday p.m.	GP surgery visits and teaching	Ward visits and continence referrals
Tuesday a.m.	Patient home visits	Investigations session
Tuesday p.m.	Hospital liaison session (link nurses)	Community hospital IV clinic
Wednesday a.m.	Community hospital II clinic	Flexible session
Wednesday p.m.	Clinical audit, training sessions	Clinical audit, training sessions
Thursday a.m.	Investigations session	Hospital assessment and specialist clinic
Thursday p.m.	GP surgery visits	Ward teaching
Friday a.m.	Community hospital III clinic	Hospital-based research session
Friday p.m.	Flexible session	Investigations session

Table 9.3 Stages of a business plan

1	Mission statement
2	Market analysis
3	Situation analysis
4	SWOT analysis (strengths, weaknesses, opportunities and threats)
5	Objectives
6	Strategy
7	Tactics
8	Implementation and control

A number of home visits are always necessary but these should be kept to a minimum.

A business plan for continence services

Changes in health services worldwide have resulted in a more business-orientated approach to healthcare. Therefore, the management of continence has to compete with other areas of concern within healthcare. Many hospital and community departments would still benefit from the establishment of an integrated continence care programme. Knowledge of how to develop a proper business plan (Table 9.3) will improve the chances of securing the necessary approval and funding. The increased use of evidence-based medicine within public health departments and the proper appraisal of unmet need within the community have given continence an enhanced profile. This is an area that is currently under-resourced and provided the appropriate case for enhanced services can be made it is likely to be successful.

This section is designed to help present the necessary case to the hospital or health authority management for an effective service. Much of this is common sense but the use of a specific plan greatly increases the scope of information collected and leads to a more logical presentation. Initially, the lead person should prepare notes on the background data to the situation and then detail the specification and demands of the service. This person should then involve all interested personnel in this exercise to further develop each of the stages of the business plan. This may need to contain a certain amount of management jargon but this should not occur at the expense of obtaining thorough data and presenting a reasoned argument.

Mission statement

The plan needs to start with the rationale for the service development, placing it in the context of the current facilities in your area. This needs to state in simple plain language the overall purpose of the development, indicating what is included (and perhaps also what is excluded). This is known as the mission statement and should state the message clearly to hospital managers, employees and patients. For example, the statement could start:

> The West Borsetshire Continence Service will provide rapid assessment of continence problems for patients of all ages, at a site close to their homes and will act as a source of information and training for interested health care professionals. Appropriate referrals for secondary advice will be made.

The statement will vary widely from region to region depending on the current facilities and needs in that area.

Market analysis

The mission statement should be followed by an analysis of the current situation with regard to the number of patients (or an assessment of the level of unmet need) and some estimation of the sources of available funding: NHS, private and commercial. The new service will generate new 'income', which should be balanced against the planned expenditure. The prevalence of continence problems within the hospital setting, primary care and institutions should be calculated. The numbers of fundholding and total-purchasing general practices may have an impact on these calculations. This is essentially an assessment of the current market or a market analysis. Information may be obtained from published national literature, departments of public health, local census data and hospital and general practice business managers, amongst others. Local surveys or pilot studies may provide powerful additional information.

Situation analysis

This should be followed by a situation analysis, which should examine the current resources and practices and include the number of providers within the hospital and community services, the number of trained staff, including their sessional availability, and the equipment currently available on different sites. This should be followed by an assessment or audit of the existing service, the numbers of patients seen and referred, the waiting lists and some estimation of the outcomes for the patients.

SWOT analysis

The next stage is the SWOT analysis, best undertaken as a brainstorming exercise with a multidisciplinary team (medical, nursing and management staff from all sectors involved in continence care) that examines the *strengths, weaknesses, opportunities* and *threats* within your local area. This can be a valuable exercise in all planning.

1   Your strengths may include high staff morale and a flexible enthusiastic team, a good local reputation, good contacts with other hospital or community departments or modern up-to-date buildings.

2   Your weaknesses may be lack of good equipment, poor communication or low expectations from local purchasers, or an absence of cooperation between community and hospital-based services.

3   The opportunities may be to improve the overall quality of patient care and patient literature, the attraction of high-calibre staff and the improvement of staff morale. Opportunities may be related to local or national health initiatives that offer sources of additional support or funding (e.g. the health gain initiative on physical disability) or relate to analyses of a large unmet need within the local community or political pressures to reduce long waiting lists. Expansion within the private sector or increased media publicity may also lead to new opportunities.

4   The threats may include strong competition from neighbouring trusts or a public health impression that this is not a high priority locally.

Objectives

Once these initial stages are complete the planning group needs to clarify the objectives or aims of the scheme. This implies a statement of the perceived benefits, which should include both the short-term gains and the long-term goals. The short-term objectives might include management-based targets, such as increased numbers of patients assessed and shorter waiting lists, while the long-term objectives should be to improve the overall quality of care to patients, reduce the number of complications of the disease and to significantly improve overall patient quality of life.

Strategy

The strategy is the means by which these stated objectives will be achieved and represents a long-term view. This may involve directing the appropriate resources to the appropriate patients, securing appropriate levels of staffing and providing education and training. In our model this would include the process of establishing community assessments with appropriate staff, to allow patients easier access to limited treatments locally. Local protocols would be developed to ensure rapid referral to hospital for the smaller numbers of patients who need specialist investigations or treatment.

Tactics

The final planning stage is to identify the specific actions or short-term tactics that will be used to implement the strategy and secure the eventual objectives. This may include taking the message to the right people at the right time (i.e. whoever the business case is being developed for) and producing publicity and patient information leaflets. Local meetings should be organized to inform and educate other healthcare professionals. Training is essential at practice nurse or ward nurse level, contacts should be established with nursing homes, community hospitals or other institutions and open days organized.

Implementation and control

Once approval is granted implementation and control needs to be set up. This includes the designation of standards for patient waiting times for first visits and subsequent referrals and the development of training programmes area by area to cover the whole geographical sector. This should be followed by systematic clinical audit to monitor patient throughput and patient satisfaction, waiting times, management, clinical outcomes and also income generation. Successful implementation of a fully integrated service that incorporates dynamic links between primary and secondary care and appropriate and timely referral and treatment of urinary and faecal incontinence should help achieve the public health goals of improving quality of care, reducing waiting times, increasing efficacy and increasing value for money.

Appendices

Appendix 1

An example of a purpose-built outpatient unit for the management of incontinence.

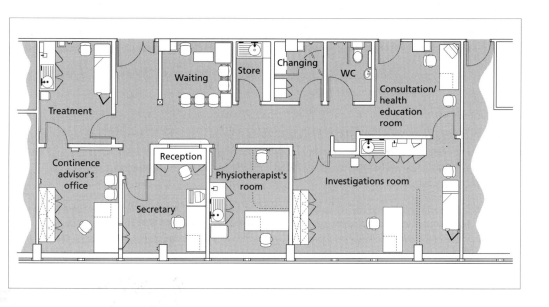

Appendix 2

Pelvic floor exercises

Introduction

Physiotherapists, doctors and nurses know that pelvic floor exercises can help you to improve your bladder control. When done correctly, pelvic floor exercises can build up and strengthen the muscles to help you to hold urine.

What is the pelvic floor?

Layers of muscle stretch like a hammock from the pubic bone in front to the bottom of the backbone (see diagram). These firm supportive muscles are called the pelvic floor. They help to hold the bladder, womb and bowel in place, and to close the bladder outlet and back passage.

How does the pelvic floor work?

The muscles of the pelvic floor are kept firm and slightly tense to stop leakage of urine from the bladder or faeces from the bowel. When you pass water or have a bowel motion the pelvic floor muscles relax. Afterwards, they tighten again to restore control.

Pelvic floor muscles can become weak and sag because of childbirth, lack of exercise, the change of life or just getting older. Weak muscles give you less control, and you may leak urine, especially with exercise or when you cough, sneeze or laugh.

How can pelvic floor exercises help?

Pelvic floor exercises can strengthen these muscles so that they once again give support. This will improve your bladder control and improve or stop leakage of urine. Like any other muscles in the body, the more you use and exercise them, the stronger the pelvic floor muscles will be.

Learning to do pelvic floor exercises

It is important to learn to do the exercises in the right way, and to check from time to time that you are still doing them correctly.

1 Sit comfortably with your knees slightly apart. Now imagine that you are trying to stop yourself passing wind from the bowel. To do this you must squeeze the muscle around the back passage. Try squeezing and lifting that muscle as if you really

do have wind. You should be able to feel the muscle move. Your buttocks and legs should not move at all. You should be aware of the skin around the back passage tightening and being pulled up and away from your chair. Really try to feel this.

2 Now imagine that you are sitting on the toilet passing urine. Picture yourself trying to stop the stream of urine. Really try to stop it. Try doing that now as you are reading this. You should be using the same group of muscles that you used before, but don't be surprised if you find this harder than exercise 1.

3 Next time you go to the toilet to pass urine, try the 'stop test' about half way though emptying your bladder. Once you have stopped the flow of urine, relax again and allow the bladder to empty completely. You may only be able to slow down the stream. Don't worry; your muscles will improve and strengthen with time and exercise. If the stream of urine speeds up when you try to do this exercise, you are squeezing the wrong muscles.

Do not get into the habit of doing the 'stop test' every time you pass urine. This exercise should be done only once a day at the most.

Now you know what it feels like to exercise the pelvic floor!

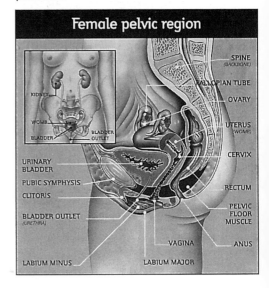

Female pelvic region

SPINE *(BACKBONE)*

FALLOPIAN TUBE

KIDNEY

OVARY

WOMB

UTERUS *(WOMB)*

BLADDER

BLADDER OUTLET

CERVIX

URINARY BLADDER

PUBIC SYMPHYSIS

RECTUM

CLITORIS

PELVIC FLOOR MUSCLE

BLADDER OUTLET *(URETHRA)*

VAGINA

ANUS

LABIUM MINUS

LABIUM MAJOR

Appendix 2 *Continued.*

Practising your exercises

1 Sit, stand or lie with your knees slightly apart. Slowly tighten and pull up the pelvic floor muscles as hard as you can. Hold tightened for at least 5 seconds if you can, then relax. Repeat at least 5 times (slow pull-ups).

2 Now pull the muscles up **quickly** and tightly, then relax immediately. Repeat at least 5 times (fast pull-ups).

3 Do these two exercises – 5 slow and 5 fast – at least 10 times every day.

4 As the muscles get stronger, you will find that you can hold for longer than 5 seconds, and that you can do more than 5 pull-ups each time without the muscle getting tired.

5 It takes time for exercise to make muscles stronger. You are unlikely to notice improvement for several weeks – so stick at it! You will need to exercise regularly for several months before the muscles gain their full strength.

Tips to help you

1 Get into the habit of doing your exercises with things you do regularly – every time you touch water if you are at home, every time you answer the phone if you are at the office ... whatever you do often.

2 Do the 'stop test' once a day when passing urine. Stopping your urine should get faster and easier.

3 If you are unsure that you are exercising the right muscle, put one or two fingers in the vagina and try the exercises, to check. You should feel a gentle squeeze if you are exercising the pelvic floor.

4 Use the pelvic floor when you are afraid you might leak – pull up the muscles before you sneeze or lift something heavy. Your control will gradually improve.

5 Drink normally – at least 6–8 cups every day. And don't get into the habit of going to the toilet 'just in case'. Go only when you feel that the bladder is full.

6 Watch your weight – extra weight puts extra strain on your pelvic floor muscles.

7 Once you have regained control of your bladder, don't forget your pelvic floor. Continue to do your pelvic floor exercises a few times each day to ensure that the problem does not come back.

You can do pelvic floor exercises wherever you are – nobody need know what you are doing!

Do you have any questions?

This information sheet is designed to teach you how to control your bladder, so that you'll be dry and comfortable. If you have problems doing the exercises, or if you don't understand any part of this information sheet, ask your doctor, nurse, continence advisor or physiotherapist for help.

Do your pelvic exercises every single day. Have faith in them. You should begin to see good results in a few weeks.

Pelvic floor exercises for men

Men have the same hammock-like sling of pelvic floor muscles as women, and if they have 'weak bladders' (particularly after treatment for an enlarged prostrate) they too can benefit from the exercises described in this leaflet – with, of course, the necessary allowances for differences in anatomy!

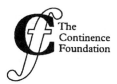

The Continence Foundation

Further information can be obtained from The Continence Foundation, 307 Hatton Square, 16 Baldwins Gardens, London EC1N 7RJ or phone the Helpline: Mon-Fri, 9.30-4.30

0171 831 9831

An educational service

UroNews
PRACTICAL SOLUTIONS IN UROLOGY

sponsored by

Lorex Synthélabo

Appendix 3

Features of the catheter.

Correct size

The smallest catheter which will adequately drain the bladder should be used (consider shape of the urethra which is elliptical and potential damage to its mucosa the larger the catheter). A 10 ml balloon is appropriate in almost all cases.

(a) Size 12–16 Fg for adults with clear urine, 12–14 female/14–16 male.

(b) Size 18–22 Fg for adults with haematuria.

(c) Size 8–10 Fg for children; (6 Fg Nelaton available also for intermittent catheterization).

The *lumen* of the catheter can vary, depending on the material used to make the catheter, e.g. Teflon or silicone coatings reduce the lumen size.

Catheters recommended for use

Indwelling (Foley):

Shot term – 'Siliconised' latex or PTFE, 4–6 weeks.

Long term – 100% Silicone up to 3 months.

– 'Hydrogel' coated latex up to 3 months.

For *Clean Intermittent Self-Catheterization (CISC) and for in/out catheterization to relieve acute retention*

Nelaton single patient use, pvc.

Nelaton single use, pvc pre-coated.

Standard/male length catheters: 40 cm.

Female length catheters: 22 cm.

Paediatric length catheters: 26 cm.

NB   Remember to use female length catheters for females unless contraindicated viz. poor thigh abduction, spasticity of lower limbs, excessive obesity.

Appendix 4(a)

Videourodynamics results (Males)

Summary of history

Preliminary void

Q_{max} :   ml/s   Trace pattern :   Normal/intermittent/prolonged/flattened

Filling study

Residual urine at start :   ml   Filling rate :   ml/min

First desire to void :   ml   Strong desire to void :   ml

Compliance :   Normal/hypocompliant throughout filling/terminal hypocompliance

End fill pressure : cmH_2O

CMG :   Stable/unstable   Detrusor pressure : cmH_2O

Incontinent :   Yes/no

Bladder neck competent? :   Yes/open throughout/opens with stress/opens at capacity

Any sphincter weakness? :

Valsalva leak point pressure : cmH_2O

Detrusor LPP (neuropaths) : cmH_2O

Any reflux? :

Voiding study

Q_{max} :   ml/s P_{det} at Q_{max} : cmH_2O

Pressure flow plot :   Normal/equivocal/obstructed   Straining? :   Yes/no

Obstruction seen on screening :   Yes/no   Bladder neck/prostate or apical/other

Stop test-plso : cmH_2O Trapping? :

Emptying? :

Summary

Date :   Investigator :

Appendix 4(b)

Swansea NHS trust. Morriston and Singleton Hospitals
Depts. of Urology and Gynaecology w\urml\doc\data\vcmgfem

Videourodynamics results (Females)

Summary of history

Preliminary void

Q_{max} :   ml/s   Trace pattern :   Normal/intermittent/prolonged/flattened

Filling study

Residual urine at start :   ml   Filling rate :   ml/min

First desire to void :   ml   Strong desire to void :   ml

Compliance :   Normal/hypocompliant throughout filling/terminal hypocompliance

End fill pressure : cmH_2O

CMG :   Stable/unstable   Detrusor pressure : cmH_2O

Incontinent :   Yes/no

Bladder neck competent? :   Yes/open throughout/opens with stress/opens at capacity

Was GSI seen? :   No/yes/gross

Bladder neck support :   Normal/mild descent/gross descent (Type 1)

Bladder base descent :   No?/<2cm = Type 2a/>2cm = Type 2b

Valsalva leak point pressure : cmH_2O Detrusor LPP (neuropaths) : cmH_2O

Any reflux ? :

Voiding study

Q_{max} :   ml/sec P_{det} at Q_{max} : cm/H_2O

Pressure flow plot :   Normal/equivocal/obstructed   Straining? :   Yes/no

Stop test-plso : cmH_2O

Emptying? :

Summary

Date :   Investigator :

Bibliography

Recommended further reading

Beck, D.E. & Wexner, S.D. (eds) (1992) *Fundamentals of Anorectal Surgery*. McGraw Hill, New York.

Cardozo, L. (ed.) (1997) *Urogynaecology: The Kings Approach*. Churchill Livingstone, Edinburgh.

Eloat, C. (1986) *Stoma Care Nursing*. Baillière Tindall, London.

Fielding, C.P. & Goldberg, S.M. (eds) (1993) *Surgery of the Colon, Rectum and Anus. Rob Smiths's Operative Surgery*, 5th edn. Butterworth-Heinemann, Oxford.

Gosling, J.A. & Dixon, J. (1982) *Functional Anatomy of the Urinary Tract: Integrated Text and Colour Atlas*. Churchill Livingstone, Edinburgh.

Henry, M. & Swash, M. (eds) (1992) *Coloproctology and the Pelvic Floor*. Butterworth-Heinemann, Oxford.

Keighley, M.R.B. & Williams, N.S. (1997) *Surgery of the Anus, Rectum and Colon*, 2nd edn. W.B. Saunders, London.

Krane, R.J. & Siroky, M.B. (1991) *Clinical Neuro-urology*, 2nd edn. Little, Brown, Boston.

Mann, C.V. & Glass, R.E. (1997) *Surgical Treatment of Anal Incontinence*, 2nd edn. Springer Verlag, London.

Mazier, W.P., Levien, D.H., Luchtffeld, M.A. & Senagore, A.J. (eds) (1995) *Surgery of the Colon, Rectum and Anus*. W.B. Saunders, Philadelphia.

Monaghan, J.M. (ed.) (1986) *Bonney's Gynaecological Surgery*, 9th edn. Baillière Tindall, London.

Morrison, J.F.B. (ed.) (1987) *The Physiology of the Lower Urinary Tract*. Springer Verlag, Berlin.

Mundy, A.R. (1993) *Urodynamics and Reconstructive Surgery of the Lower Urinary Tract*. Churchill Livingstone, Edinburgh.

Mundy, A.R., Stephenson, T.P. & Wein, A.J. (eds) (1994) *Urodynamics. Principles, Practice and Application*, 2nd edn. Churchill Livingstone, Edinburgh.

Myers, C. (1996) *Stoma Care Nursing: A Patient Centred Approach*. Arnold, London.

Norton, C. (1986) *Nursing for Continence*. Beaconsfield Publishers Ltd, Beaconsfield.

Stanton, S.L. & Tanagho, E.A. (1986) *Surgery of Female Incontinence*, 2nd edn. Springer Verlag, Berlin.

Wall, L.L., Norton, P.A. & DeLancey, J.O. (1993) *Practical Urogynaecology*. Williams and Wilkins, Baltimore.

References

Abrams, P.H. & Yande, S.D. (1988) Stamey endoscopic bladder suspension. In J.C. Gingell & P.H. Abrams (eds) *Controversies and Innovations in Urological Surgery*, pp. 153–159. Springer Verlag, London.

Abrams, P., Blaivas, J.G., Stanton, S.L. & Anderson, J.T. (1988) The Standardisation of terminology of lower urinary tract function. *Scandinavian Journal of Urology and Nephrology* (Suppl. 114), 5–19.

Abrams, P.H., Farrar, D.J., Turner Warwick, R.T., Whiteside, C.G. & Feneley, R.C.L. (1979) The results of prostatectomy: a symptomatic and urodynamic analysis of 152 patients. *Journal of Urology* 121, 640–642.

Anderson, W. (1971) *Practical Management of the Elderly*, 2nd edn. Blackwell Scientific Publications, Oxford.

Badger, F., Drummond, M.F. & Isaacs, B. (1983) Some issues in the clinical, social and economic evaluation of new nursing services. *Journal of Advanced Nursing* 8, 487–494.

Barrington, J.W., Fern Davies, H., Adams, R.J., Evans, W.D., Woodcock, J.P. & Stephenson, T.P. (1995) Bile acid dysfunction after clam enterocystoplasty. *British Journal of Urology* 76, 169–171.

Barua, J.M., Byrne, D.J., Goodman, C.M. & Wheeler, J.P.A. (1993) A dynamic anti-incontinence procedure medium term follow-up. *Proceedings of the British Association of Urological Surgeons 1993*. Harrogate, p. 90, abstract 90. Royal College of Surgeons, London.

Black, N.A., Griffiths, J., Pope, C., Bowling, A. & Abel, P. (1997) Impact of surgery for stress incontinence on morbidity: cohort study. *British Medical Journal* 315, 1493–1498.

Blaivas, J.G. (1998) Outcome measures for urinary incontinence. *Urology* 51 (Suppl. 2A), 11–19.

Blaivas, J.G. & Barbalias, G.A. (1983) Characteristics of neural injury after abdominoperineal resection. *Journal of Urology* 129, 84–87.

Blaivas, J.G., Appell, R.A., Fantl, J.A. *et al.* (1997a) Definition and classification of urinary incontinence: recommendations of the Urodynamic Society. *Neurourology and Urodynamics* 16, 149–151.

Blaivas, J.G., Appell, R.A., Fantl, J.A. *et al.* (1997b) Standards of efficacy for evaluation of treatment outcomes in urinary incontinence: recommendations of the Urodynamic Society. *Neurourology and Urodynamics* 16, 145–147.

Blannin, J.P. (1989) The sooner the better! Teaching continence promotion to women. *Professional Nurse* December, 149–152.

Borirakchanyavat, S., Aboseif, S.R., Carroll, P.R., Tanagho, E.A. & Lue, T.F. (1997) Continence mechanism of the isolated female urethra: an anatomical study of the intrapelvic somatic nerves. *Journal of Urology* 158, 822–826.

Brading, A.F. & Turner, W.H. (1994) The unstable bladder: towards a common mechanism. *British Journal of Urology* 73, 3–8.

Bramble, F.J. (1982) The treatment of adult enuresis and urge incontinence by enterocystoplasty. *British Journal of Urology* 54, 693–696.

Breakwell, S.L. & Walker, S.N. (1988) Differences in physical health, social interaction and personal adjustment between continent and incontinent homebound aged women. *Journal of Community Health Nursing* 5, 19–31.

Bricker, E.M. (1950) Bladder substitution after pelvic evisceration. *Surgical Clinics of North America* 30, 1511.

Brocklehurst, J. (1993) Urinary incontinence in the community: analysis of a MORI poll. *British Medical Journal* 306, 832–834.

Brown, M. & Wickham, J.E.A. (1969) The urethral pressure profile. *British Journal of Urology* 41, 211–217.

Bump, R.C., Mattiasson, A., Bo, K. *et al.* (1996) The standardisation of terminology of female pelvic organ prolapse and pelvic floor dysfunction. *American Journal of Obstetrics and Gynecology* 175, 10–17.

Burch, J.C. (1961) Urethrovesical fixation to Cooper's ligament for correction of stress incontinence, cystocele and prolapse. *American Journal of Obstetrics and Gynecology* 81, 281–290.

Buson, H., Diaz, M.C., Marivel, J.C. *et al.* (1993) The development of tumours in experimental gastroenterocystoplasty. *Journal of Urology* 150, 730–733.

Cartwright, P.C. & Snow, B.W. (1989) Bladder autoaugmentation. Partial detrusor excision to augment the bladder without the use of bowel. *Journal of Urology* 142, 1050–1053.

Chandiramani, V.A., Palace, J. & Fowler, C.J. (1997) How to recognise patients with parkinsonism who should not have urological surgery. *British Journal of Urology* 80, 100–104.

Chapple, C.R., Hampson, S.J., Turner Warwick, R.T. & Worth, P.H. (1991) Subtrigonal phenol injection. How safe and effective is it? *British Journal of Urology* 68, 483–486.

Cosisky Marana, H.R., Moreira de Andrade, J., Matheus de Sala, M., Duarto, G., Fonzar Maraua, R.R. (1996) Evaluation of long term results of surgical correction of stress urinary incontinence. *Gynecologic and Obstetric Investigation* 41, 214–219.

Das, S. (1998) Comparative outcome analysis of laparoscopic colosuspension, abdominal colosuspension and vaginal needle suspension for female urinary incontinence. *Journal of Urology* 160, 368–371.

Dasgupta, P., Haslam, C., Goodwin, R. & Fowler, C.J. (1997) The Queen Square bladder stimulator: a device for assisting emptying of the neurogenic bladder. *British Journal of Urology* 80, 234–237.

Deen, K.I., Kumar, D., Williams, J.G., Olliff, J. & Keighley, M.R. (1993) The prevalence of anal sphincter defects in faecal incontinence: a prospective endoscopic study. *Gut* 34, 685–688.

Dietzen, C.D. & Pemberton, J.H. (1989) Perineal Approaches in Treatment of Complete Rectal Prolapse. *Netherland Journal of Surgery* 41, 140–144.

Diokno, A.C., Brock, B.M., Brown, M.B. & Herzog, A.R. (1986) Prevalence of urinary incontinence and other urological symptoms in the noninstitutionalized elderly. *Journal of Urology* 136, 1022–1025.

Diokno, A.C., Brown, M.B., Brock, B.M., Herzog, A.R. & Normolle, D.P. (1988) Clinical and cystometric characteristics of continent and incontinent noninstitutionalized elderly. *Journal of Urology* 140, 567–571.

Diseth, T.H. & Emblem, R. (1996) Somatic function, mental health, and psychosocial adjustment of adolescents with anorectal anomalies. *Journal of Pediatric Surgery* 31, 638–643.

Drummond, M.F., Stoddart, G.L. & Torrance, G.W. (1990) *Methods for the Economic Evaluation of Health Care Programmes*. Oxford University Press, Oxford.

Dunn, M., Smith, J.C. & Ardran, G.M. (1974) Prolonged bladder distension as a treatment of urgency and urge incontinence of urine. *British Journal of Urology* 46, 645–652.

Elbadawi, A. & Schneck, E.A. (1974) A new theory of the innervation of bladder musculature. Part 4. Innervation of the vesicourethral junction and external urethral sphincter. *Journal of Urology* 111, 613–615.

Elbadawi, A., Yalla, S.V. & Resnick, N.M. (1993) Structural basis of geriatric voiding dysfunction. III. Detrusor overactivity. *Journal of Urology* 150, 1668–1680.

Essenhigh, D.M. & Yeates, K. (1973) Transection of the bladder with particular reference to enuresis. *British Journal of Urology* 45, 299–305.

Ewing, R., Bultitude, M.I. & Shuttlewoth, K.E.D. (1983) Subtrigonal phenol injection therapy for incontinence in female patients with multiple sclerosis. *Lancet* i, 1304–1306.

Fantl, J.A., Newman, D.K. & Colling, J. (1996) *Urinary Incontinence in Adults: Acute and Chronic Management. Clinical Practice Guideline No. 2 1996 Update*. AHCPR Publication 96–0682. Agency for Health Care Policy and Research, US Public Health Service, Washington, DC.

Fisher, S.E., Breckon, H.A., Andrews, H.A. & Keighly, M.R.B. (1989) Psychiatric screening for patients with faecal incontinence or chronic constipation referred for surgical treatment. *British Journal of Surgery* 76, 352–355.

Fliegner, J.R. & Glenning, P.P. (1979) Seven years experience in the evaluation and management of patients with urge incontinence of urine. *Australian and New Zealand Journal of Obstetrics and Gynaecology* 19, 42–44.

Foster, C.D., Speakman, M.J., Fujii, K. & Brading, A.F. (1989) The effects of Cromakalim on the detrusor muscle of human and pig urinary bladder. *British Journal of Urology* 63, 284–294.

Freeman, R.M., McPherson, F.M. & Baxby, K. (1985) Psychological features of women with idiopathic detrusor instability. *Urologia Internationalis* 40, 257–259.

Frewen, W.K. (1978) An objective assessment of the unstable bladder of psychometric origin. *British Journal of Urology* 50, 246–249.

Fujii, K. (1987) Electrophysiological evidence that adenosine triphosphate (ATP) is a co-transmitter with acetylcholine (ACh) in isolated guinea-pig, rabbit and pig urinary bladder. *Journal of Physiology* 394, 26P.

Fulford, S., Flynn, R. & Stephenson, T.P. (1997) A subjective and urodynamic assessment of the rectus fascial sling with particular reference to the urge syndrome. *British Journal of Urology* 79 (Suppl. 4), 57.

Gittes, R.F. & Loughlin, K.R. (1987) No incision pubovaginal suspension for stress incontinence. *Journal of Urology* 138, 568–570.

Grimby, A., Milsom, I., Molander, U., Wiklund, I. & Ekelund, P. (1993) The influence of urinary incontinence on the quality of life of elderly women. *Age and Ageing* 22, 82–89.

Gunasena, K.T., Nimmo, A.J., Morrison, J.F.B. & Whitaker, E.M. (1995) Effects of denervation on muscarinic receptors in the rat bladder. *British Journal of Urology* 76, 291–296.

Hadelman, S. (1982) Pudendal Evoked Responses. *Archives of Neurology* 39, 280–283.

Harzmann, R. & Weckerman, D. (1992) Problem of secondary malignancy after urinary diversion and enterocystoplasty. *Scandinavian Journal of Urology and Nephrology* 142 (Suppl.), 56.

Herzog, A.R., Diokno, A.C. & Fultz, N.H. (1989) Urinary Incontinence: Medical and Psychosocial Aspects. *Annual Review of Gerontology and Geriatrics*, 9, 74–119.

Herzog, A.R., Fultz, N.H., Brock, B.M., Brown, M.B. & Diokno, A.C. (1988) Urinary incontinence and psychological distress among older adults. *Psychology and Aging* 3, 115–121.

Heslington, K. & Hilton, P. (1996) Ambulatory urodynamic monitoring. *British Journal of Obstetrics and Gynaecology* 103, 393–399.

Hickey, A.M., Bury, G., O'Boyle, C., Bradley, F. & O'Kelly, F.D. (1996) A new short form individual quality of life measure (SEIQoL-DW): application in a cohort of individuals with HIV/AIDS. *British Medical Journal* 313, 29–33.

Higson, R.H. & Smith, J.C. (1981) Prolonged bladder distension. *Recent Advances in Urology/Andrology* 3, 145–154.

Hinman jnr, F. (1989) *Atlas of Urological Surgery*. W.B. Saunders, Philadelphia.

Ho, Y.H., Chang, J.M., Tan, M. & Low, J.Y. (1996) Biofeedback therapy for excessive stool frequency and incontinence following anterior resection or total colectomy. *Diseases of the Colon and Rectum* 39, 1289–1292.

Hunskaar, S. & Sandvik, H. (1993) One hundred and fifty men with urinary incontinence. *Scandinavian Journal of Primary Health Care* 11, 193–196.

Hunskaar, S. & Vinsnes, A. (1991) The quality of life in women with urinary incontinence as measured by the Sickness Impact Profile. *Journal of the American Geriatrics Society*, 39, 378–382.

Huppe, D., Enck, P., Kruskemper, G. & May, B. (1992) Psychosocial aspects of fecal incontinence. *Leber, Magen, Darm* 22, 138–142.

Ingelman-Sundberg, A. (1980) Denervation of the bladder. In S.L. Stanton & E.A. Tanagho (eds) *Surgery of Female Incontinence*, 2nd edn, pp. 93–97. Springer Verlag, Berlin.

International Continence Society (1976) First report on the standardisation of terminology of lower urinary tract function. *British Journal of Urology* 48, 39–42.

Iosif, S., Henriksson, L. & Ulmsten, U. (1981) The frequency of disorders of the urinary tract, urinary incontinence in particular, as evaluated by a questionnaire survey in a gynaecological health control population. *Acta Obstetricia et Gynecologica Scandinavica* 60, 71–76.

Isaacs, B. (1992) Incontinence. In *The Challenge of Geriatric Medicine*, pp. 102–122. Oxford University Press, Oxford.

Jackson, S.R., Avery, N.C., Tarlton, J.F., Eckford, S.D., Abrams, P. & Bailey, A.J. (1996) Changes in metabolism of collagen in genitourinary prolapse. *Lancet* 347, 1658–1661.

Jarvis, G.J. (1994a) Stress incontinence. In A.R. Mundy, T.P. Stephenson & A.J. Wein (eds) *Urodynamics. Principles, Practice and Application*, 2nd edn., pp. 299–326. Churchill Livingstone, Edinburgh.

Jarvis, G.J. (1994b) Surgery for genuine stress incontinence. *British Journal of Obstetrics and Gynaecology* 101, 371–374.

Johannesson, M., O'Conor, R.M. & Kobelt-Nguyen, G. (1997) Willingness to pay for reduced incontinence symptoms. *British Journal of Urology* 80, 557–562.

Johnson, D. (1998) Observations on the uninhibited bladder of the common wombat. *British Journal of Urology* 81, 641–642.

Jolleys, J. (1988) Reported prevalence of urinary incontinence in women in a general practice. *British Medical Journal* 296, 1300–1302.

Kaufman, J.J. & Raz, S. (1979) Urethral compression procedure for the treatment of male urinary incontinence. *Journal of Urology* 121, 605–608.

Keane, D.P., Sims, T.J., Abrams, P. & Bailey, A.J. (1997) Analysis of collagen status in premenopausal nulliparous women with genuine stress incontinence. *British Journal of Obstetrics and Gynaecology* 104, 994–998.

Kelleher, C.J., Khullar, V. & Cardozo, L.D. (1993) The impact of urinary incontinence on quality of life. *Neurourology and Urodynamics* 12, 388–389.

Kenaki, T. (1997) *Molecular Pharmacology: A Short Course*. Blackwell Science, Oxford.

Kobelt, G. (1997) Economic considerations and outcome measurement in urge incontinence. *Urology* 50 (Suppl. 6A), 100–107.

Lagro-Janssen, A.L.M., Smits, A.J.A. & Van Weel, C. (1991) Women with urinary incontinence: self perceived worries and general practitioners' knowledge of the problems. *British Journal of General Practice* 40, 331–334.

Laycock, J. (1992) Assessment and Treatment of Pelvic Floor Dysfunction. PhD Thesis, University of Bradford. 145–177.

Laycock, J. (1994) Clinical Evaluation of the Pelvic Floor. In: (Eds.) B. Schussler, J. Laycock, P. Norton & S. Stanton. Pelvic Floor Re-education: Principles and Practice. Springer-Verlag, London. 42–48.

Levin, R.M. & Wein, A.J. (1982) Response of *in vitro* whole bladder preparation to autonomic agonists. *Journal of Urology* 128, 1087–1090.

Lindsttom, S. & Fall, M. (1983) The neurophysiological basis of bladder inhibition in response to intravaginal electrical stimulation. *Journal of Urology* 129, 405–410.

Ludman, L. & Spitz, L. (1996) Coping strategies of children with fecal incontinence. *Journal of Pediatric Surgery* 31, 563–567.

Macaulay, A.J., Stern, R.S., Holmes, D.M. & Stanton, S.L. (1987) Micturition and the mind: psychological factors in the aetiology and treatment of urinary symptoms in women. *British Medical Journal* **294**, 540–543.

McGhee, M., O'Neill, K., Major, K. & Twaddle, S. (1997) Evaluation of a nurse led continence service in the south west of Glasgow. *Journal of Advanced Nursing* **26**, 723–728.

McGrother, C.W., Castleden, C.M., Duffin, H. & Clarke, M. (1987) Do the elderly need better incontinence services? *Community Medicine* **9**, 62–67.

McGuire, E.J. & Savastano, J.A. (1984) Stress incontinence and detrusor instability/urge incontinence. *Neurourology and Urodynamics* **4**, 313.

McGuire, E.J., Woodside, J.R., Borden, T.A. & Weiss, R.M. (1981) Prognostic value of urodynamic testing in myelodysplastic patients. *Journal of Urology* **126**, 205–209.

McInerney, P.D., Vanner, T.F., Harris, S.A.B. & Stephenson, T.P. (1991) Ambulatory urodynamics. *British Journal of Urology* **67**, 272–274.

Madersbacher, H. & Jilg, G. (1991) Control of detrusor hyperreflexia by the intravesical instillation of oxybutynin hydrochloride. *Paraplegia* **29**, 84–90.

Madersbacher, H. & Knoll, M. (1995) Intravesical application of oxybutynin: mode of action in controlling detrusor hyperreflexia. *European Urology* **28**, 340–344.

Mahone, D.T. & Lafferte, R.O. (1972) Multiple detrusor myotomy: a new operation for the rehabilitation of severe detrusor hypertrophy and ahypercontractility. *Journal of Urology* **107**, 1064–1067.

Marshall, V.T., Marchetti, A.A. & Krantz, K.E. (1949) The correction of stress incontinence by simple vesicourethral suspension. *Surgery, Gynecology and Obstetrics* **88**, 509–518.

Meadow, S.R. & Evan, J.H. (1989) Desmopressin for Enuresis. *British Medical Journal* **298**, 1596–7.

Mills, R., Persad, R. & Handley Ashken, M. (1996) Long term follow up results with the Stamey operation for stress incontinence of urine. *British Journal of Urology* **77**, 86–88.

Moisey, C.U., Stephenson, T.P. & Brendler, C.B. (1980) The urodynamic and subjective results of treatment of detrusor instability with oxybutynin chloride. *British Journal of Urology* **52**, 472–475.

Montgomery, B.S.I. & Fry, C.H. (1992) The action potential and net membrane currents in isolated human detrusor smooth muscle cells. *Journal of Urology* **147**, 176–184.

Mundy, A.R. (1993) *Urodynamics and Reconstructive Surgery of the Lower Urinary Tract.* Churchill Livingstone, Edinburgh.

Noelker, L.S. (1987) Incontinence in elderly cared for by family. *Gerontologist* **27**, 194–200.

Norgaard, J.P., Djurhuus, J.C. & Watanabe, H., Stenberg, A. & Lettgen, B. (1997) Experience and current status of research into the pathophysiology of nocturnal enuresis. *British Journal of Urology* **79**, 825–835.

Norton, C. (1986) *Nursing for Continence.* Beaconsfield Publishers Ltd, Beaconsfield.

Norton, C. (1996) Providing appropriate services for continence: an overview. *Nursing Standard* **10**, 41–45.

Norton, P.A., MacDonald, P.M., Sedgwick, S.L. & Stanton, S.L. (1988) Distress and delay associated with urinary incontinence, frequency and urgency in women. *British Medical Journal* **297**, 1187–1189.

Norton, P., Karram, M., Well, L.L., Rosenzweig, B., Benson, J.T. & Fantl, J.A. (1994) Randomised double blind trial of terodiline in the treatment of urge incontinence in women. *Obstetrics and Gynecology* **84**(3), 386–91.

Nurse, D.E. & Mundy, A.R. (1989) Metabolic complications of cystoplasty. *British Journal of Urology* **63**, 165–170.

Nurse, D.E., Restorick, J.M. & Mundy, A.R. (1991) The effect of cromakalim on normal and hyperreflexic detrusor muscle. *British Journal of Urology* **68**, 27–31.

O'Brien, J., Austin, M., Sefini, P. *et al.* (1991) Urinary incontinence: prevalence, need for treatment and effectiveness of intervention by nurses. *British Medical Journal* 303, 1308–1312.

Ory, M.G., Wyman, J.F. & Yu, L. (1986) Psychosocial factors in urinary incontinence. *Clinics in Geriatric Medicine* 2, 657–671.

Palmer, L.S., France, I., Kogan, S.J., Reda, E., Gill, B. & Levitt, S.B. (1993) Urolithiasis in children following augmentation cystoplasty. *Journal of Urology* 150, 726–729.

Parsons, K.F., Machin, D.G., Woolfenden, K.A., Walmsley, B., Abercrombie, G.F. & Vinnicombe, J. (1984) Endoscopic bladder transection. *British Journal of Urology* 56, 625–628.

Payne, C.K. (1998) Epidemiology, pathophysiology and evaluation of urinary incontinence and overactive bladder. *Urology* 51 (Suppl. 2A), 3–10.

Peet, S.M., Castleden, C.M. & McGrowther, C.W. (1995) Prevalence of urinary and faecal incontinence in hospitals and residential and nursing homes for older people. *British Medical Journal* 311, 1063–1064.

Peyreyra, A.J. (1959) A simplified surgical procedure for the correction of stress incontinence in women. *Western Journal of Surgery* 67, 223–226.

Raz, S. (1981) Modified Bladder Neck Suspension for Female Stress Incotninence. *Urology* 17, 82–85.

Raz, S., Caine, M. & Ziegler, M. (1972) The vascular component in the production of urethral pressure. *Journal of Urology* 108, 93–96.

Raz, S., Klutke, C.G. & Colomb, J. (1989) Four corner bladder and urethral suspension for moderate cystocele. *Journal of Urology* 142, 712–715.

Reymert, J. & Hunskaar, S. (1994) Why do only a minority of perimenopausal women with urinary incontinence consult a doctor? *Scandinavian Journal of Primary Health Care* 12, 180–183.

Rogers, J., Levy, D.M., Henry, M.M. & Misiewicz, J.J. (1988) Pelvic floor neuropathy: a comparative study of diabetes mellitus and idiopathic faecal incontinence. *Gut* 29, 756–761.

Rosen, M. (1976) A simple artificial implantable sphincter. *British Journal of Urology* 48, 675–680.

Rovner, E.S., Ginsberg, D.A. & Raz, S. (1997) The UCLA approach to sphincteric incontinence in women. *World Journal of Urology* 15, 280–294.

Schwartz, M.S. & Stanton, A.H. (1950) A social psychological study of incontinence. *Psychiatry* 13, 399–416.

Simons, J. (1985) Does incontinence affect your client's self concept? *Journal of Gerontological Nursing* 11, 37–42.

Singh, G., Wilkinson, J.M. & Thomas, D.G. (1997) Supravesical diversion for incontinence: a long term follow-up. *British Journal of Urology* 79, 348–53.

Siroky, M.B. (1984) Electromyography: Needle. In: *Controversies in Neurology* (eds D.M. Barrett & A. Wein). Churchill Livingstone, London.

Snooks, S.J., & Swash, M. (1986) Innervation of the muscles of continence. *Annals of the Royal College of Surgeons of England* 68, 45–49.

Snooks, S.J., Setchell, M., Swash, M. & Henry, M.M. (1984) Injury to innervation of pelvic floor sphincter musculature in childbirth. *Lancet* ii, 546–550.

Snow, B.W. & Cartwright, P.C. (1996) Bladder Autoaugmentation. *Urological Clinics of North America* 23, 323–331.

Stamey, T. (1973) Endoscopic suspension of the vesical neck for urinary incontinence. *Surgery, Gynaecology and Obstetrics* 136, 547–554.

Stanton, S.L., Cardozo, L.D., Williams, J.E. *et al.* (1978) Clinical and urodynamic features of failed incontinence surgery in the female. *Obstetrics and Gynaecology* 51, 515–520.

Stothers, L., Johnson, H. & Arnold, W. (1994) Bladder autoaugmentation by vesicomyotomy in paediatric neurogenic bladder. *Urology* **44**, 110–113.

Sutherst, J.R. (1979) Sexual dysfunction and urinary incontinence. *British Journal of Obstetrics and Gynaecology* **86**, 387–388.

Tarrier, N. & Larner, S. (1983) The effects of manipulation of social reinforcement on toilet requests on a geriatric ward. *Age and Ageing* **12**, 234–239.

Thuroff, J.W., Bunke, B., Ebner, A. *et al.* (1991) Randomised double blind multicentre trial on treatment of frequency, urgency and incontinence related to detrusor hyperactivity: oxybutynin versus propantheline versus placebo. *Journal of Urology* **145**, 813–816.

Torrens, M.J. & Griffith, H.B. (1974) The control of the uninhibited bladder by sacral neurectomy. *British Journal of Urology* **46**, 639–644.

Turner Warwick, R.T. & Ashken, M.H. (1969) Functional results of partial and total cystoplasty with special reference to ureterocaecocystoplasty, selective sphincterotomy and cystocystoplasty. *British Journal of Urology* **39**, 3.

Vetter, N.J., Jones, D.A. & Victor, C.R. (1981) Urinary incontinence in the elderly at home. *Lancet* ii, 1275–1277.

Wan, J., McGuire, E.J. & Ritchey, M.L. (1993) Stress leak point pressure: a diagnostic tool for incontinent children. *Journal of Urology* **150**, 700–702.

Warzak, W.J. (1993) Psychosocial implications of nocturnal enuresis. *Clinical Pediatrics* Special Edition, 38–40.

Wassef, R. & Rothenberger, D.A. (1986) Rectal Prolapse. *Current Problems in Surgery* **23**, 402–451.

Weese, D.L., Roskamp, D.A., Leach, G.E. & Zimmern, P.E. (1993) Intravesical oxybutynin chloride: experience with 42 patients. *Urology* **41**, 527–530.

Wein, A.J. & Barrett, D.W. (1988) *Voiding Function and Dysfunction: A Logical and Practical Approach*. Year Book Medical Publishers, Chicago.

Wells, T. (1984) Social and psychological implications of incontinence. In *Urology in the Elderly* (ed. J.C. Brocklehurst), pp. 74–92. Churchill Livingstone, New York.

Whiteside, C.G. & Arnold, E.P. (1975) Persistent primary enuresis: a urodynamic assessment. *British Medical Journal* **1**, 364–367.

Williams, M.E. & Pannill, F.C. (1982) Urinary incontinence in the elderly: physiology, pathophysiology, diagnosis and treatment. *Annals of Internal Medicine* **97**, 895–907.

Wise, B.G., Cardoza, L.D., Cutner, A., Benness, C.J. & Burton, G. (1993) Prevalence and significance of urethral instability in women with detrusor instability. *British Journal of Urology* **72**, 26–29.

Woodhouse, C.R. (1996) The Mitrofanoff principle for continent urinary diversion. *World Journal of Urology* **14**, 99–104.

Wyman, J.F., Harkins, S.W., Choi, S.C., Taylor, J.R. & Fantl, J.A. (1987) Psychosocial impact of urinary incontinence in women. *Obstetrics and Gynecology* **70**, 378–381.

Wyman, J.F., Harkins, S.W. & Fantyl, J.A. (1990) Psychosocial impact of urinary incontinence in the community dwelling population. *Journal of the American Geriatrics Society* **38**, 282–288.

Yu, L.C. & Kaltreider, D.L. (1987) Stressed nurses dealing with incontinent patients. *Journal of Gerontological Nursing.* **13**, 27–30.

Index

Page references in *italics* refer to Figures; those in **bold** refer to Tables